THE YEAR IN
INFECTION
VOLUME 2

THE YEAR IN INFECTION

VOLUME 2

Edited by

MARK WILCOX

CLINICAL PUBLISHING

OXFORD

Distributed worldwide by
CRC Press
Boca Raton   London   New York   Washington, DC

Clinical Publishing

an imprint of Atlas Medical Publishing Ltd

Oxford Centre for Innovation
Mill Street, Oxford OX2 0JX, UK

Tel: +44 1865 811116
Fax: +44 1865 251550
Web: www.clinicalpublishing.co.uk

Distributed by:

CRC Press LLC
2000 NW Corporate Blvd
Boca Raton, FL 33431, USA
E-mail: orders@crcpress.com

CRC Press UK
23–25 Blades Court
Deodar Road
London SW15 2NU, UK
E-mail: crcpress@itps.co.uk

ISBN 1 904392 32 6
ISSN 1479-5361

**The publisher makes no representation, express or implied, that the dosages in this book are correct.
Readers must therefore always check the product information and clinical procedures with the most
up-to-date published product information and data sheets provided by the manufacturers and the
most recent codes of conduct and safety regulations. The authors and the publisher do not accept
any liability for any errors in the text or for the misuse or misapplication of material in this work**

Project manager: Rosemary Osmond
Typeset by Footnote Graphics Limited, Warminster, Wiltshire, UK
Printed in Spain by T G Hostench SA, Barcelona

Contents

Part III
Emerging infections

Editor

Mark H Wilcox, MD, MRCPath, Reader/Consultant, Head of Medical Microbiology, Leeds General Infirmary and University of Leeds, Old Medical School, Leeds, UK

Contributors

Amanda J Barnes, MRCP, FRCPath, Consultant Microbiologist, Lancashire Teaching Hospitals Trust, Fulwood, Preston, UK

Robert N Davidson, MD, FRCP, DTM&H, Department of Infection and Tropical Medicine, Lister Unit, Northwick Park Hospital, Harrow, Middlesex, UK

Jeremy N Day, MA, MRCP, DTM&H, Senior Research Fellow, Liverpool School of Tropical Medicine, Visiting Fellow, Oxford University Clinical Research Unit, Hospital for Tropical Diseases, Ho Chi Minh City, Viet Nam

Miles Denton, MD, MRCPath, Consultant Microbiologist, Department of Microbiology, Leeds General Infirmary, Leeds, UK

Christiane Dolecek, MD, University of Oxford Clinical Research Unit, The Hospital for Tropical Diseases, Ho Chi Minh City, Viet Nam

Jane Freeman, PhD, Senior Post-Doctorate Research Scientist, Microbiology, University of Leeds, Leeds, UK

Vanya Gant, PhD, FRCP, MRCPath, Clinical Director and Head of Department, The Division of Infection and Microbiology, University College NHS Hospitals NHS Foundation Trust, The Windeyer Institute of Clinical Sciences, London, UK

Frédérique Gouriet, MD, Unité des Rickettsies, Faculté de Médecine and Hopital de la Timone, Marseille, France

ROBIN HOWE, MA, MBBS, MRCPath, Consultant Senior Lecturer in Clinical Microbiology, Department of Medical Microbiology, Southmead Hospital, North Bristol NHS Trust, Bristol, UK

ALAN P JOHNSON, BSc, PhD, Consultant Clinical Scientist, Department of Healthcare-associated Infection and Antimicrobial Resistance, HPA Communicable Disease Surveillance Centre, Colindale, London, UK

IAN KERRIDGE, BA, BMed(Hons), MPhil, FRACP, FRCPA, Associate Professor, Haematology Department, Westmead Hospital, Sydney, New South Wales, Australia

E DAVID G McINTOSH, MBBS, MPH, PhD, FAFPHM, FRACP, FRCP&CH, DRCOG, DCH, Senior Medical Adviser, Wyeth; and Honorary Clinical Senior Lecturer, Imperial College, London, UK

BERYL A OPPENHEIM, FRCPath, West Midlands Public Health Laboratory, Health Protection Agency, Birmingham Heartlands and Solihull NHS Trust (Teaching), Bordesely Green East, Birmingham, UK

PHILIPPE PAROLA, MD, PhD, Unité des Rickettsies, Faculté de Médecine and Hopital Nord, Marseille, France

DIDIER RAOULT, MD, PhD, Unité des Rickettsies, Faculté de Médecine and Hôpital de la Timone, Marseille, France

NEIL WIGGLESWORTH, BSc, Senior Infection Control Nurse, Leeds Teaching Hospital NHS Trust, Leeds, UK

MARK H WILCOX, MD, MRCPath, Reader/Consultant, Head of Medical Microbiology, Leeds General Infirmary and University of Leeds, Old Medical School, Leeds, UK

Foreword

ROBERT A SALATA, MD, FACP, FIDSA
Professor and Vice-Chairman
Department of Medicine
Director, Division of Infectious Diseases
Case Western Reserve University
University Hospitals of Cleveland
Cleveland, Ohio, USA

The field of infectious diseases continues to evolve with emerging and re-emerging infections globally, as well as continued problems with antimicrobial resistance. This year's issue of *The Year in Infection* focuses on drug resistant infections in *Staphylococcus aureus* (including the worrisome appearance of community-acquired methicillin-resistant and vancomycin-resistant infections), *Burkholderia cepacia* (which has primarily remained a health-care-associated infection and in certain patient populations), *Salmonella* typhi and drug-resistant strains worldwide, and vancomycin-resistant enterococcal infections.

This issue also discusses the currently available 23 polyvalent pneumococcal vaccination and addresses issues of its use in stem cell transplant recipients and HIV infected persons as well as the impact of vaccination on otitis media in children. Broader issues of infections in stem cell transplant patients are also discussed. New information about the benefit of the use of adjunctive corticosteroids in bacterial meningitis is also reviewed. The persistent problem with *Clostridium difficile*-associated disease is also highlighted with focus on issues of pathogenesis, management of relapsing disease, healthcare-associated outbreaks, environmental contamination and metronidazole failures.

It will be my pleasure to edit next year's edition of *The Year in Infection (Volume 3)*. In the meantime, I congratulate Professor Wilcox and contributors on a timely and well-researched volume which will enable all those interested in the field to keep up to date.

Part I

Mycology

1

Epidemiology and diagnosis of invasive fungal infections

AMANDA BARNES

Introduction

Over the past 20 years, the incidence of invasive fungal infection has increased steadily. This increase has affected both patients heavily immunosuppressed because of their underlying disease or treatment modality—HIV-positive individuals, solid organ transplant recipients and neutropenic cancer patients; and also patients, both adults and neonates, receiving intensive care. Some of these problems are 'diseases of medical progress', reflecting increasing use of therapeutic immunosuppression, indwelling intravascular devices, and also broad-spectrum antibacterial antibiotics in the care of critically ill patients.

Candida infections remain the most significant challenge in terms of numbers of patients affected. Overall, invasive *Candida* infection affects 1–8% of patients admitted to hospital but about 10% of intensive care unit patients |**1**|.

Gudlaugsson and colleagues from the University of Iowa recently published a re-examination of the attributable mortality of nosocomial candidaemia, 15 years after their original paper showing an attributable mortality of 38%. The attributable mortality in their recent series was 49% |**2**|. Data from the US National Nosocomial Infections system has shown that *Candida* species are now the fourth most commonly isolated bloodstream pathogens. In terms of the *Candida* species involved, a number of centres have reported a shift, non-albicans *Candida* (NAC) species causing an increasing proportion of invasive infections. This has considerable implications, particularly for the empirical therapy of candidaemia, so attention remains keenly focused on this area |**1–3**|.

Invasive aspergillosis is numerically less common, but is often associated with very high mortality, particularly in neutropenic patients and patients who have undergone haematopoietic stem cell transplantation (HSCT). Recent reports highlight the changing pattern of infection, with a trend towards later occurrence of invasive aspergillosis. Moulds other than *Aspergillus* are also causing more frequent infections in HSCT patients. As the recent review by Nina Singh details, some of the changes in epidemiology are due to changing practices in transplantation, in both HSCT patients and the recipients of solid organ transplants |**4**|.

Finally, as the number of people infected with the HIV virus increases, there have been dramatic increases in fungal opportunistic infections—particularly cryptococcal meningitis and disseminated infection due to *Penicillium marneffei*.

The papers selected for inclusion inevitably cover only a fraction of the field of fungal epidemiology, but include recent data on *Aspergillus*, *Candida* bloodstream infection and invasive fungal infection in solid organ transplant recipients.

Epidemiology of *Aspergillus terreus* at a university hospital

Baddley JW, Pappas PG, Smith AC, Moser SA. *J Clin Microbiol* 2003; **41**: 5525–9

BACKGROUND. Invasive fungal infections due to *Aspergillus* species have become a major cause of morbidity and mortality among immunocompromised patients. *Aspergillus terreus*, a less common pathogen, appears to be an emerging cause of infection at the authors' institution, the University of Alabama Hospital, Birmingham. They therefore investigated the epidemiology of *A. terreus* over the past 6 years by using culture data; antifungal susceptibility testing with amphotericin B, voriconazole and itraconazole; and molecular typing with random amplification of polymorphic DNA-polymerase chain reaction (RAPD-PCR). During the study period, the percentage of *A. terreus* isolates relative to those of other *Aspergillus* species significantly increased, and *A. terreus* isolates were frequently resistant to amphotericin B. Molecular typing with the RAPD technique was useful in discriminating between patient isolates, which showed much strain diversity. Further surveillance of *A. terreus* may better define epidemiology and determine whether this organism is becoming more frequent in relation to other *Aspergillus* species.

INTERPRETATION. The authors identified 41 patients with cultures positive for *Aspergillus terreus*. Over the 6-year period 1996–2001 they demonstrated an increase in the percentage of *A. terreus* isolates relative to the total number of *Aspergillus* isolates, from 1.5% in 1996 to 15.4% in 2001 (P <0.001) (Fig. 1.1). Clinical data were collected for 41 patients, of whom 20 were immunocompromised. Among 11 patients with invasive

Table 1.1 *In vitro* susceptibilities of 23 isolates of *A. terreus* to amphotericin B, itraconazole and voriconazole

Antifungal agent	MIC (μg/ml)*			% of isolates susceptible at an MIC (μg/ml) of:				
	Range	50%	90%	0.25	0.5	1	2	4
Amphotericin B	1–4	2	4	0	0	13	87	100
Itraconazole	0.06–1	0.5	1	48	83	100	100	100
Voriconazole	0.25–1	0.5	0.5	30	96	100	100	100

* 50% and 90%, MICs at which 50 and 90% of isolates are inhibited, respectively.
Source: Baddley *et al.* (2003).

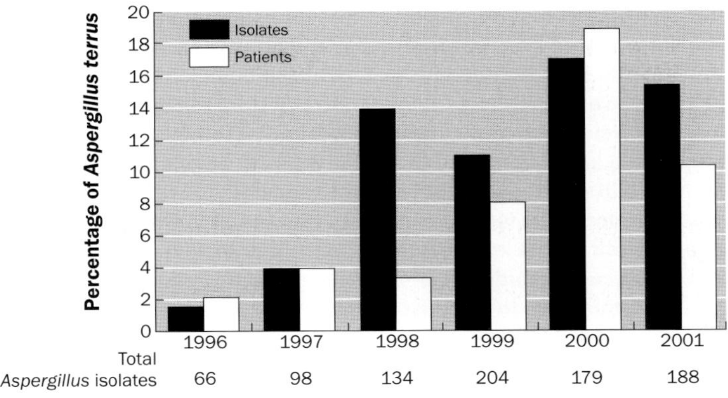

Fig. 1.1 Graph depicting the frequency of isolation of *A. terreus* isolates relative to that of all *Aspergillus* species during the study period (black bars) and the percentage of patients with *A. terreus* isolates relative to the total number of patients with *Aspergillus* species (white bars). Total numbers of *Aspergillus* isolates are listed below the *x* axis. The *y* axis represents percentages of *A. terreus* isolates or patients. Source: Baddley *et al.* (2003).

aspergillosis, eight deaths were attributed to *A. terreus* infection. Antifungal susceptibility testing was performed on 23 isolates, demonstrating that only 13% of isolates were susceptible to amphotericin B at a minimum inhibitory concentration (MIC) of <1 μg/ml. Itraconazole and voriconazole were highly active against *A. terreus* (Table 1.1). Molecular genotyping using RAPD-PCR identified 19 distinct strains and was not felt to suggest a common source.

Comment

The authors conclude that, at their hospital, *A. terreus* appears to be an emerging pathogen, particularly among immunocompromised patients, in whom it is associated with a rapidly progressive clinical course. As in previous reports, MICs of amphotericin B were higher for *A. terreus* than for *A. fumigatus*. Typing suggested that in this instance isolates of *A. terreus* were highly diverse and unlikely to come from a common source.

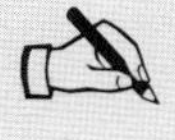

Molecular epidemiology of *Aspergillus fumigatus* isolates recovered from water, air, and patients show two clusters of genetically distinct strains

Warris A, Klaassen CH, Meis JF, *et al. J Clin Microbiol* 2003; **41**: 4101–6

BACKGROUND. There has been an increase in data suggesting that, besides air, hospital water is a potential source of transmission of filamentous fungi, in particular

Aspergillus fumigatus. Molecular characterization of environmental and clinical *A. fumigatus* isolates, collected prospectively during an 18-month period, was performed to establish if waterborne fungi play a role in the pathogenesis of invasive aspergillosis. Isolates recovered from water (*n* = 54) and air (*n* = 21) at various locations inside and outside the hospital and from 15 patients (*n* = 21) with proven, probable or possible invasive aspergillosis were genotyped by amplified fragment length polymorphism analysis. Based on genomic fingerprints, the environmental *A. fumigatus* isolates could be grouped into two major clusters primarily containing isolates recovered from either air or water. The genotypic relatedness between clinical and environmental isolates suggests that patients with invasive aspergillosis can be infected by strains originating from water or from air. In addition, twelve clusters with genetically indistinguishable or highly related strains were differentiated, each containing two to three isolates. In two clusters, clinical isolates recovered from patients matched those recovered from water sources, while in another cluster the clinical isolate was indistinguishable from one cultured from air. This observation might open new perspectives in the development of infection control measures to prevent invasive aspergillosis in high-risk patients. The genetic variability found between airborne and waterborne *A. fumigatus* strains might prove to be a powerful tool in understanding the transmission of invasive aspergillosis and in outbreak control.

INTERPRETATION. The authors performed molecular typing studies on environmental and clinical isolates of *Aspergillus fumigatus* from a Norwegian hospital that houses two bone marrow transplant units. The method used for genomic fingerprinting was amplified fragment length polymorphism. A total of 66 environmental isolates (Table 1.2) and 19 clinical isolates, from 13 patients, were evaluated in this way. Twelve clusters were found, of which seven contained genetically indistinguishable strains. Two clusters each contained a clinical isolate and an isolate obtained from water.

Table 1.2 *A. fumigatus* isolates recovered from environmental samples

Recovery location	Total no. of samples	Total no. of A. *fumigatus* isolates recovered
Water	226	192
Lake	14	7
Untreated water	22	34
Treated water	22	28
Main pipe	36	30
Tap	96	91
Shower	36	2
Air	68	88
Inside	43	51
Outside	13	20
Shower effect	12	17
Total	294	280

Source: Warris *et al*. (2003).

Comment

Nosocomial aspergillosis is a particular problem in neutropenic and bone marrow transplant patients, although other immunosuppressed hosts are occasionally affected. It is traditionally regarded as airborne, the initial stage of pathogenesis involving the inhalation of *Aspergillus* conidia. The mainstay of prevention for high-risk patients is air filtration (as laminar flow and high efficiency particulate airflow [HEPA] filtration) to prevent exposure to spores. Data emerging from several centres over the last 5 years have suggested that water is another potential source of *Aspergillus* species and other filamentous fungi.

Warris and colleagues suggest that environmental *A. fumigatus* strains may consist of two distinct subgroups, leading them to speculate that one group is adapted to an aqueous environment and the other to transmission via air. They conclude that additional measures may be warranted to control *Aspergillus* exposure, targeted at water quality and aerosol formation.

Opportunistic mycelial fungal infection in organ transplant recipients: emerging importance of non-*Aspergillus* mycelial fungi

Husain S, Alexander BD, Munoz P, *et al. Clin Infect Dis* 2003; **37**: 221–9

BACKGROUND. To determine the spectrum and impact of mycelial fungal infections, particularly those due to non-*Aspergillus* moulds, 53 liver and heart transplant recipients with invasive mycelial infections were prospectively identified in a multicentre study. Invasive mycelial infections were due to *Aspergillus* species in 69.8% of patients, to non-*Aspergillus* hyalolyphomycetes in 9.4.%, to phaeohyphomycetes in 9.4%, to zygomycetes in 5.7%, and to other causes in 5.7%. Infections due to mycelial fungi other than *Aspergillus* species were significantly more likely to be associated with disseminated (*P* = 0.005) and central nervous system (*P* = 0.07) infection than were those due to *Aspergillus* species. Overall mortality at 90 days was 54.7%. The associated mortality was 100% for zygomycosis, 80% for non-*Aspergillus* hyalohyphomycosis, 54% for aspergillosis and 20% for phaeohyphomycosis. Thus, non-*Aspergillus* moulds have emerged as significant pathogens in organ transplant recipients. These moulds are more likely to be associated with disseminated infections and to be associated with poorer outcomes than aspergillosis.

INTERPRETATION. This study involved patients admitted between December 1998 and July 2002; it was limited to liver and heart recipients, because of the perceived difficulty in making the diagnosis of probable invasive aspergillosis in lung transplant recipients. Thirty-six of the patients were liver transplant recipients (including two recipients of liver/kidney and one liver/small-bowel recipient), and 17 heart transplant recipients (including one heart/lung transplant recipient). The causative agents are shown in Table 1.3. As detailed above, the risk of disseminated infection differed between specific types of infection; infections due to mycelial fungi other than *Aspergillus* species were more likely to be disseminated than were infections due to *Aspergillus* species (50% of 14 infections vs 10.8% of 37 infections; $P = 0.005$).

Comment

This study documents the growing importance of infection due to non-*Aspergillus* mycelial fungi in solid organ transplant recipients, and the higher mortality associated with these infections. This poorer outcome is probably attributable to the higher rate of dissemination but also to ineffective antifungal therapy in the case of some of the unusual pathogens implicated.

Table 1.3 Types of invasive fungal infections in the 53 organ transplant recipients

Fungus	No. (%) of patients, $n = 53$
Aspergillus species	
All	37 (69.8%)
A. fumigatus	29
A. flavus	5
A. terreus	2
A. niger	1
Non-Aspergillus hyalohyphomycetes	
All	5 (9.4)
Scedosporium apiospermum	3
Fusarium species	2
Phaehyphomycetes	
All	5 (9.4)
Cladophialophora bantiana	1
Scedosporium prolificans	1
Exophiala jeanselmei	1
Pyrenochaeta romeroi	1
Cladosporium species	1
Zygomycetes	
All	3 (5.7)
Rhizopus species	2
Mucor species	1
Other	
All	3 (5.7)
Trichophyton rubrum	1
Unidentified	2

Source: Husain *et al.* (2003).

Incidence of bloodstream infections due to *Candida* species and *in vitro* susceptibilities of isolates collected from 1998 to 2000 in a population-based active surveillance program

Hajjeh RA, Sofair AN, Harrison LH, *et al. J Clin Microbiol* 2004; **42**: 1519–27

BACKGROUND. To determine the incidence of *Candida* bloodstream infections and antifungal drug resistance, population-based active laboratory surveillance was conducted from October 1998 to September 2002 in two areas of the USA (Baltimore, MD, and the state of Connecticut; combined population 4.7 million). A total of 1143 cases were detected, giving an average adjusted annual incidence of 10 per 100 000 population or 1.5 per 10 000 hospital days. In 28% of patients, *Candida* bloodstream infections developed prior to or on the day of admission; only 36% of patients were in an intensive care unit at the time of diagnosis. No fewer than 78% of patients had a central catheter in place at the time of diagnosis, and 50% had undergone surgery within the previous 3 months. *C. albicans* constituted 45% of the isolates, followed by *C. glabrata* (24%), *C. parapsilosis* (13%) and *C. tropicalis* (12%). Only 1.2% of *C. albicans* isolates were resistant to fluconazole (MIC 64 μg/ml), compared with 7% of *C. glabrata* and 6% of *C. tropicalis* isolates. Only 0.9% of *C. albicans* isolates were resistant to itraconazole (MIC 1 μg/ml), compared with 19.5% of *C. glabrata* isolates and 6% of *C. tropicalis* isolates. Only 4.3% of *C. albicans* isolates were resistant to flucytosine (MIC 32 μg/ml) compared with <1% of *C. parapsilosis* and *C. tropicalis* isolates and no *C. glabrata* isolates.

INTERPRETATION. As determined by E-test, the MICs of amphotericin B were 0.38 μg/ml for 10% of *Candida* isolates, 1 μg/ml for 1.7% of isolates and 2 μg/ml for 0.4% of isolates. These findings highlight changes in the epidemiology of *Candida* bloodstream infections in the 1990s and provide a basis on which to conduct further studies of selected high-risk populations.

Comment

This type of detailed analysis of individual patients with candidaemia yields very valuable data. The method provides robust data regarding levels of antifungal drug resistance among *Candida* isolates causing invasive infection. As stated in the introduction, since the widespread use of fluconazole began, some centres have observed a shift in the spectrum of invasive candidiasis. The surveillance data show that the proportion of candidaemia due to *C. albicans* is falling, but also that the level of fluconazole resistance among *C. albicans* isolates is low. Other important conclusions drawn include the major importance of indwelling intravascular devices (almost 80% of patients had a catheter in place at diagnosis of their infection), and that candidaemia is increasingly occurring in non-intensive care unit, and even outpatient settings (the latter reflecting the trend towards delivery of healthcare in the patient's home).

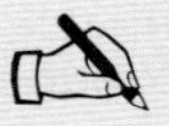

A prospective observational study of candidemia: epidemiology, therapy and influences on mortality in hospitalised adult and pediatric patients

Pappas PG, Rex JH, Lee J, *et al*.; NIAID Mycoses Study Group. *Clin Infect Dis* 2003; **37**: 634–43

BACKGROUND. The authors conducted a prospective multicentre observational study of adults (*n* = 1447) and children (*n* = 144) with candidaemia at tertiary care centres in the US in parallel with a candidaemia treatment trial that included non-neutropenic adults. *Candida albicans* was the most common bloodstream isolate recovered from adults and children (45 vs 49%), and was associated with high mortality (47% among adults vs 29% among children). Three-month survival was better among children than among adults (76 vs 54%; *P* <0.001). Most children received amphotericin B as initial therapy, whereas most adults received fluconazole. In adults, *Candida parapsilosis* fungaemia was associated with lower mortality than was non-*parapsilosis* candidaemia (24 vs 46%; *P* <0.001). Mortality was similar among subjects with *Candida glabrata* or non-*glabrata* candidaemia; mortality was also similar among subjects with *C. glabrata* fungaemia who received fluconazole rather than other antifungal therapy. Subjects in the observational cohort had higher Acute Physiology and Chronic Health Evaluation II scores than did participants in the clinical trial (18.6 vs 16.1), which suggests that the former subjects are more often excluded from therapeutic trials.

INTERPRETATION. This large-scale trial provides another source of valuable data on patients with candidaemia. All were hospital inpatients (91% adults and 9% children).

Comment

Several conclusions can be drawn about the data. First, in terms of the *Candida* species causing invasive infection, *C. albicans* is still the most common pathogen, but NAC species are also emerging. As a group, NAC species constituted over half of infections. *C. glabrata* caused about 20% of bloodstream infections in adults but was uncommon in infants and children (as others have reported); *C. parapsilosis* was commoner in children. Overall mortality 3 months after the initial positive blood culture was 40%.

Recent progress in the diagnosis of invasive fungal infection

In patients at risk of invasive fungal infection (IFI), the diagnosis may be problematic, requiring a combined approach of clinical assessment, interpretation of microbiology and histopathology results, and diagnostic imaging. A particular challenge is the diagnosis of invasive aspergillosis in neutropenic patients, which has historically been associated with mortality rates of 80–90% in some series, the diagnosis often being unsuspected in life and made only at post mortem. Difficulties in making a firm diagnosis of IFI led to the approach of initiating empirical antifungal therapy in neutropenic patients with fever unresponsive to broad-spectrum antibiotics.

If it were possible to make a more precise diagnosis, therapy could be tailored more precisely; but the stumbling block we still face is the lack of sensitive and specific methods for the early diagnosis of IFI.

Conventional laboratory methods for diagnosis involve microscopy of fluids for fungal material and culture plus identification of the fungus, and, crucially, histological examination of biopsy material plus culture of the organism. Positive histology remains the gold standard, but many of the patients at highest risk are unfit for lung or brain biopsy.

The British Society for Medical Mycology working party report published in 2003 provides very useful standards, including recommendations for the diagnostic laboratory in processing specimens from patients at risk for IFI |**5**|.

Non-culture methods for the diagnosis of invasive fungal infection offer great promise, particularly nucleic acid-based methods of diagnosis. This area has recently been comprehensively reviewed by Yeo and Wong |**6**|.

To summarize briefly, various approaches to non-culture diagnosis have been described. Fungal antigens may be measured in blood or other samples. In the diagnosis of invasive aspergillosis, measurement of galactomannan has been studied extensively and used widely to monitor patients at risk of aspergillosis (particularly in European haematology centres). The format developed by Platelia, of a sandwich enzyme-linked immunosorbent assay (ELISA), has improved sensitivity and this test has recently received a licence for use in the US.

For diagnosis of candidiasis, antigen detection methods include: measurement of circulating beta-(1,3)-D-glucan, the cell wall component of *Candida*—this test is commercially available as the 'Fungitec G-test'; and the detection of mannan. The paper from Sendid and colleagues included here is an example of this type of approach.

Finally, detection of fungal DNA or RNA is potentially the most powerful technique of all. Numerous reports have now been published describing methods for detection in blood and other specimens, such as bronchoalveolar lavage (BAL), but they are not yet part of routine care for the majority of high-risk patients. The report of Sanguinetti *et al.* includes real-time PCR performed on BAL fluid for the diagnosis of invasive pulmonary aspergillosis.

The challenge facing us now is to translate the research tools, particularly nucleic acid-based detection methods for fungal pathogens, into the routine diagnostic service.

The Expert Group meeting in 2002 had the remit of considering the design of studies on deep mycoses, but considered issues in the evaluation of diagnostic tests as part of that remit |**7**|. They concluded that trials of diagnostic tests must define the population appropriate for testing and the clinical question being asked. In essence, we have to understand the kinetics of the markers studied, for instance serum galactomannan, before we can use those results effectively |**7,8**|.

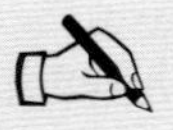

Direct isolation of *Candida* spp from blood cultures on the chromogenic medium CHROMagar candida

Horvath LL, Hospenthal DR, Murray CK, Dooley DP. *J Clin Microbiol* 2003; **41**: 2629–32

BACKGROUND. CHROMagar *Candida* is a selective and differential chromogenic medium that has been shown to be useful for identification of *Candida albicans*, *C. krusei*, *C. tropicalis* and perhaps *C. glabrata*. Colony morphology and colour have been well defined when CHROMagar *Candida* has been used to isolate yeast directly from clinical specimens, including stool, urine, respiratory, vaginal, oropharyngeal and oesophageal sources. Direct isolation of yeast on CHROMagar *Candida* from blood cultures has not been evaluated. The authors evaluated whether the colour and colony characteristics produced by *Candida* species on CHROMagar *Candida* were altered when yeasts were isolated directly from blood cultures. Fifty clinical isolates of *Candida* were inoculated into aerobic and anaerobic blood culture bottles and incubated at 35°C in an automated blood culture system. When growth was detected, an aliquot was removed and plated on to CHROMagar *Candida*. As a control, CHROMagar *Candida* plates were inoculated with the same isolate of yeast grown on Sabouraud dextrose agar simultaneously. No significant difference was detected in colour or colony morphology between the blood and control isolates in any of the tested organisms. All *C. albicans* ($n = 12$), *C. tropicalis* ($n = 12$), *C. glabrata* ($n = 9$) and *C. krusei* ($n = 5$) isolates exhibited the expected species-specific colony characteristics and colour, whether isolated directly from blood or from control cultures. CHROMagar *Candida* can be reliably used for the direct isolation of yeast from blood cultures. Direct isolation could allow mycology laboratories to identify *Candida* species more rapidly, to enable clinicians to make antifungal agent selections more quickly, and to potentially decrease patient morbidity and mortality.

INTERPRETATION. The use of a chromogenic medium for direct isolation appears robust in this evaluation.

Comment

As NAC species cause an increasing proportion of invasive infections, identification to species level is a key priority. This method provides a potentially simple technique based on conventional isolation from blood cultures, but speeding up the process for identification. This could dictate initial antifungal therapy for candidaemia for the majority of bloodstream isolates.

Contribution of the Platelia *Candida*-specific antibody and antigen tests to early diagnosis of systemic *Candida tropicalis* infection in neutropenic adults

Sendid B, Caillot D, Baccouch-Humbert B, *et al. J Clin Microbiol* 2003; **41:** 4551–8

BACKGROUND. The Platelia *Candida*-specific antigen and antibody assays (Bio-Rad Laboratories, Hercules, CA, US) were used to test serial serum samples from seven neutropenic adult patients with haematological malignancies who had developed systemic *Candida tropicalis* infections. The diagnosis of candidiasis was based on a positive blood culture (all seven patients) and the isolation of *C. tropicalis* from a normally sterile site (six patients). All patients received early antifungal therapy with amphotericin B and/or an azole derivative and had successful outcomes. When the combined assays were applied to sera collected at different time-points before and after the first positive blood culture, all patients tested positive. In six patients, at least one positive test was obtained with sera collected on average 5 days (range 2–10 days) prior to the first positive blood culture, while blood cultures were persistently negative. High and persistent mannanaemias were detected in all patients during the neutropenic period. In five patients, an increased antibody response was detected when the patients recovered from aplasia. Controls consisted of 48 serum samples from twelve febrile neutropenic patients with aspergillosis ($n = 4$), bacteraemia ($n = 4$), or no evidence of infection ($n = 4$). A low level of mannanaemia was detected in only one serum sample, and none showed significant *Candida* antibody titres. These data thus confirm the value of the combined detection of mannanaemia and antimannan antibodies in individuals at risk of candidaemia and suggest that, in neutropenic patients, an approach based on the regular monitoring of both markers could contribute to the earlier diagnosis of systemic infection with *C. tropicalis*.

INTERPRETATION. As outlined, this small series of patients with candidaemia involved testing for both mannan and antimannan antibodies and yielded promising results.

Comment

Testing for mannan, a polysaccharide component of the *Candida* cell wall, in body fluids offers a method of non-culture diagnosis in patients at risk of invasive candidiasis. The approach described, of using assays for both mannan and antimannan antibodies, is of interest not least because the results relate to a group of candidaemic patients with confirmed infection (clinical details of infected patients, Table 1.4). One of these patients had hepatosplenic candidiasis, often a very difficult diagnosis to confirm; and detection of mannanaemia and/or anti-mannan antibodies may be useful in this subset of patients.

Table 1.4 Underlying diseases and mycological culture findings for infected patients*

Patient no. (age [yr], sex)	Haematological malignancy	Other diagnostic site of *Candida* isolation or infection	Antifungal therapy (dose) and duration	Outcome at day 30	Treatment and comments
1 (71, F)	AML		Day 15, Abelcet (300 mg/day) + itraconazole (400 mg/day) for 5 weeks	Survived	Day 17, chemotherapy; day 15, invasive pulmonary aspergillosis
2 (48, M)	Refractory anaemia with an excess of blasts	Urine, throat, cutaneous (biopsy specimen)	Day 0, AMB (1 mg/kg of body wt/day); day 2, Abelcet (300 mg/day) + fluconazole (1200 mg/day) + 5FC (7.5 g/day); day 14, itraconazole (200 mg/day) + 5FC (7.5 g/day); >day 30, itraconazole (200 mg/day)	Survived	Day 10, chemotherapy; >day 0, cutaneous metastasis and myosite
3 (61, M)	AML	Cutaneous, renal, endophthalmitis	Day 1, AMB (1 mg/kg); day 0 to day 9, Abelcet (300 mg/day) + itraconazole (60 mg/day); day 10 to day 22, itraconazole (600 mg/day); day 23 to day 50, voriconazole (400 mg/day) i.v.; day 50 to day 70, voriconazole (400 mg/day) per os	Survived	Day 19, chemotherapy; day 1, invasive pulmonary aspergillosis
4 (40, F)	ALL	Cutaneous, renal, occular, liver, spleen (biopsy specimens)	Day 0 to day 22, abelcet (300 mg per day); day 23 to day 94, Ambisome® (400 mg per day)	Survived	Day 7, chemotherapy
5 (70, F)	AML, breast cancer	Cutaneous (biopsy specimen)	Day 0 to day 25: AMB and then Abelcet (total dose, 7180 mg)	Survived (recovery)	Day 6, chemotherapy
6 (28, M)	AML	Septicaemic metastasis	Day 2 to day 21, AMB (1 mg/kg per day) + fluconazole (1200 mg/day) per os >day 21, itraconazole (600 mg/day) per os	Survived (recovery)	Day 12, chemotherapy; day 10, septicaemia due to *E. faecium* and *S. epidermidis*
7 (55, F)	ALL	Cerebrospinal fluid, cutaneous (biopsy specimen)	Day −2 to day 0, AMB (60 mg/day) i.v.; Day 1 to day 7, fluconazole (800 mg/day) per os + Abelcet (300 mg/day) i.v.; >day 7, Ambisome (300 mg/day)	Survived	Day 22, chemotherapy; day 7, infection relapse with isolation of *C. tropicalis* from blood and liver biopsy specimen

* *C. tropicalis* was isolated from the blood of all patients. F, female; M, male; AML, acute myeloid leukaemia; ALL, acute lymphocytic leukaemia; AMB, amphotericin B; 5FC, flucytosine; i.v., intravenous injection. Abelcet and Ambisome are liposomal amphotericin B.
Source: Sendid *et al.* (2003).

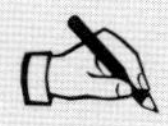

Improved outcomes associated with limiting identification of *Candida* spp in respiratory secretions

Barenfanger J, Arakere P, Dela Cruz R, *et al. J Clin Microbiol* 2003; **41**: 5645–9

BACKGROUND. Pneumonia due to infection with *Candida* species is extremely rare, though these yeasts are commonly cultured from respiratory secretions. The diagnosis of pneumonia due to *Candida* species should be made only by demonstrating tissue invasion of a biopsy specimen. Physicians might misinterpret the presence of *Candida* species in respiratory secretions as being the aetiological agent of pneumonia. This study describes the practice of limiting identification (ID) of rapidly growing yeasts (i.e. *Candida* species) in respiratory secretions and its impact on patients. Before November 2001, rapidly growing yeasts found in respiratory secretions were identified to the species level. After November, rapidly growing yeasts were reported as 'yeasts, not *Cryptococcus*'. The group of patients with respiratory secretions processed before November 2001 was called the 'full ID' group ($n = 267$); the group with samples processed after that date was called the 'limited ID' group ($n = 77$). Full ID patients had an average length of hospital stay of 12.1 days/patient; that of limited ID patients was 10.1 days/patient, a decrease of 2 days/patient ($P = 0.02$). The full ID patients had an average cost of $9407 per patient; that of limited ID patients was $6973 per patient ($P = 0.03$) a decrease of $2434 per patient ($P = 0.03$). Antifungal medications were used in 103 of 267 (39%) of full ID patients and in 16 of 77 (21%) limited ID patients, a decrease of 18 percentage units ($P = 0.004$). Limited ID patients had a mortality rate of 14.3% and that of full ID patients was 18.7%, a decrease of 4.4 percentage units ($P = 0.37$). This policy of limiting yeast ID did not impair the diagnosis of pneumonia. Rather, decreases in lengths of stay, costs and administration of unnecessary antifungal therapy were observed after instituting this policy.

Table 1.5 Clinicians' interpretation of the significance of *Candida* species in respiratory specimens

Physicians' opinion or action	No. (%) of patients in:	
	Full ID group	Limited ID group
Pathogen	45 (16.9)	7 (9.1)
Colonization	8 (3.0)	4 (5.2)
Contamination	7 (2.6)	4 (5.2)
No mention	207 (77.5)	62 (80.5)
Initiation of empiric antifungal agent in response to microbiology report	38 (14.2)	6 (7.8)
Obtain tissue diagnosis	0	0

Source: Barenfanger *et al.* (2003).

INTERPRETATION. This study was performed in a 450-bed hospital in the US and involved inpatients who had respiratory specimens submitted for fungal culture. As shown in Table 1.5, limiting identification led to differences in the clinician's interpretation.

Comment

A key question in optimizing the diagnosis of invasive fungal infection is that of 'significance'. This is a particular problem with *Candida* species, present as a commensal in the oropharynx, so that its isolation from sputum, for example, often reflects that colonization state. The approach described is in some ways a draconian solution. The policy of limiting identification must include (as the authors do) a means of screening for *Cryptococcus neoformans*. These caveats aside, the approach of tailoring the diagnostic service as described could potentially decrease the unnecessary use of antifungal agents.

Comparison of real-time PCR, conventional PCR, and galactomannan antigen detection by enzyme-linked immunosorbent assay using bronchoalveolar lavage fluid samples from hematology patients for diagnosis of invasive pulmonary aspergillosis

Sanguinetti M, Posteraro B, Pagano L, *et al*. *J Clin Microbiol* 2003; **41**: 3922–5

BACKGROUND. An iCycler iQ real-time PCR assay targeting 18S rRNA *Aspergillus*-specific sequences was developed for the diagnosis of invasive pulmonary aspergillosis (IPA). Positive findings were obtained for 18 of 20 (90%) BAL fluid specimens from patients with probable or confirmed IPA and were obtained for none of the 24 BAL samples from patients with no clinical evidence of aspergillosis. These results were concordant with those of a nested PCR assay, which detected 90% of the patients with IPA, while galactomannan ELISA revealed positivity for 100% of these patients, suggesting that the combined use of methods might improve the diagnosis of IPA.

INTERPRETATION. The authors developed a new real-time PCR assay for the diagnosis of IPA, based on iCycler iQ (Bio-Rad Laboratories) and assessed its performance on BAL fluids from haematology patients, comparing results with those of a conventional PCR assay and the measurement of galactomannan. Their results are shown in Table 1.6.

Comment

The use of real-time PCR as described offers the potential benefit of quantification of the fungal burden in the respiratory tree. The authors suggest that this could help to distinguish colonization from true invasive infection due to *Aspergillus* species.

Table 1.6 Results of real-time PCR, conventional PCR, and GM ELISA of BAL fluid specimens from patients with IPA

Patient no.	Sex, age (yr)	Primary disease*	Outcome	IPA diagnosis (EORTC criteria†)	BAL fungal culture	GM ELISA	BAL PCR result Real time (copies/ml)	Conventional
1	F, 47	NHL	Survival	Probable	*C. albicans*	Positive	Negative	Negative
2	F, 72	NHL	Death	Probable	*C. glabrata*	Positive	3000	Positive
3	F, 65	ML	Death	Probable	Negative	Positive	4500	Positive
4	M, 41	AML	Survival	Probable	Negative	Positive	8000	Positive
5	M, 50	ALL	Death	Proven	*A. fumigatus*	Positive	60 000	Positive
6	M, 65	SAA	Death	Proven	*A. flavus*	Positive	45 000	Positive
7	M, 68	AML	Survival	Probable	Negative	Positive	4200	Positive
8	M, 48	SAA	Death	Proven	*A. fumigatus*	Positive	75 000	Positive
9	F, 72	ML	Survival	Probable	*C. albicans*	Positive	2000	Positive
10	M, 65	AML	Death	Probable	Negative	Positive	3900	Positive
11	M, 60	AML	Death	Probable	Negative	Positive	9800	Positive
12	F, 60	AML	Death	Probable	Negative	Positive	10 500	Positive
13	M, 67	ALL	Survival	Probable	Negative	Positive	8700	Positive
14	F, 42	NHL	Death	Proven	*A. fumigatus*	Positive	85 000	Positive
15	M, 77	ALL	Death	Probable	Negative	Positive	5400	Positive
16	M, 70	AML	Death	Probable	*A. fumigatus*	Positive	23 000	Positive
17	M, 70	NHL	Death	Proven	*A. flavus*	Positive	100 000	Positive
18	M, 74	AML	Death	Probable	Negative	Positive	7600	Positive
19	F, 39	AML	Survival	Probable	*C. albicans*	Positive	Negative	Negative
20	M, 54	ALL	Survival	Probable	*C. albicans*	Positive	3200	Positive

*NHL, non-Hodgkin's lymphoma; ML, malignant lymphoma; AML, acute myeloblastic leukaemia; ALL, acute lymphoblastic leukaemia; SAA, severe aplastic anaemia.
†EORTC, European Organization for Research and Treatment of Cancer.
Source: Sanguinetti *et al.* (2003).

False identification of *Coccidioides immitis*—do molecular methods always get it right?

Millar BC, Jiru X, Walker MJ, Evans JP, Moore JE. *J Clin Microbiol* 2003; **41**: 5578–80

BACKGROUND. rRNA sequence analysis of a partial region of the 18S and 5.8S internal transcribed spacer 2 (ITS2) region of *Chrysosporium keratinophilum* highlights its potential misidentification as *Coccidioides immitis*. Molecular identification of medically important fungi should not be based solely on sequence analysis of the 18S rRNA gene but should be confirmed by sequence analysis of an additional rRNA gene locus, such as the ITS region(s).

INTERPRETATION. The authors describe a potential major problem with using a molecular method to identify fungal isolates. Use of a sequencing method alone led to misidentification of *C. keratinophilum* (a soil fungus) as the pathogen *Coccidioides immitis*, which requires category 3 isolation facilities for its handling.

Comment

They conclude that the 18S rRNA gene database is currently incomplete for medically important and environmental fungi, so laboratory identification should not reply on this gene locus alone.

Conclusion

Invasive fungal infection is a major challenge for all involved in the care of immuno-compromised patients. It is vital that trends in invasive infection continue to be monitored, particularly in the area of invasive infection due to *Candida* species, but also less common opportunistic pathogens, so that when antifungal treatment is needed the most appropriate choice of agent can be made.

The diagnosis of invasive fungal infection remains difficult—it requires a combination of astute clinical assessment, radiology and laboratory methods. While advances are being made continually, many of the basic questions about the pathogenesis and the kinetics of diagnostic markers are still unanswered.

References

1. Eggiman P, Garbino J, Pittet D. Epidemiology of Candida species infections in critically ill non-immunosuppressed patients. *Lancet Infect Dis* 2003; 3: 685–702.
2. Gudlauggsson O, Gillespie S, Lee K, Vande Berg J, Hu J, Messer S, Herwaldt L, Pfaller M, Dikema D. Attributable mortality of nosocomial candidema, revisited. *Clin Infect Dis* 2003; 37: 1172–7.
3. Hobson RP. The global epidemiology of invasive candida infections—is the tide turning? *J Hosp Infect* 2003; 55: 159–68.
4. Singh N. Impact of current transplantation practices on the changing epidemiology of infections in transplant recipients. *Lancet Infect Dis* 2003; 3: 156–61.
5. Denning DW, Kibbler CC, Barnes RA; British Society for Medical Mycology. British Society for Medical Mycology proposed standards of care for patients with invasive fungal infection. *Lancet Infect Dis* 2003; 3: 230–40.
6. Yeo SF, Wong B. Current status of nonculture methods for diagnosis of invasive fungal infections. *Clin Microbiol Rev* 2002; 15: 465–84.

7. Bennett JE, Kaufmann C, Walsh T, de Pauw B, Dismukes W, Galgiani J, Glauser M, Herbrecht R, Lee J, Pappas P, Powers J, Rex J, Verweij P, Viscoli C. Forum report: issues in the evaluation of diagnostic tests, use of historical controls, and merits of the current multi-centre collaborative groups. *Clin Infect Dis* 2003; **36**(Suppl 3): S123–7.

8. Severens JL, Donnelly JP, Meis JF, De Vries Robbe PF, Pauw BE, Verweij PE. Two strategies for managing invasive aspergillosis: a decision analysis. *Clin Infect Dis* 1997; **25**: 1148–54.

2

Diagnostic methods for fungal infections

BERYL OPPENHEIM

Introduction

Invasive fungal infections remain an important cause of morbidity and mortality. In developed countries the majority of infections occur in the setting of the immuno-compromised host, and this patient group is on the increase because major developments in high-technology medicine allow treatment for an ever-increasing range of medical and surgical conditions. In particular, high-dependency care for neonates, the elderly and a range of critically ill individuals, cytotoxic chemotherapy for an increasing range of malignancies, and bone marrow and solid organ transplantation are all contributing to increasingly large numbers of patient groups at risk of developing an invasive fungal infection.

Candida and *Aspergillus* infections continue to form the majority of infections encountered, but, although there is some overlap, the risk factors for these infections differ. *Candida* has become predominantly associated with treatment in high-dependency areas where the widespread use of central venous catheters and multiple courses of antibiotics are important risk factors. Invasive aspergillosis, on the other hand, is particularly noted in association with neutropenia and bone marrow and solid organ transplantation, and in this setting mortality remains high [1]. Other fungal infections include cryptococcosis, zygomycosis and some emerging agents, such as *Fusarium*, but infection due to these remains relatively rare.

The diagnosis of fungal infections is problematic and this results in difficulties in designing and evaluating treatment regimens and a continuing high mortality from invasive fungal infections. In many vulnerable patients the only early sign of infection may be a fever and more specific signs and symptoms occur late, when opportunities for successful treatment are limited. This has led to a number of different strategies for therapy; for example, using prophylactic and empiric regimens. Both result in large numbers of patients receiving treatment unnecessarily, with attendant high costs and unwanted adverse affects. The desire for using pre-emptive therapy (that is, initiating therapy in only those individuals with infection) at the earliest stage in infection, preferably before signs and symptoms are manifest, has provoked a large amount of research into improved methods of fungal diagnosis [2].

In the past, the mainstay of diagnosis of fungal infection has been the isolation or identification of pathogenic fungi from sterile body sites, such as blood or tissue. While this approach remains the gold standard, it is now well recognized that this would result in many fungal infections being undiagnosed until late in the infective process, or, in many cases, after death, and this has led to a considerable amount of research into more non-invasive methods of diagnosis.

Radiological imaging has advanced in recent years and it is becoming clear that newer methods can make significant contributions to earlier diagnosis of fungal infection. High-resolution computed tomography (CT) scanning is well recognized as being able to detect typical lesions of invasive aspergillosis at a stage when the chest X-ray may be entirely normal. Similarly, both CT and magnetic resonance imaging are also valuable in the diagnosis of chronic disseminated candidiasis, which is a condition in which culture methods often prove negative.

Because many of the patients suffering from invasive fungal infection are highly immunosuppressed, they are often unable to produce an immune response, and this has meant that antibody detection has generally not proved useful in identifying or monitoring fungal infections. However, the concept of antigen detection has been attractive for a number of reasons, and systems for detecting both *Candida* and *Aspergillus* are well advanced. There are now a number of studies evaluating their utility in a variety of clinical settings.

Molecular methods for the detection of a number of otherwise difficult to diagnose infections have become well established over recent years, and it is therefore not surprising that this route has been studied extensively for the early diagnosis of invasive fungal infections. Despite the increasingly large number of studies in this area, a number of important questions remain unanswered. These include such critical issues as the optimal DNA or RNA targets to be chosen, the best methods for extracting fungal DNA from various clinical samples, and even the choice of sample to be tested such as whole blood, plasma, serum or other samples such as bronchoalveolar lavage (BAL) fluid.

This review will focus particularly on the early or improved diagnosis of *Candida* and *Aspergillus* infections in the setting of the immunocompromised or otherwise susceptible host.

The radiological spectrum of invasive aspergillosis in children: a 10 year review

Thomas KE, Owens CM, Veys PA, Novelli V, Costoli V. *Pediatr Radiol* 2003; **33**: 453–60

BACKGROUND. Invasive pulmonary aspergillosis is an important cause of opportunistic infection in children with a variety of underlying diseases, including neutropenia following chemotherapy for haematological malignancy, bone marrow and solid organ transplantation and primary immunodeficiency syndromes. Despite aggressive treatment, mortality remains high. One reason for this may be delays in the institution of treatment because of difficulty in making an early diagnosis. The respiratory tract is the main portal of entry for infection and most cases will present first with symptoms referable to the lungs, although disseminated infection can occur in up to 30% of patients. Chest X-ray findings are often late, variable and non-specific. CT of the chest has been well described as a useful tool in improving the early detection of pulmonary aspergillosis, and in adults two lesions in particular have been shown to be associated with this condition. The first, the halo sign, is associated with a zone of lower attenuation surrounding a nodule or pulmonary mass, and is usually the earliest specific feature noted. The air-crescent sign occurs later and is associated with the development of cavitation |3|. Most of the series detailing these features have focused on adult patients but there are few large paediatric series available to draw conclusions about the CT appearance of pulmonary aspergillosis in children.

INTERPRETATION. Twenty-seven consecutive cases of invasive aspergillosis diagnosed in children over a 10-year period were reviewed, correlating all available imaging material with clinical and microbiological data. Ages ranged from 7 months to 18 years and all patients had an underlying disease associated with immunodeficiency or had received immunosuppressive therapy. Disease appeared confined to a single site in 12 children, in 10 there was evidence of multisystem disease, while in the remaining five there was probable multisystem disease. Chest radiographs were available in 18 cases with documented respiratory disease. X-ray findings were varied, but the major findings were segmented consolidation, multilobar consolidation, perihilar infiltrate, multiple small nodules, large peripheral nodular masses and pleural effusions. In no case was convincing radiographic evidence of cavitation or air crescent formation seen. Chest CT was available in eight cases. Multiple small nodules were seen in four, and in two of these central cavitation of a number of the nodules was observed. None demonstrated the halo sign.

Comment

Invasive aspergillosis is becoming more important in children because of the increasing use of radiotherapy, high doses of chemotherapy, and bone marrow transplantation for a variety of underlying diseases. In adults, respiratory disease is associated with radiological evidence of cavitation in approximately 50% of cases and air crescent formation in 40%. The CT halo sign is said to be highly predictive of pulmonary aspergillosis in the appropriate clinical setting.

This study has shown that X-ray changes are often extremely non-specific in children with invasive pulmonary aspergillosis and that multiple small nodules are an important pointer to the diagnosis. No signs of cavitation were seen. The reasons for these differences remain unclear. Cavitation tends to occur later in disease, often coinciding with recovery of neutropenia. However, paediatric cases often occur in children with primary immunodeficiency, where recovery of the underlying risk factor does not occur, so differences in host response may be at least partly responsible for this finding. This study highlights the problems with relying on clinical or radiological findings to make the diagnosis of invasive aspergillosis, and underscores the necessity for improved diagnostic tools.

Detection of fungal antigens

Antigen detection is an attractive option for fungal diagnosis. The test may be performed on a variety of patient samples, such as serum, urine, cerebrospinal fluid (CSF) or BAL fluid. If appropriate antigens are chosen, they could be highly specific for a particular infection. The typical formats used are easy to perform in a routine laboratory. In addition, dilution or quantitation techniques may allow for assessment of fungal load and monitoring response to therapy. Antigen detection for fungal infection is already well established for organisms such as *Cryptococcus*.

This approach has been more problematic in the diagnosis of *Candida* and *Aspergillus* infections. For *Candida,* a number of target antigens have been considered, but the most widely studied is the mannan antigen. Mannan is a major component of the cell wall of *Candida* and is able to induce a strong antibody response. A variety of studies have shown an association between a positive mannan assay and invasive candidiasis, rather then colonization or transient infection. Two assays for detection of mannan antigenaemia have been marketed, a latex agglutination test and a double sandwich enzyme immunoassay, which is the more sensitive. While it is becoming clear that these assays have some utility in diagnosing invasive candidiasis, they do have limitations involving sensitivity, specificity, and a continued lack of experience of timing of sampling and interpretation of results.

Antigen detection for the diagnosis of *Aspergillus* infection has been of particular interest in the light of the considerable difficulties in making a diagnosis early enough to influence effective treatment. The most extensively studied antigen for *Aspergillus* diagnosis has been galactomannan and a commercially available sandwich enzyme immunoassay is now widely available |4|. A number of studies have shown good sensitivity and specificity of the test and its use in monitoring the success of treatment has also been demonstrated. However, results of its use as an early marker of infection before the advent of clinical signs and symptoms have varied. In addition, some studies have yielded fairly high rates of false positives, possible explanations including cross-reactivity with other bacterial or fungal antigens, and the absorption of galactomannan from foodstuffs into the circulation in patients with a damaged gastrointestinal mucosa.

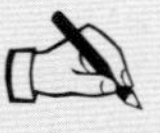

Contribution of the Platelia *Candida*-specific antibody and antigen tests to early diagnosis of systemic *Candida tropicalis* infection in neutropenic adults

Sendid B, Caillot D, Baccouch-Humbert B, *et al*. *J Clin Microbiol* 2003; **41**: 4551–8

BACKGROUND. Mannan antigen induces a strong antibody response towards a large repertoire of oligomannose epitopes, some of which may be protective to the host. A new diagnostic approach, based on the combined detection of both mannan and antimannan antibodies, has been suggested to improve the diagnosis of invasive candidiasis, and with regular sampling good sensitivity and specificity for most pathogenic *Candida* species has been demonstrated. In this study, retrospective serum samples from seven neutropenic patients were studied to assess the value of this approach in *Candida tropicalis*.

INTERPRETATION. Subjects consisted of a cohort of seven patients with proven *C. tropicalis* infection. The Platelia *Candida*-specific antigen and antibody assays (Bio-Rad Laboratories) were used on 83 samples from this group of patients and four samples each from 12 controls. All study patients tested positive and in six of the seven at least one positive result was obtained on average 5 days (range 2–10 days) prior to the first positive culture. High persistent mannanaemia was noted in all patients during the neutropenic period, while in five patients an increased antibody response was detected when they recovered from aplasia. A low level of mannanaemia was detected in only one of 48 serum samples from control patients and none showed significant antibody titres.

Comment

C. tropicalis was isolated from blood cultures in all the subjects in this study, so in many ways this was not a particularly challenging diagnostic group. However, it is of great interest that mannanaemia was detected in all but one case at a time when blood cultures had been taken but had not yet become positive. Also of interest was the detection of mannanaemia in an individual who subsequently presented with proven hepatosplenic candidiasis, as this is well recognized as a condition that is difficult to diagnose. The contribution of antibody detection to early diagnosis is less clear-cut in this setting, as antibodies tended to be detected later, after bone marrow recovery.

Detection of the *Candida* antigen mannan in cerebrospinal fluid specimens from patients suspected of having *Candida* meningitis

Verduyn Lunel FM, Voss A, Kuijper EJ, *et al*. *J Clin Microbiol* 2004; **42**: 867–70

BACKGROUND. Meningitis caused by *Candida* is both rare and difficult to diagnose. The majority of cases occur in very-low birth weight neonates but infection has also been detected in patients with HIV and in individuals with ventricular shunts. While CSF findings are often abnormal, culture may be negative because the number of fungal cells in the CSF is extremely low. The recommendation is that large volumes of CSF be cultured, but this may not always be possible. In addition, the significance of a positive culture is not always clear because contamination of the sample may have occurred.

INTERPRETATION. This study looks at the role of mannan antigen detection in five patients from whom *Candida* was cultured in CSF and who were treated for *Candida* meningitis. Ages ranged from 4 days to 76 years and all had underlying diseases causing

Table 2.1 Results of detection of *Candida* mannan in CSF compared with culture

Case no. or group	Classification	Culture result* (no. positive/ total)	Mean OD (range)	Interpretation† (no. positive/ total)
1	Proven infection	4/4	2.999‡	3/3
2	Proven infection	2/5	0.571 (0.489–0.779)	7/7
3	Proven infection	3/9	1.721 (1.057–2.935)	4/4
4	Proven infection	1/2	3.500‡	2/2
5	No infection	1/6	0.297 (0.259–0.331)	0/3
A§	Control	0/28	0.264 (0.211–0.365)	0/28
B	Control	10/10	0.163 (0.112–0.228)	0/10
C	Control	0/16	0.211 (0.160–0.270)	0/16

* Culture for yeasts.
† Cut-off value = 0.440.
‡ ODs out of range.
§ Control group: A, patients with clinically suspected bacterial meningitis and negative fungal cultures; B, patients with cultures positive for *C. neoformans* and CSF positive for cryptococcal antigen; C, patients CSF positive for *Aspergillus* antigen.
Source: Verduyn Lunel *et al.* (2004).

severe immunosuppression. Four of the cases had good supporting evidence of *Candida* meningitis, including repeated positive candidal culture from CSF, while the fifth had a single positive CSF culture, which was subsequently considered to be a contaminant (Table 2.1). Mannan was detected in the CSF in all four of the cases with proven CNS candidiasis, but not in the case where the culture was considered to be a contaminant. In addition, 54 CSF samples from a variety of control patients, including a number with cryptococcal or *Aspergillus* infection, were tested and none was positive.

Comment

These results show high specificity for the mannan antigen in the diagnosis of *Candida* meningitis. The negative result in a patient for whom a positive culture was subsequently considered to be a contaminant is of interest as the test may be useful in discriminating between infection and contamination.

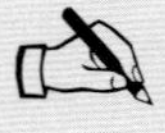

Detection of *Aspergillus* galactomannan by enzyme immunoabsorbent assay in recipients of allogeneic hematopoietic stem cell transplantation: a prospective study

Rovira M, Jimenez M, De La Bellacasa JP, *et al. Transplantation* 2004; **77**: 1260–4

BACKGROUND. The introduction of a commercially available assay for the detection of galactomannan has allowed a number of evaluations of its use in various settings,

Table 2.2 Characteristics of patients with invasive aspergillosis

Patient no.	Sex/age (yr)	Underlying disease	Acute GVHD grade	Dose steroids at time of IA	Type of IA	Time of diagnosis of IA post-HSCT (d)	Organ involvement by IA	Site(s) of *Aspergillus* isolation	ELISA samples	Death in relation with IA
1	F/33	sAA	I	1 mg/kg	Probable	135	Lung, sinus	BAL: *A. fumigatus*	2+	No
2	F/41	NHL	0	No	Proven	32	Brain, lung, liver thyroid gland	BAL: *A. flavus* Autopsy specimen	2+	Yes
3	F/30	AML	I	2 mg/kg	Possible	53	Lung	Non-isolation	1+	Yes
4	M/50	AML	I	2 mg/kg	Probable	38	Lung, brain	BAL: *A. fumigatus*	1+	Yes
5	M/48	AML	I	1 mg/kg	Probable	90	Lung	BAL: *A. flavus*	–	Yes
6	M/35	MDS	0	No	Probable	180	Lung	BAL: *A. fumigatus*	–	No
7	M/50	MM	III	1 mg/kg	Probable	106	Lung	BAL: *A. terreus* and *A. flavus*	6+	Yes
8	M/35	ALL	I	2 mg/kg	Possible	62	Lung	Non-isolation	2+	No

BAL, bronchoalveolar lavage; GVHD, graft-versus-host disease; ELISA, enzyme-linked immunosorbent assay; IA, invasive aspergillosis; HSCT, haematopoietic stem cell transplantation.
Source: Rovira *et al.* (2004).

and to date varying results have been obtained, relating particularly to sensitivity of the assay and whether antigen could be detected before diagnosis could be made by other means. Another controversial issue is the optimum cut-off value for a positive result. Initially a cut-off ratio of 1.5 was recommended, but subsequently many investigators moved to using 1.0 or even 0.7. In the US, approval is for a ratio as low as 0.5. This study prospectively analysed the value of galactomannan in the allogeneic haematopoietic stem cell transplantation setting, using a relatively high cut-off for positivity.

INTERPRETATION. Seventy-four patients, with a total of 832 samples, were studied. Galactomannan testing was performed twice weekly from admission until death or discharge. Strict criteria were employed to define categories of infection. Overall, seven of the patients had proven, probable or possible aspergillosis, and all 14 positive samples occurred in this patient group. Distribution of positivity is shown in Table 2.2. In the six patients with positive results, four were already receiving antifungal treatment because of persistent fever when the result became positive, and two showed a positive galactomannan at the time that antifungals were initiated.

Comment

This study, in line with a number of others, shows a high specificity of the galacto-mannan assay, and considerable use in providing corroborating evidence of infection in possible or probable cases. Disappointingly, however, the sensitivity was relatively poor and the positive tests did not precede other evidence of fungal infection to allow earlier initiation of therapy. This study used a relatively high cut-off for positivity and it would be of interest to know whether improved results could be obtained by lowering the cut-off. In addition, account will need to be taken of the cost–benefits of adding an additional test to the diagnostic armamentarium where a large proportion of the results are negative, and even the small number of positives do not appear to significantly influence patient management.

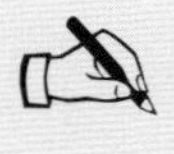

Prospective assessment of Platelia™ *Aspergillus* galactomannan antigen for the diagnosis of invasive aspergillosis in lung transplant recipients

Husain S, Kwak EJ, Obman A, *et al. Am J Transplant* 2004; **4**: 796–802

BACKGROUND. *Aspergillus* galactomannan has been widely evaluated as a tool for improving early diagnosis of invasive aspergillosis. However, the majority of the evaluations have focused on patients with haematological malignancies or undergoing bone marrow transplantation. Aspergillosis is an important complication of lung or heart–lung transplantation, but the clinical presentation and course of the infection are different and patients are seldom neutropenic. The aim of this study was to evaluate the utility of the Platelia galactomannan assay in the early diagnosis of invasive aspergillosis in a cohort of lung transplant recipients.

Table 2.3 Sensitivity of galactomannan test according to clinical syndromes of invasive aspergillosis

Systemic aspergillosis	100%	(1/1)
Aspergillus tracheobronchitis	0%	(0/4)
Pulmonary aspergillosis	28.5%	(2/7)
Pulmonary and systemic aspergillosis	37.5%	(3/8)

Source: Husain *et al.* (2004).

INTERPRETATION. Seventy consecutive lung transplant recipients were prospectively enrolled in this study and serum samples were collected twice weekly during their post-transplant hospital stay and subsequent hospitalizations. The most common indications for transplantation were chronic obstructive pulmonary disease, cystic fibrosis and idiopathic pulmonary fibrosis. Nine patients had proven and three had probable invasive aspergillosis. Of the 12, seven had pulmonary aspergillosis, four had tracheobronchitis, and one had systemic aspergillosis. A total of 891 sera from the 70 patients were analysed. Galactomannan was positive in three of the 12 patients with invasive aspergillosis (Table 2.3) Fourteen patients without invasive aspergillosis had 36 false-positive test results. False-positive tests did not correlate with colonization with *Aspergillus*, use of antifungal prophylaxis, or prior rejection episodes.

Comment

These results suggest that galactomannan testing may be of less value in the lung transplant population than in the setting of neutropenia or bone marrow transplantation. The authors speculate that the lower sensitivity of the test in this non-neutropenic population may reflect the lower fungal burden in individuals able to clear antigens from the bloodstream. A possible reason for the false-positive results could be low-level respiratory tract colonization with *Aspergillus* in patients with chronic obstructive pulmonary disease or cystic fibrosis.

False-positive galactomannan platelia *Aspergillus* test results for patients receiving piperacillin–tazobactam

Viscoli C, Machetti M, Cappellano P, *et al. Clin Infect Dis* 2004; **38**: 913–16

BACKGROUND. In many centres, routine screening of high-risk bone marrow transplant or leukaemia patients for galactomannan is now taking place. A letter |5|, this paper and a further brief report |6| have now become available, suggesting false-positive results for this test in patients receiving piperacillin/tazobactam.

INTERPRETATION. This report is from a centre where twice-weekly monitoring of galactomannan in at-risk patients has been common practice since 1999. In April 2003, during routine review of this procedure, it was recognized that the proportion of samples which were positive was increasing, and a full evaluation of the process was instituted. During the period from January 1999 until May 2003 a total of 4702 serum samples from 420 patients were tested. Figure 2.1 shows the median positivity rate per month. The overall proportion of patents classified as positive for invasive aspergillosis increased from 10% to 36%. The authors reviewed patient case notes to exclude the possibility of a true outbreak of aspergillosis and also reviewed the method of performance of the test to exclude a technical problem. What was noted, however, was a strong correlation between galactomannan positivity and piperacillin–tazobactam administration. The authors then tested 30 piperacillin–tazobactam vials from 15 batches and were able to show that 12 (80%) of the batches had positive galactomannan results, with a median galactomannan index of 4.6.

Comment

There have now been three recent reports of false-positive galactomannan results occurring in patients receiving piperacillin–tazobactam therapy, and positive results of galactomannan testing can be reproduced in testing certain batches of the antimicrobial. The precise reason for this occurrence is not yet known, but it is known that the rat monoclonal antibody used to detect galactomannan can recognize moulds of other genera, such as *Penicillium* species. Piperacillin and tazobactam are semisynthetic drugs derived from natural compounds produced by moulds of the *Penicillium* genus and it is hypothesized that this may be causing contamination

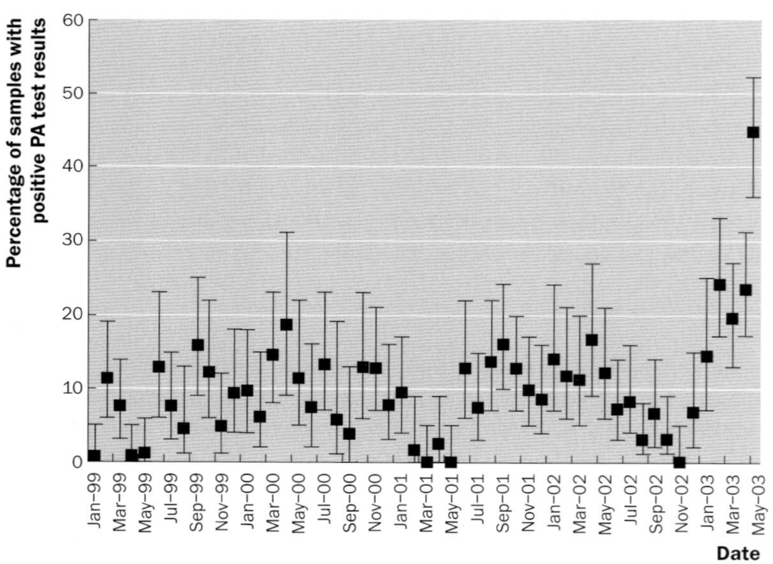

Fig. 2.1 Percentage of samples with positive galactomannan results. Source: Viscoli *et al.* (2004).

of certain batches of the drug. The published studies suggest that this is a new phenomenon, possibly related to some modification in the drug production process. Regardless of whether this particular issue can be resolved by the manufacturers, these incidents highlight the requirement for continued vigilance when using galactomannan and other similar diagnostic tests, and careful review and surveillance of results is essential.

Molecular methods for fungal diagnosis

Molecular methods have been widely employed for the diagnosis of a large number of infections that are otherwise difficult to detect, so it is not surprising that interest has focused on their utility in fungal diagnosis. Despite the very large literature that has become available on the subject since the first reports |7|, it is becoming clear that there are limitations of the techniques.

Studies continue to use a variety of in-house techniques. The polymerase chain reaction (PCR) is the most frequently used amplification procedure, but a very large number of DNA and RNA targets have been exploited. It has become clear that specimen choice and preparation can have a significant impact on results, but to date no universal specimen type or extraction method appears to have emerged as optimal.

With the advent of a number of platforms offering the possibility of real-time quantitative PCR, the attraction of being able to both detect and quantify fungal nucleic acid has become clear.

Development of a LightCycler PCR assay for detection and quantification of *Aspergillus fumigatus* DNA in clinical samples from neutropenic patients

Spiess B, Buchheidt D, Baust C, *et al. J Clin Microbiol* 2003; **41**: 1811–18

BACKGROUND. A number of studies looking at PCR methodology for detection of *Aspergillus* species have been described, some showing good sensitivity and specificity. However, the optimal method is still not clear, as many of the methods described use different targets and methods of extraction and there is still some controversy over which clinical samples yield the most clinically useful results. To aid in interpretation and possibly assist in monitoring the severity, course, and prognosis of infection, quantitation of the fungal load would be an important additional piece of information. A number of commercial platforms are now available which allow real-time quantitative PCR assays to be performed, and studies assessing the clinical utility of these for fungal diagnosis are required.

INTERPRETATION. This study used a LightCycler™-based real-time PCR assay to detect and quantify *Aspergillus fumigatus* DNA in blood and BAL from high-risk patients. The primers

Table 2.4 PCR results for patient blood and BAL samples

Patient no.	Sample	Time sample was taken (day after date of diagnosis)	Diagnosis*	Diagnostic significance†	LightCycler PCR gene copy no./ml‡	Corresponding no. of CFU/ml‡	Nested PCR result	Outcome
1	1(BAL)	+2	AML	Proven	37 ± 9	15 ± 4	+	Death, AML
1	2(blood)	+3	AML	Proven			+	Death, AML
2	BAL	+3	Hodgkin's disease	Proven	17 837 ± 1605	5270 ± 474	+	Death, HD[d] relapse
3	BAL	+3	AML	Proven	13 670 ± 2324	4038 ± 686	+	Death, AML
4	BAL	+1	ALL	Proven	910 525 ± 81 947	269 018 ± 24 211	+	Death, IPA
5	BAL	+4	AML	Proven	597 ± 280	176 ± 83	+	Death/bacteraemia
6	BAL	+4	AML	Probable	385 ± 254	114 ± 75	+	Death, IPA
7	I (BAL)	+4	CML blast crisis	Proven	922 ± 396	272 ± 117	+	Death, IPA
7	2(BAL)	+13	CML blast crisis	Proven	2697 ± 863	797 ± 255	+	Death, IPA
8	BAL	+3	AML	Probable	920 ± 223	271 ± 66	+	Death, IPA
9	BAL	+1	AML	Probable	44 687 ± 6740	13 202 ± 1991	+	Survival
10	1(BAL)	+2	Chronic neutropenia	Proven	55 171 ± 26 157	16 300 ± 7727	+	Death, IPA
10	2(blood)	+2	Chronic neutropenia	Proven	1010 ± 707	298 ± 208	+	Death, IPA
11	BAL	+4	AML	Probable	2704 ± 243	799 ± 72	+	Survival
12	blood	+8	ALL	Probable	11 790 ± 6930	3483 ± 2047	+	Survival
13	1(blood)	+5	CLL	Proven			+	Death, IPA
13	2(blood)	+10	CLL	Proven	28 491 ± 8262	8418 ± 2441	+	Death, IPA
14	1(blood)	+9	ALL relapse	Proven			+	Death, ALL
14	2(blood)	+11	ALL relapse	Proven			+	Death, ALL
14	3 (blood)	+15	ALL relapse	Proven			+	Death, ALL
15	blood	+8	AML	Probable			+	Death, AML
16	1(blood)	+9	AML relapse	Proven			+	Death, AML
16	2(blood)	+13	AML relapse	Proven	78 000 ± 3013	23 045 ± 890	+	Death, AML
17	blood	+5	AML	Probable			+	Survival
18	1(blood)	+8	AML	Probable	106 360 ± 27 654	31 424 ± 8170	+	Death, AML
18	2(blood)	+10	AML	Probable	352 388 ± 96 671	104 114 ± 28 561	+	Death, AML

* AML, acute myeloid leukaemia; ALL, acute lymphoblastic leukaemia; CML, chronic myeloid leukaemia; CLL, chronic lymphoblastic leukaemia.
† Data represent means ± standard deviations from three separate experiments. Where no value is given, the result was negative.
‡ HD, Hodgkin's disease.
Source: Spiess *et al.* (2003).

and hybridization probes were derived from an *A. fumigatus*-specific sequence of the mitochondrial cytochrome *b* gene. The assay was able to detect between 3 and 300 000 colony-forming units (c.f.u.) per ml. Clinical samples were taken from patients with proven or probable invasive aspergillosis and had all been previously positive using a nested PCR assay developed by the same group. Twelve of 12 BAL samples which had been positive using the nested PCR were positive on the LightCycler PCR and quantification of fungal burden showed 37–910 525 copies of the mitochondrial cytochrome *b* gene, corresponding to 15–269 018 c.f.u./ml of BAL (Table 2.4). Fourteen blood samples from nine patients, all of which had been positive by the nested PCR, were also tested. Eight of these were negative, giving a sensitivity rate for these samples of 43%. Quantification of fungal burden showed 298–104 114 c.f.u./ml of blood. Twenty BAL samples from non-immunocompromised patients and 50 blood samples from healthy volunteers were subjected to testing by the LightCycler PCR and all were negative.

Comment

A rapid, sensitive PCR assay for both detection and quantification of fungal load in invasive aspergillosis would be of major clinical benefit. It is therefore disappointing, although perhaps not surprising, that this assay proved less sensitive than the nested PCR already developed by this group. The authors speculate that this could be due to the fact that the fungal load was below the limit of detection by the quantitative assay, or that the specificity of the assay for *A. fumigatus* may have led to infections due to other species being missed. The latter appears to be an unlikely explanation for such a high proportion of false negatives, given that most infections are caused by *A. fumigatus.*

The LightCycler assay matched the nested PCR for BAL specimens, in which it is likely that fungal load is higher. However, in the case of BAL, which is usually taken as a one-off diagnostic sample, quantitative monitoring is less likely to be of use in assessing the response to treatment. The authors suggest that the LightCycler PCR might find a use in the diagnostic armamentarium as a follow-on to the nested PCR in those individuals who are positive, for monitoring the success of therapy. It would be of interest to see an evaluation of such a strategy, including cost-effectiveness, given the likely high cost of the assay and the high rates of negativity even in those individuals who were shown to be positive in the nested PCR. While this study establishes the feasibility of such an approach, the search must continue for a sensitive, specific quantitative assay which can be used for both diagnosis and monitoring.

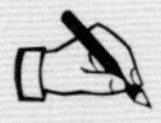

Prospective clinical evaluation of a LightCycler™-mediated polymerase chain reaction assay, a nested-PCR assay and a galactomannan enzyme-linked immunosorbent assay for detection of invasive aspergillosis in neutropenic cancer patients and haematological stem cell transplant recipients

Buchheidt D, Hummel M, Schleiermacher D, *et al. Br J Haematol* 2004; **125**: 196–202

BACKGROUND. While the literature abounds with studies describing the development and limited evaluation of a number of different PCR assays for *Aspergillus*, there is still a dearth of evidence regarding strategies for bringing the various tests into routine clinical use. Particular areas which have not been addressed include the timing and frequency of sampling, and the influence on the results of the use of antifungals, either for prophylaxis or treatment. This study, from the same centre as the one reviewed above, attempts to address some of these issues in a prospective evaluation of their strategy of using a sensitive nested PCR for diagnosis and a LightCycler-based PCR for quantitation. In addition, they compare these results with those obtained from galactomannan testing on the same patient group.

INTERPRETATION. Five university hospitals contributed samples from 165 patients with haematological malignancies undergoing intensive chemotherapy or haematopoietic stem cell transplantation. Samples were obtained over the course of an episode (mean, every 3 days) and at least three samples were required for inclusion in the study. Samples were tested using a previously described nested PCR and serum samples were tested for galactomannan using enzyme immunoassay (Bio-Rad). Only the nested PCR samples that were positive were then submitted for quantitative PCR, using a previously described LightCycler assay. In total, 205 patient episodes from 165 patients were analysed. An interesting finding related to the correlation between the number of samples tested and PCR positivity, the frequency of positive PCR results being associated with the number of samples tested (Fig. 2.2). If more than 25 samples per episode were tested, 100% of episodes had at least one positive result. Looking at patients with proven and probable invasive aspergillosis, for at least one positive PCR, sensitivity was 63.6% and specificity 63.5%. If two or more positive PCRs were required for positivity, sensitivity became 36.4% and specificity 92.3%. For galactomannan testing, sensitivity was 33.3% and specificity was 98.9%. One hundred and seventeen nested PCR-positive samples were analysed by the LightCycler quantitative PCR. Twenty-five of these were positive, with ranges from 37 to 4 410 667 copies/ml.

Comment

This study provides a fascinating insight into the complexities associated with using non-culture methods of diagnosis of invasive aspergillosis in the routine clinical setting. Although the study was prospective, there did not appear to be rigid criteria for the timing of sampling, and clearly those patients with ongoing and unresolving

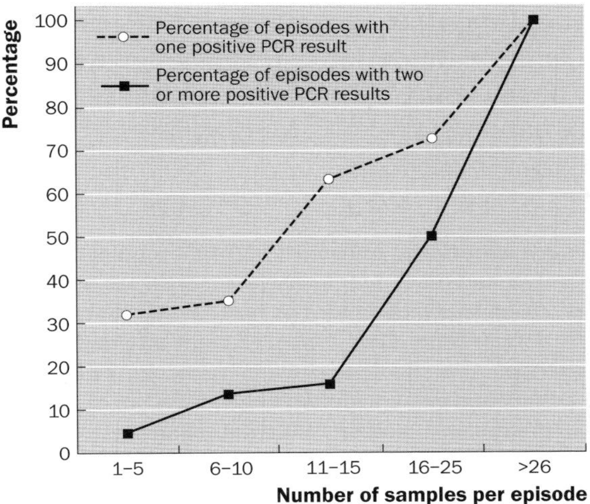

Fig. 2.2 Correlation between number of samples obtained per episode and percentage of PCR positive episodes. Source: Buchheidt *et al.*, 2003.

infections, which were more likely to be fungal in origin, would have been more likely to have more samples submitted.

In addition, those patients considered to have proven or probable invasive aspergillosis would have been treated with high doses and possibly combinations of antifungal agents. The influence of antifungal treatment on PCR or galactomannan assay results has not been studied systematically, but it is likely that this may influence positivity significantly.

Both false-positive and false-negative PCR results proved problematic in this cohort of patients. The reasons for positive *Aspergillus* PCR results in patients with no features of invasive disease remain unclear. It will be difficult to establish whether these positive results represent transient episodes of fungal DNA entering the circulation, either with no adverse effects to the patient or as part of early infection which never becomes clinically detectable, or are manifestations of contamination occurring during sampling or processing of specimens. False negatives may reflect poor sensitivity of the test, or it may be that even in the presence of invasive infection fungal DNA is only present in the circulation transiently.

In this study the addition of a quantitative PCR to attempt to aid in distinguishing between contamination, colonization and true infection was not particularly helpful, largely because the poor sensitivity of the quantitative PCR allowed quantification in less than one-quarter of the positive samples. In the very few samples that were able to be quantified, an obvious differentiation between categories of infection on the basis of fungal load did not seem apparent.

Comparison of real-time PCR, conventional PCR, and galactomannan antigen detection by enzyme-linked immunosorbent assay using bronchoalveolar lavage fluid samples from hematology patients for diagnosis of invasive pulmonary aspergillosis

Sanguinetti M, Posteraro B, Pagano L, *et al*. *J Clin Microbiol* 2003; **41**: 3922–5

BACKGROUND. Many of the studies undertaken previously highlight problems with poor sensitivity of PCR and galactomannan testing for invasive aspergillosis when blood and serum samples are used. One explanation for this may be that, because it is primarily a pulmonary infection, neither *Aspergillus* DNA nor fungal antigens are consistently present in the bloodstream. Other biological fluids, particularly BAL, may be more reliable in terms of the continuous presence of *Aspergillus* DNA or galactomannan, but are fraught with problems relating to the detection of contamination or colonization and the differentiation of these from true invasive infection. Quantitation of the fungal load appears to be an attractive adjunct to PCR testing which might be able to distinguish true infection from other causes of positive PCR, as well as being used for assessing the severity of infection and the response to treatment. Studies to date, however, have proved disappointing because of the low sensitivity of these assays in blood samples. This study sought to evaluate the performance of a new real-time quantitative PCR on BAL samples and compare this with conventional PCR and galactomannan testing.

INTERPRETATION. For this study, a new iCycler iQ (Bio-Rad) real-time PCR was developed. The nucleic acid target was a conserved region from the 18S RNA genes of several *Aspergillus* species. This new quantitative assay was compared with a nested PCR and galactomannan enzyme immunoassay on 44 BAL fluid samples from patients for whom full details of infection status were available. Twenty-four of the patients showed no evidence of aspergillosis, and specimens from these patients yielded negative results in all these assays and in cultures. For the remaining 20 patients who had proven (5) or probable (15) invasive aspergillosis, all 20 were galactomannan-positive, and 18 of the 20 were positive in both PCR assays (Table 2.5). Those samples with the highest estimated fungal loads were also confirmed by culture.

Comment

While studies on *Aspergillus* PCR on blood samples appear to give conflicting and often disappointing results, this and other studies looking at non-culture methods on BAL fluids in the setting of neutropenia and haematological malignancy seem more promising. The addition of a quantitative result may give further useful information and, if a relevant threshold can be established, may enable differentiation between contamination, colonization and true infection.

Although the search must continue for a reliable test using non-invasive sampling, BAL fluid is an attractive option for a number of reasons. Although not truly non-invasive, it is generally considered to be a safe technique, even in the setting of

Table 2.5 Results of real-time PCR, conventional PCR, and GM ELISA of BAL fluid specimens from patients with IPA

Patient no.	Sex, age (yr)	Primary disease*	Outcome	IPA diagnosis (EORTC criteria†)	BAL fungal culture	GM ELISA	BAL PCR result	
							Real-time (copies/ml)	Conventional
1	F,47	NHL	Survival	Probable	C. albicans	Positive	Negative	Negative
2	F, 72	NHL	Death	Probable	C. glabrata	Positive	3000	Positive
3	F, 65	ML	Death	Probable	Negative	Positive	4500	Positive
4	M, 41	AML	Survival	Probable	Negative	Positive	8000	Positive
5	M, 50	ALL	Death	Proven	A. fumigatus	Positive	60 000	Positive
6	M, 65	SAA	Death	Proven	A. flavus	Positive	45 000	Positive
7	M,68	AML	Survival	Probable	Negative	Positive	4200	Positive
8	M, 48	SAA	Death	Proven	A. fumigatus	Positive	75 000	Positive
9	F, 72	ML	Survival	Probable	C. albicans	Positive	2000	Positive
10	M, 65	AML	Death	Probable	Negative	Positive	3900	Positive
11	M, 60	AML	Death	Probable	Negative	Positive	9800	Positive
12	F, 60	AML	Death	Probable	Negative	Positive	10 500	Positive
13	M, 67	ALL	Survival	Probable	Negative	Positive	8700	Positive
14	F, 42	NHL	Death	Proven	A. fumigatus	Positive	85 000	Positive
15	M, 77	ALL	Death	Probable	Negative	Positive	5400	Positive
16	M, 70	AML	Death	Probable	A. fumigatus	Positive	23 000	Positive
17	M, 70	NHL	Death	Proven	A. flavus	Positive	100 000	Positive
18	M, 74	AML	Death	Probable	Negative	Positive	7600	Positive
19	F, 39	AML	Survival	Probable	C. albicans	Positive	Negative	Negative
20	M, 54	ALL	Survival	Probable	C. albicans	Positive	3200	Positive

* NHL, non-Hodgkin's lymphoma; ML, malignant lymphoma; AML, acute myeloblastic leukaemia; ALL, acute lymphoblastic leukaemia; SAA, severe aplastic anaemia.
† EORTC, European Organization for Research and Treatment of Cancer.
Source: Sanguinetti et al. (2003).

pancytopenia. The fluid can also be subjected to microscopy and culture, so that other potential pathogens can be sought at the same time. However, repeated sampling is unlikely to be acceptable, so quantitative PCR in BAL could not be used for monitoring the response to therapy.

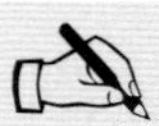

Diagnosing and monitoring of invasive aspergillosis during antifungal therapy by polymerase chain reaction: an experimental study in mice

Lass-Florl C, Speth C, Mayr A, *et al. Diagn Microbiol Infect Dis* 2003; **47**: 569–72

BACKGROUND. As has been shown previously, results of PCR assays for invasive aspergillosis are extremely variable, and most workers have demonstrated negative results in the face of proven or probable disease. Varying sensitivity of the assay, disagreement about the optimal sample for testing and the possibility of transient periods of DNA in the bloodstream have all been put forward as explanations for this, but the confounding factor of antifungal therapy has not yet been studied carefully. In clinical practice, most patients with suspected fungal infections will be receiving an antifungal agent, but this has rarely been documented or included in analysis in the studies performed to date. A simpler method of studying the effect of antifungal treatment on PCR monitoring may be to use an animal model. This study looked at the effect on a PCR assay of amphotericin B treatment in mice experimentally infected with *Aspergillus*.

INTERPRETATION. The PCR assay used was based on the 18S r RNA of various fungal pathogens, and detection was by enzyme-linked immunosorbent assay. Forty-two female BALB/c mice were infected with either *A. fumigatus* (28) or *A. terreus* (14). One group of mice was treated with amphotericin B by once daily injection, whereas glucose injection was given to the other group. Blood samples were taken on days 1, 3 and 8, and kidneys, brain and lung were removed after the animals had been killed for microscopy, culture and PCR. Over the 8 days following treatment, 72% of samples in the control group and 41% in the treatment group were PCR-positive in blood (Table 2.6). Based on at least one positive PCR result, the sensitivity was 77% for the treatment group and 92% for the untreated group.

Comment

There are a number of problems in extrapolating the results of this study to the clinical setting. The route of infection and course of disease are different. Only amphotericin B treatment was evaluated, whereas in the clinic a variety of agents may be used. The PCR assay employed may not have been as sensitive as some described in the literature, and it is disappointing that a real-time quantitative PCR was not studied.

Despite these shortcomings, this study is of interest for a variety of reasons. The authors were able to show a difference in PCR positivity in blood between the treated and untreated groups, as well as inconsistent results even in the mice that did not receive any antifungal. This study highlights the importance of frequent serial

Table 2.6 Distribution of results of blood monitoring using *Aspergillus* PCR in treated and untreated mice with proven infection

PCR results from blood

	During antifungal therapy			**Without antifungal therapy**		
A. fumigatus						
Mice	Day 1	Day 3	Day 8	Day 1	Day 3	Day 8
1	+	–	–	+	+	+
2	+	–	–	+	–	–
3	–	–	–	–	–	+
4	–	+	+	+	–	+
5	–	–	+	+	+	–
6	+	–	–	–	+	+
7	–	–	–	+	–	–
8	+	–	–	+	+	–
A. terreus						
Mice	Day 1	Day 3	Day 8	Day 1	Day 3	Day 8
1	+	–	–	+	+	+
2	+	–	–	+	–	–
3	–	–	–	–	–	–
4	–	+	+	+	–	+
5	–	–	+	+	–	–

Source: Lass-Florl *et al.* (2003).

sampling of blood for PCR in any future studies. Similarly, it will be essential to document and analyse the effect of any antifungal therapy being administered to subjects in such studies.

Conclusion

While there continues to be a pool of susceptible patients, the problem of fungal infection will continue to challenge infection specialists. It is clear that invasive fungal infections carry a high mortality, and that early and appropriate treatment is required to minimize this. A number of promising new antifungal agents have become available recently, but because it is so difficult to make a definitive diagnosis of fungal infection, much of their evaluation has been in the empirical setting, and this makes it more difficult to develop clear guidelines for their use in invasive infection. The agents are often extremely costly and may have significant side effects or toxicities. The dilemma remains, therefore, that their use should be limited to only those who are likely to benefit, but in the early stages of infection signs and symptoms are non-specific, and there is a great need for improved diagnostic tests.

Imaging, particularly computed tomography scanning of the chest for pulmonary aspergillosis, is well described as a useful adjunct. The paper reviewed here inserts a note of caution in reporting that the typical findings may be absent in paediatric patients. While the use of imaging should be encouraged for patients with the earliest signs of possible fungal infection, logistical reasons dictate that it is unlikely to be feasible for screening for early infection in at-risk groups.

Antigen detection is a promising option and it is encouraging that standardized, commercially produced assays are now available. Galactomannan testing appears well established in the setting of haematological malignancies but it may not be possible to extrapolate this usage directly to other groups at risk of aspergillosis. Results of studies of detection of mannan in the diagnosis of candidiasis are also encouraging and it will be of interest to see where this test finds its role in clinical practice, given the very large numbers of patient groups at risk of candidaemia.

Despite a decade of study, molecular methods for fungal diagnosis have not yet established a routine role in clinical practice. If this approach is to move forward, the temptation to develop further tests based on slightly different technologies with small evaluations must be resisted. What is now required are multicentre studies using standardized sampling regimens in which the administration of antifungal agents is carefully documented and included in any analysis of results.

References

1. Lin SJ, Schranz J, Teutsch SM. Aspergillosis case-fatality rate: systematic review of the literature. *Clin Infect Dis* 2001; **32**: 358–66.

2. Yeo SF, Wong B. Current status of non-culture methods for diagnosis of invasive fungal infections. *Clin Microbiol Rev* 2002; **15**: 465–84.

3. Kuhlman JE, Fishman EK, Siegelman SS. Invasive pulmonary aspergillosis in acute leukemia: characteristic findings on CT, the CT halo sign, and the role of CT in early diagnosis. *Radiology* 1985; **157**: 611–14.

4. Mennink-Kersten MA, Donnelly JP, Verweij PE. Detection of circulating galactomannan for the diagnosis and management of invasive aspergillosis. *Lancet Infect Dis* 2004; **4**: 349–57.

5. Sulahian A, Touratier S, Ribaud P. False-positive test for aspergillus antigenemia related to concomitant administration of piperacillin and tazobactam. *N Engl J Med* 2003; **349**: 2366–7.

6. Adam O, Auperin A, Wilquin F, Bourhis JH, Gachot B, Chachaty E. Treatment with piperacillin-tazobactam and false-positive Aspergillus galactomannan antigen test results for patients with hematological malignancies. *Clin Infect Dis* 2004; **38**: 917–20.

7. Einsele H, Hebart H, Roller G, Loffler J, Rothenhofer I, Muller CA, Bowden RA, van Burik J, Engelhard D, Kanz L, Schumacher U. Detection and identification of fungal pathogens in blood by using molecular probes. *J Clin Microbiol* 1997; **35**: 1353–60.

3

What's new in antifungal therapy?

VANYA GANT

Introduction

Fungal infection represents an increasingly important clinical entity for first-world clinicians. Despite the enormous impact of highly active antiretroviral therapy on opportunistic fungal infection, mucocutaneous infection with *Candida* spp. or life-threatening conditions subsequent to *Cryptococcus* or *Pneumocystis jiroveci* var. carinii continues apace.

On another front, our ability to keep people alive for longer in intensive care units and the increasing burden of chronic disease often controlled by immunosuppressive agents also contribute to the burden imposed on us by yeasts and moulds.

Finally, the treatment of haematological malignancy continues to become ever more aggressive, with intentionally induced periods of neutropenia, often extending beyond 3 or 4 weeks. Haematologists are increasingly limited not by their failure to cure cancer but by the death of their patients through infection, very often of a fungal nature.

The need for more effective antifungal agents has therefore risen in parallel with these developments, and until recently there has been little choice. Whilst on the one hand the development of the family of triazole antifungals such as fluconazole (and to a lesser extent the less well tolerated but fascinating itraconazole) heralded a new dawn for the treatment of both superficial and deep *Candida* infections, the treatment of moulds – *Aspergillus* in particular – seemed more limited. The gold standard agent, amphotericin B, was undoubtedly effective against most moulds, but its renal toxicity and infusion side effects limit its usefulness and have earned it a reputation as an effective but difficult and toxic drug to use. Its packaging into various lipid formulations, either as lamellae or liposomes, seemed to result in a drug with at least equivalent efficacy and far better tolerability: infusion reactions, at least for some of these preparations, essentially disappeared and renal toxicity became far less of a problem. These lipid formulations of amphotericin remain the gold standard treatment for invasive mould infection to this day. Two factors, however, continued to bicker on this horizon: that no trial had ever demonstrated that lipid formulations could achieve mycological and treatment cure in all patients with infection; and price. The UK market leader liposomal preparation, Ambisome, for example, could cost up to £20 000 for a reasonable treatment course; and it is not uncommon for haematology units to spend in excess of a million pounds a year on this agent. This is because in the setting of haematological malignancy the price of failure (to treat invasive fungal infection effectively) is almost always death, with quoted mortality figures for invasive aspergillosis of over 90%. Whilst Ambisome and similar agents ruled as the unique class of agents active against moulds (as the ill-fated and little-understood itraconazole seemed to be receding into the distance for little-known reasons), development continued apace, and new agents have now reached the clinic. Pfizer continued developing congeners of its phenomenally successful product fluconazole, unfortunately devoid of activity against moulds, and has now launched voriconazole, available in both intravenous and oral forms. Merck Sharp and Dohme built on its success in invasive candidosis for its drug, caspofungin, to trial the drug in invasive mould infection. Caspofungin is particularly interesting because it represents a completely novel class of molecule (an echinocandin), with a novel target (α1,4 demethylase). These two drugs have in the last 2 years started to challenge the supremacy of amphotericin B-based products and have given clinicians a choice, at least in several landmark trial-based clinical indications. The papers I have chosen are those landmarks. I have also included in other papers a glimpse of things to come, as well as those elements of these new drugs which are either interesting or of concern to clinicians. The idea is to fast-track knowledge and to give a balance; to allow clinicians treating such patients to have a feel for exactly where each one might fit when invasive fungal infection appears and optimal treatment is necessary.

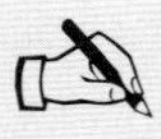

Combination antifungal therapies in HIV-associated cryptococcal meningitis: a randomised trial

Brouwer AE, Rajanuwong A, Chierakul W, *et al*. *Lancet* 2004; **363**: 1764–7

BACKGROUND. Sixty-four patients with a first episode of HIV-associated cryptococcal meningitis were randomized to receive either amphotericin B (0.7 mg/kg/day), amphotericin B plus fluconazole (400 mg daily) or triple therapy with amphotericin B, fluconazole and flucytosine. The primary end-point of fungicidal activity was defined as the comparative ability of these various drug regimens to reduce cerebrospinal fluid (CSF) colony counts of *Cryptococcus* in serial CSF samples taken 3, 7 and 14 days after institution of therapy. The authors found initial cryptococcal count density to be an important prognostic factor. Clearance of cryptococci was exponential. The combination of amphotericin B and flucytosine produced significantly more rapid clearance from the CSF than amphotericin alone, amphotericin plus fluconazole, or triple therapy (*P* <0.02).

INTERPRETATION. This paper from Nick White's group in a Thai regional hospital set out to compare four antifungal drug regimens for their ability to eliminate cryptococci from the CSF of HIV infected individuals. None of the subjects were started on antiretroviral drugs at the time of the study, and therefore the results accurately reflect the activity of the drugs alone, especially given the almost agonal CD4 counts at presentation. The authors chose to perform quantitative colony counts on the CSF throughout a 2-week study period—a simple, but (until this study) as yet unpublished technique which yielded highly relevant results. Despite the relatively small numbers of patients, quantitative colony counting demonstrated that (with deterioration of conscious level) the density of *Cryptococcus* in CSF at presentation was an important determinant of in-hospital mortality (Fig. 3.1). Whilst a little under half of the patients died, no patient with a decreased conscious level and more than 5 million colonies of *Cryptococcus* per ml of CSF survived. Curves of colony count against time (Fig. 3.2) show that none of the four regimens reliably sterilized CSF in less than 10 days or so. Furthermore, the additional speed with which CSF was sterilized in the amphotericin/flucytosine group compared with all other regimens (including triple therapy) seems very clear. Whether this group's suggestion of the value of quantitative colony counts in determining prognosis will be taken up by units treating such patients remains to be seen.

Comment

This is yet another excellent paper from a very well established group. I chose this paper because it demonstrates that three drugs are not necessarily better than two (and, in fact, are inferior). Many doctors fail to resist the temptation to add antifungal drugs to each other in the (completely non-evidence-based) belief that this will be of benefit. This paper clearly demonstrates that quite the opposite applies, and this was to some degree predictable from *in vitro* data on the possible interference of two drug classes acting on the same fungal target. This study reaffirms the combination of

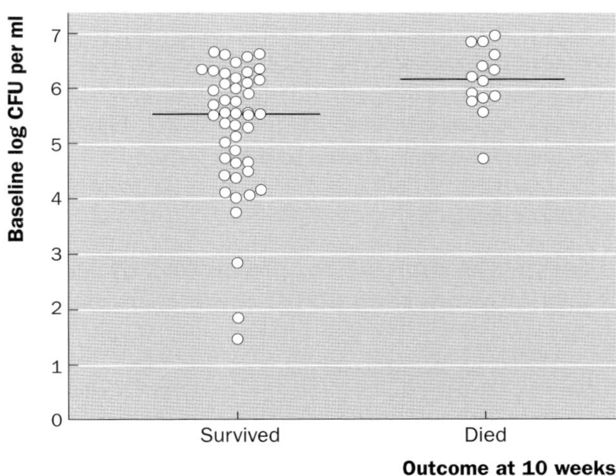

Fig. 3.1 Baseline quantitative CSF culture and death at 10 weeks. Source: Brouwer *et al.* (2004).

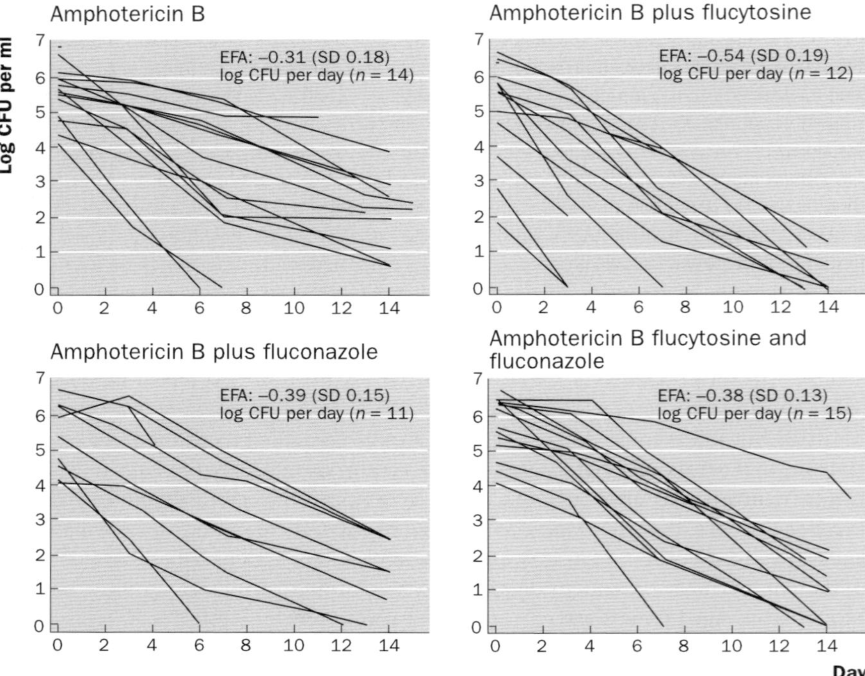

Fig. 3.2 Fall in colony-forming units in CSF over time in the different treatment groups. Source: Brouwer *et al.* (2004).

amphotericin B and flucytosine (in my opinion an unjustifiably neglected and effective drug) as setting the gold standard for therapy in this condition, which remains very common in countries unable to roll out effective antiretroviral therapy programmes. The 'more is better' clinical fraternity should read and learn.

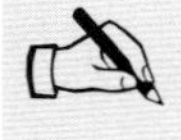

Itraconazole versus fluconazole for prevention of fungal infections in patients receiving allogenenic stem cell transplants

Marr KA, Crippa F, Leisenring W, *et al. Blood* 2004; **103**: 1527–33

BACKGROUND. A total of 304 patients receiving allogeneic stem cell transplants were entered into a randomized trial to determine whether prophylactic itraconazole would afford additional protection against invasive mould infection when compared with fluconazole.

INTERPRETATION. Both drugs were continued for 180 days after stem cell transplantation, or until 4 weeks after discontinuation of anti-graft-versus-host disease therapy. Proven or probable invasive fungal disease was evaluated by intent-to-treat and 'on treatment' analysis. The result showed a higher incidence of toxicity (usually hepatic) and gastrointestinal intolerance in the itraconazole arm (36 versus 16%). Whilst there was no difference in the incidence of invasive fungal infection during the intended study period (fluconazole 16%, itraconazole 13%), fewer patients given itraconazole developed invasive fungal infection on treatment (fluconazole 15%, itraconazole 5%, P <0.03). A further breakdown revealed that itraconazole provided better protection against invasive mould infections (fluconazole 12%, itraconazole 5%, P <0.03), but similar protection against candidiasis. No difference in overall or fungal-free survival was found. Itraconazole therefore appears to offer some advantage over fluconazole, but efficacy seems to be significantly limited by intolerance or toxicity.

Comment

Invasive fungal infection remains an important contributor to mortality and morbidity in the treatment of haematological malignancy. Furthermore, there seems to be little doubt that some therapeutic procedures, diseases and clinical states (acute myeloid leukaemia, allogeneic transplantation, graft-versus-host disease and prolonged neutropenia) are predictive of invasive fungal infection. Whilst fluconazole remains an excellent and well-tolerated agent for the treatment of most *Candida* infections, it is ineffective against moulds, such as *Aspergillus*. The latter infection in the context of haematological malignancy carries a particularly poor prognosis. Prophylactic antifungal therapy for high-risk diseases and procedures is now the norm, but individual units worldwide differ in their choice of whether this should be fluconazole (better tolerated, inactive against *Aspergillus*) or itraconazole (greater toxicity and intolerance, active against *Aspergillus*). Accordingly, this study has much relevance. It demonstrates and reaffirms the superiority of itraconazole against invasive mould infection, but it also documents the high rate of intolerance to this drug, mostly related to the diarrhoea which its oral formulation carrier, cyclodextrin (essential for absorption), induces. Itraconazole seems to be in danger of being left by the wayside in the brave new world of far more expensive and trendier antifungal agents, especially since its makers (in the UK at least) no longer seem to be interested in marketing it. This does not detract from its potential efficacy in reducing the number of (often lethal) mould infections in high-risk haematological malignancy therapy. Perhaps this baby should not be thrown out with the bathwater, especially since this study (and my personal experience) demonstrates that most patients develop diarrhoea, not hepatotoxicity, on the oral formulation whose major drawback beyond this seems to be an unutterably foul taste.

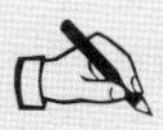

Comparison of caspofungin and amphotericin B for invasive candidiasis

Mora-Duarte J, Betts R, Rostein C, *et al. N Engl J Med* 2002; **347**: 2020–30

BACKGROUND. A total of 224 patients with invasive candidiasis (as designed by culture of *Candida* from either blood or another sterile site within the previous

4 days) were randomly assigned to receive either intravenous caspofungin or amphotericin B. The study's design was double-dummy and included patients with neutropenia. Modified intention-to-treat analysis demonstrated that the effectiveness of caspofungin was similar to that of amphotericin B, with successful outcomes (defined by complete resolution of the signs and symptoms of *Candida* infection, together with mycological eradication) in the caspofungin arm of 73.4% and of 61.7% with amphotericin B. Eligibility for analysis according to prespecified clinical criteria demonstrated a significantly better performance for caspofungin than for amphotericin B (80.7 versus 64.9%). All toxicity criteria were also seen less often in the caspofungin group.

INTERPRETATION. This paper proved to be very important for the continued success of caspofungin. The data are particularly interesting in several ways. *Candida albicans* accounted for only a third to a half of the isolates; indeed, there was a discrepancy between the proportions of these isolates in the two groups, with a preponderance in the amphotericin group. The relative paucity of albicans isolates was also commented on by the authors, who surmised that the authors may have excluded eligible patients with *C. albicans* from the study and simply treated them up front with fluconazole. The other observation – that most of the non-albicans isolates came from South America – is also consistent with the known geographical distribution of this organism. There are other interesting points of note, such as the fact that the presence of neutropenia lowers the chances of success by 10% in both drug arms, and that the major cause of failure and relapse arose from the development of metastatic hepatosplenic candidiasis. This is a particularly ominous development, as those of us who have to treat it can all attest. Caspofungin was also clearly and very impressively less toxic on all counts. Whilst this might be expected for predictable side effects (such as infusion-related toxicity and renal toxicity), the lower adverse effect profile right across the board might not have been predicted.

Table 3.1 Baseline *Candida* isolates*

Isolate	Caspofungin	Amphotericin B
	Percentage of patients	
Candida albicans	35.6	54.1
C. parapsilosis	19.8	18.3
C. tropicalis	19.8	12.8
C. glabrata	12.8	9.2
C. krusei	4.0	0.9
C. guilliermondii	3.0	0.9
C. lipolytica	1.0	0
C. rugosa	1.0	0
Multiple species†	3.0	3.7

* Differences between the treatment groups were not statistically different except for the proportion of patients with *C. albicans* isolates ($P = 0.009$).
† Two patients in the caspofungin group had *C. albicans* and *C. glabrata*, and one patient had *C. parapsilosis* and *C. guilliermondii*. In the amphotericin B group, one patient each had *C. albicans* and *C. glabrata*, *C. albicans* and *C. lusitaniae*, *C. albicans* and *C. tropicalis*, and *C. krusei, C, glabrata*, and *C. tropicalis*.
Source: Mora-Duarte *et al.* (2002).

Table 3.2 Drug-related adverse events and other safety end-points

Variable	Casofungin (*n* = 114)	Amphotericin B (*n* = 125)	*P* value
	no./total no. (%)		
Clinical events	33/114 (28.9)	73/125 (58.4)	0.002
Chills	6/114 (5.3)	33/125 (26.4)	0.003
Fever	8/114 (7.0)	29/125 (23.2)	0.01
Hypertension	2/114 (1.8)	8/125 (6.4)	
Phlebitis or thrombophlebitis	4/114 (3.5)	6/125 (4.8)	
Tachycardia	2/114 (1.8)	13/125 (10.4)	
Nausea	2/114 (1.8)	7/125 (5.6)	
Vomiting	4/114 (3.5)	10/125 (8.0)	
Tachypnoea	0/114	13/125 (10.4)	
Rash	1/114 (0.9)	4/125 (3.2)	
Laboratory abnormalities	27/111 (24.3)	67/124 (54.0)	0.002
Elevated serum alanine aminotransferase	4/109 (3.7)	10/123 (8.1)	
Elevated serum aspartate aminotransferase	2/108 (1.9)	11/122 (9.0)	
Elevated serum alkaline phosphatase	9/109 (8.3)	19/122 (15.6)	
Elevated total serum bilirubin	3/109 (2.8)	11/124 (8.9)	
Elevated blood urea nitrogen	2/108 (1.9)	19/120 (15.8)	0.02
Elevated serum creatinine	4.109 (3.7)	28/124 (22.6)	0.05
Decreased serum potassium	11/111 (9.9)	29/124 (23.4)	0.04
Decreased haemoglobin	1/111 (0.9)	13/124 (10.5)	
Clinical event or laboratory abnormality	48/114 (42.1)	94/125 (75.2)	0.002
Withdrawal because of adverse event	3/114 (2.6)	29/125 (23.2)	0.003
Infusion-related event	23/114 (20.2)	61/125 (48.8)	0.002
Hypokalaemia requiring supplementation within 72 hr after onset	13/114 (11.4)	33/125 (26.4)	0.02
Nephrotoxic effect†	8/95 (8.4)	26/105 (24.8)	0.02

* The denominator for each laboratory abnormality is dependent on the number of patients who had at least one evaluation for that laboratory test following the start of intravenous therapy.
† A nephrotoxic effect was defined as a serum creatinine level that was twice the baseline value or higher, or an increase of at least 1 mg per decilitre (88.4 μmol per litre) in patients with a baseline serum creatinine level above the upper limit of the normal range. Patients with a creatinine clearance of less than 30 ml per minute were excluded from this analysis.
Source: Mora-Duarte *et al.* (2002).

Comment

I have included this paper (now several years old) because it was at the time a landmark for antifungal therapy: for the first time there seemed to be an effective and far better-tolerated alternative to amphotericin B. The paper's major flaw was, of course, its choice of comparator—amphotericin B, which is known to be far more toxic than its lipid formulations. It is interesting to note that even in 2002 (despite the widespread use, experience with and availability of, Ambisome) the US Food and Drug Administration still considered the original product to represent the appropriate gold standard for treatment. I remember well all of us asking 'I wonder whether a head to head with Ambisome would have looked as good? What a shame they compared caspofungin to the wrong drug'.

Safety and efficacy of caspofungin and liposomal amphotericin B, followed by voriconazole in young patients affected by refractory invasive mycosis

Cesaro S, Toffolutti T, Messina C, *et al*. *Eur J Haematol* 2004; **73**: 50–5

BACKGROUND. This group from Padua in Italy assessed ten patients with various haematological malignancies who developed as defined by proven (3), probable (6) and possible (1) invasive mycosis apparently refractory to liposomal amphotericin B. Combination therapy with caspofungin and liposomal amphotericin was well tolerated, hypokalaemia and thrombophlebitis being the most common side effect. Therapy was administered for a median of 19 days, with a range of 6–40 days. One patient was censored from subsequent analysis because of massive haemoptysis. Voriconazole was well tolerated, although interactions were noted with methotrexate and digoxin. Nine out of 10 patients were alive at 125 days. A 'favourable response' was observed in eight out of ten patients.

INTERPRETATION. This study's only merit is that it suggests that polypharmacy with a variety of antifungals in a small group of patients was well tolerated with no unpredictable and serious side effects. Like so many other similar studies, this paper does little to advance the state of knowledge. No conclusions can be drawn concerning whether or not combination therapy is more effective than single-agent therapy. I was interested to note that failure of previous therapy was defined (amongst other soft criteria) thus: 'failure to improve was defined as persistent fever *and/or* the lack of significant reduction (at least 50%) of the number and/or the size of significant lesions'. One patient had cardiac surgery for *Aspergillus* endocarditis! However, the paper acquits itself by demonstrating that the antifungal book can literally be thrown at desperately ill patients, with relatively minor and certainly non-lethal drug-related problems. It is hardly surprising that there is no association between giving combination therapy and either increased efficacy or better outcome. The authors cautiously conclude that 'medical antifungal treatment may be intensified in severely ill patients with refractory invasive mycosis without significant compromise of safety'. This appears to be an increasingly well-established observation. Whether this is of any relevance to mitigating against loss of a chance of life is certainly not demonstrated, and the paper is presented as a typical example of an entirely clinical viewpoint in this difficult field of possible invasive mycosis. This would be fine if it did not give the example to other units to also administer combination antifungal therapy for purely emotional reasons with no basis in evidence.

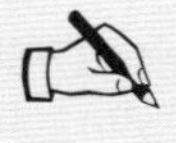

A multicenter open-label clinical study of micafungin in the treatment of deep-seated mycosis in Japan

Shigeru K, Toru M, Hideyo Y, *et al*. *Scand J Infect Dis* 2004; **36**: 372–9

BACKGROUND. Micafungin is the second example in the lipopeptide class of antifungal agents, active against both *Candida* and *Aspergillus* species.

Micafungin was administered intravenously to 70 patients with deep-seated mycosis in doses of 12.5–150 mg/day. Overall clinical response rates were assessed as 60% (6/10 patients) for invasive pulmonary aspergillosis, 67% (6/9) in chronic necrotizing pulmonary aspergillosis, 55% (12/22 in pulmonary aspergilloma), 100% (6/6) in candidaemia and 71% (5/7) in oesophageal candidiasis.

INTERPRETATION. Response rates for patients who had been previously treated but had failed with other antifungal agents for reasons of either toxicity or ineffectiveness were identical to those for patients who had received no prior treatment. Mycological eradication was achieved for those patients infected with *Aspergillus fumigatus*, *A. flavus*, *A. terreus*, *A. niger*, *Candida albicans*, *C. glabrata* or *C. krusei*. There was a 30% rate of adverse events, none of which was dose-related. It was concluded that micafungin monotherapy seems to be effective in patients with deep-seated mycosis.

Comment

This is essentially an observational study of caspofungin's nearest immediate rival, performed in the country of its manufacture. Its open-label nature opens up a whole treasure-trove of potential confounding bias. I found it interesting that the local ethics committees considered it acceptable to treat patients with life-threatening disease with an untried and untested agent without prior exposure to agents with established efficacy. The dose range (ten-fold!) also suggests that this work was somewhat experimental, and that not enough preclinical data existed for a rationally based decision on a narrower dose range. The figures for 'cure' (if we assume that the study represents the truth despite the limitations of its open-label design) are essentially similar to those seen with caspofungin, with lower success rates for *Aspergillus* than for *Candida*. Possibly the most constructive message is that micafungin in this very limited study does not appear to be overtly and unpredictably toxic; if it had been we would never have seen the publication.

Cutaneous infection by *Fusarium*: successful treatment with voriconazole

Guimerá M, García-Bustín D, Noda-Cabrera A, Sánchez-González R, Montelongo RG. *Br J Dermatol* 2004; **150**: 770–95

BACKGROUND. **Infections with *Fusarium* spp. are fortunately very rare and tend to develop only in the disastrously immunosuppressed. They have justifiably acquired a particularly nasty reputation because most severe and invasive infections appear to be completely refractory to conventional antifungal treatment, including all amphotericin formulations. Mortality in disseminated infection therefore approaches 100%. I include this vignette as an example of the very real difference that new antifungal agents can make in such situations.**

INTERPRETATION. A 65-year-old Caucasian with Evans syndrome (haematological autoimmune disorder with haemolytic anaemia and thrombocytopenia) treated with 30 mg of

prednisolone and 150 mg of azathioprine a day, presented with a 1-month history of
multiple nodular lesions on the left arm. Figure 3.3 clearly shows an 8 to 10 mm nodule on
the left elbow, some of which then progressed to black eschars. The number and size of
these nodules progressed relentlessly; at the time of presentation there was minor
neutropenia (0.7 × 10^9 per litre). Biopsy material demonstrated invasive fungal infection and
Fusarium was isolated. Not surprisingly, 1 month's treatment with intravenous liposomal
amphotericin produced nothing but nephrotoxicity. Initiation of oral voriconazole, however,
produced dramatic improvement and the *Fusarium* was completely eliminated within
6 weeks.

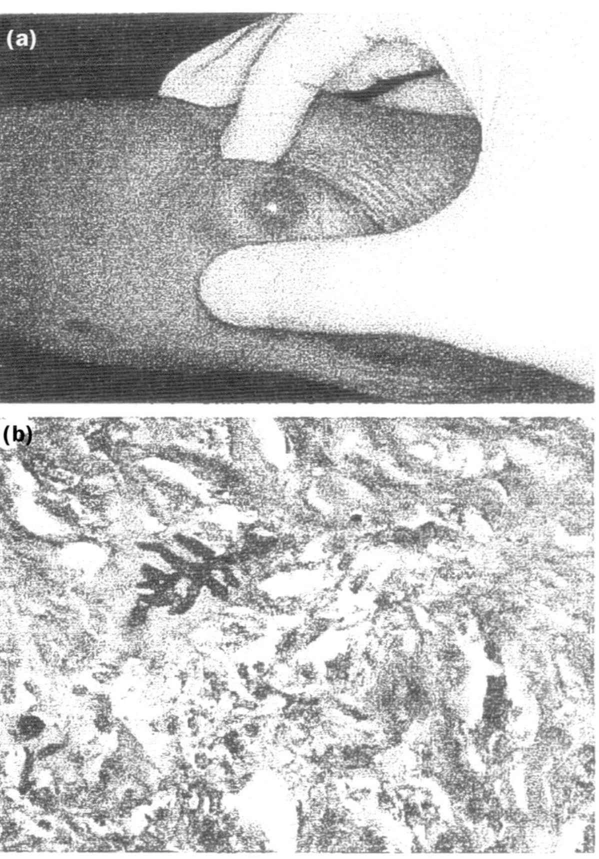

Fig. 3.3 (a) Painful nodule on left elbow and (b) branching hyaline septate hyphae in the
dermis. Periodic acid–Schiff; original magnification × 400. Source: Guimerá *et al.* (2004).

Comment

There is no doubt that the clinical course of this case was radically altered by voriconazole. It might be argued that subcutaneous infection is not particularly disseminated, but the case report clearly states that multiple non-contiguous nodules appeared on this patient's arm at different times and none resolved spontaneously. Whilst I suspect that this patient's neutrophil count, although low, was adequate to have helped mitigate against disaster, I also suspect that voriconazole's ability to penetrate most if not all tissues was also highly relevant for cure.

Case histories are often pooh-poohed by the profession in these days of the supremacy of the randomized controlled trial. As far as I am concerned, they often give the first clues as to possibilities for new therapy; for rare presentations of rare diseases, such as this, there can be no better evidence.

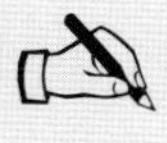

Successful treatment of chronic meningitis caused by *Scedosporium apiospermum* with oral voriconazole

Danaher PJ, Walter EA. *Mayo Clin Proc* 2004; **79**: 707–8

BACKGROUND. *Scedosporium apiospermum* (also know as teleomorph *Pseudallescheria boydii*) is a ubiquitous saprophyte found worldwide. Reports of disseminated infection, usually (but not always) in the immunosuppressed, continue to appear. Cutaneous infection is the norm; disseminated infection is often lethal and intracerebral infection is particularly disastrous.

INTERPRETATION. This is a case history of a 59-year-old woman with diabetes, hyperlipidaemia and a distant history of idiopathic autoimmune thrombocypenic purpura who presented with malaise, severe headache and mild focal one-sided neurological weakness. Lumbar puncture over a 6-month period revealed a variable but definitely abnormal lymphocytic CSF pleocytosis, which yielded on one occasion *S. apospermum*. Therapy was originally initiated with 600 mg/day itraconazole oral solution, with no effect. Voriconazole was then initiated, and rapid resolution of headache and other symptoms ensued over 4 weeks. CSF indices were normal at 4 months. The voriconazole concentration in serum was 6.14 µg/ml, with a corresponding CSF concentration of 2.14 µg/ml. The patient made a complete recovery.

Comment

I chose this short report, which probably does represent a true case of *Scedosporium* meningitis, because it illustrates very well the unique niche which voriconazole occupies subsequent to, on the one hand, its excellent bioavailability and, on the other hand, its particularly broad spectrum of action. This makes it quite unique; to my knowledge, no other broad-spectrum antifungal drug can so effectively penetrate the central nervous system, and whilst this case is certainly as rare as rocking horse manure, the same cannot be said for cerebral aspergillosis, a particularly ominous and lethal complication of haematological malignancy. Voriconazole might make the difference.

Aspergillus

Infection of the central nervous system with *Aspergillus* is fatal in about 90% of patients treated with conventional antifungal therapy. This presumably relates to a combination of the uniquely destructive properties of the mould itself as well as to the relative inefficiency of therapy with conventional antifungals, compromised even further by their dubious penetration into the central nervous system. Not surprisingly, clinicians faced with relatively hopeless situations will try just about anything. Whilst these one-off cases can never rely on an evidence base by clinical trial criteria, they nevertheless provide interesting results – and lest we forget it, this 'case law' approach has served the UK justice system well since its inception several hundred years ago. The following papers demonstrate possibilities and pitfalls.

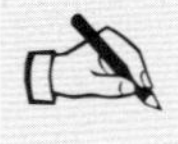

Resolution of orbitocerebral aspergillosis during combination treatment with voriconazole and amphotericin plus adjunctive cytokine therapy

Bethell D, Hall G, Goodman TR, Klein N, Pollard AJ. *J Paediatr Hematol Oncol* 2004; **26**: 304–7

BACKGROUND. A 30-month-old girl presented with common acute T-lymphoblastic leukaemia and was treated with regimen B of the Medical Research Council's ALL/97/01 protocol, with a subsequent 3-week period of neutropenia. She developed a right-sided facial swelling with marked periorbital orbital oedema and erythema. Ophthalmoscopy demonstrated endophthalmitis. *Aspergillus fumigatus* was cultured from an intravitreal sample, at which time total retinal detachment was also noted. Figure 3.4 shows marked preseptal tissue swelling, proptosis, scleritis, soft tissue involvement of the right maxillary and ethmoid sinuses, and multiple ring-enhancing lesions throughout the brain.

INTERPRETATION. The child received liposomal amphotericin 10 mg/kg/day, as well as voriconazole at a daily dose of 6 mg/kg/day after loading. Some improvement was seen after 2 weeks. In view of the slow improvement, γ-interferon (50 μg three times a week) and subsequently GM-CSF (granulocyte-macrophage colony-stimulating factor) (5 μg /kg/day) were also started after an original period of interferon-related toxicity, which did not recur when it was reintroduced. The patient was discharged home 6 weeks after starting definitive antifungal treatment and 4 weeks after starting antifungal chemotherapy, and continued both combination antifungal and cytokine therapy as an outpatient. Voriconazole levels were monitored and were noted to be dropping. Dosage was increased in a stepwise fashion up to 25 mg/kg/day. Vincristine toxicity developed, as did a florid facial rash, ascribed to the voriconazole. The child was subsequently taken through subsequent intensification blocks of chemotherapy, and (apart from having lost the eye) has no signs of continuing *Aspergillus* infection.

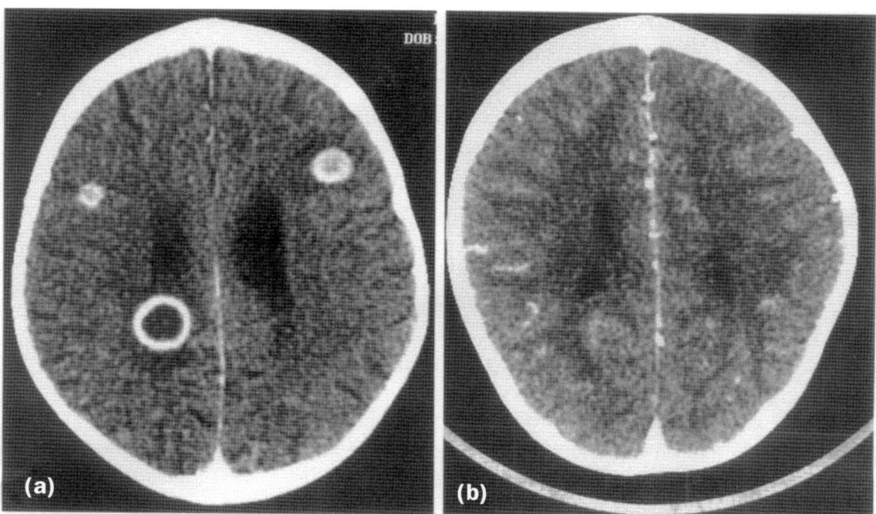

Fig. 3.4 (a) Contrast-enhanced CT scans of the brain showing multiple ring-enhancing lesions consistent with invasive cerebral aspergillosis. (b) Contrast-enhanced CT scan sections of the brain 4 months later, showing complete resolution of the previously demonstrated lesions. Source: Bethell *et al.* (2004).

Comment

Orbitocerebral aspergillosis carries a disastrous and dire prognosis. When faced with such a difficult case, the treating physicians quite justifiably opted to combine antifungal therapy and biological response modifiers. Denning *et al.* |**1**| found a very low (16%) response rate to voriconazole in patients with cerebral aspergillosis; and this presumably drove the above authors to add in cytokines in this desperate situation. In view of the scans demonstrating extensively disseminated and established infection, I would have put this child's chances of death in excess of 95% with antifungal treatment alone. Voriconazole-related side effects in this case seem to have been related to a facial acneiform rash—a recognized side effect that is usually seen in sunlit countries.

Combination therapy with caspofungin and either voriconazole or amphotericin preparations has been advocated following increased clearance in animal models |**2**| as well as better *in vitro* killing of *Aspergillus* |**3**|, and this presumably prompted the therapy used in this case.

Cytokines were also added in the second case because of its appalling prognosis. Furthermore, the addition of cytokines has been reported as efficacious |**4**|, especially in the treatment of fungal infection on a background of chronic granulomatous disease |**5**|.

It is unfortunately not possible to dissect out those specific components (or which combination of therapeutic agents) which made the difference in this case, a familiar scenario with all such case histories, where multiple therapeutic agents are prescribed simultaneously. Unfortunately, each and every case of intracerebral infection with mould is different in nature, in terms of both the infection itself and the extent and reversibility of underlying immunosuppression.

Caspofungin versus liposomal amphotericin B for empiric antifungal therapy in patients with persistent fever and neutropenia

Walsh J, Teppler H, Donowitz GR, *et al*. *N Engl J Med* 2004; **351**: 1391–402

BACKGROUND. Neutropenic patients who remain feverish despite adequate broad-spectrum antimicrobial therapy often receive empirical antifungal therapy in order to prevent, or treat, invasive fungal infection. The choice for such empirical therapy has essentially been limited to amphotericin-based compounds. This large trial is the first to compare the safety and efficacy of liposomal amphotericin to those of caspofungin, the first echinocandin to reach the market.

INTERPRETATION. This was a very large, multinational, randomized double-blind trial in which patients were stratified according to risk and prior antifungal prophylaxis at entry. Successful outcome was defined as fulfilling all the components of a five-part composite endpoint. The majority of these patients had a disease diagnosis predictive of a high risk of fungal infection. Efficacy was evaluated in 1095 patients, with overall success rates of 33.7% for liposomal amphotericin B and 33.9% for caspofungin, satisfying the statistical test of non-inferiority. A higher proportion of patients with baseline fungal infection treated with caspofungin had a successful outcome (51.9 versus 25.9%; $P = 0.04$). The proportion of patients in the caspofungin group surviving to 7 days was also greater (92.6 versus 89.2%; $P < 0.05$), and premature drug discontinuation was necessary in a smaller number of patients treated with caspofungin (10.3 versus 14.5%; $P < 0.03$). All drug-related adverse events were lower for the caspofungin group, and this was especially significant for nephrotoxicity (2.6 versus 11.5%; $P < 0.001$).

Comment

This is a landmark paper for all those physicians deliberately inducing neutropenia through cytotoxic chemotherapy. There seems little doubt that (especially for haematological malignancy, specifically acute myeloid leukaemia and allogeneic bone marrow transplantation) our ability to induce long-lasting remission of a tumour, if not clinical cure, is constantly improving. Patients nevertheless continue to die from invasive fungal infection: this is the payback for increasingly aggressive chemotherapeutic regimens, with ever-longer neutropenic periods. Amphotericin-based compounds (and, increasingly, liposomal amphotericin) have remained the cornerstone of the empirical treatment of non-bacterial neutropenic fever for almost a decade now.

Table 3.3 Demographic characteristics of the patients in the modified intention-to-treat population*

Characteristic	Caspofungin (n = 556)	Liposomal amphotericin B (n = 539)
Female sex—no. (%)	238 (42.8)	247 (45.8)
Age—yr		
Median	51	49
Range	17–83	16–83
Age group—no. (%)		
≤17 yr	3 (0.5)	8 (1.5)
18–40 yr	158 (28.4)	160 (29.7)
41–65 yr	307 (55.2)	297 (55.1)
>65 yr	88 (15.8)	74 (13.7)
Race—no. (%)†		
White	502 (90.3)	476 (88.3)
Black	21 (3.8)	19 (3.5)
Other	35 (5.9)	44 (8.2)
High-risk group—no. (%)	146 (26.3)	122 (22.6)
Allogenic haematopoietic stem cell transplantation‡	36 (6.5)	39 (7.2)
Relapse of acute leukaemia	110 (19.8)	83 (15.4)
Prior antifungal prophylaxis—no. (%)§	313 (56.3)	304 (56.4)
Primary diagnosis—no. (%)		
Acute myelogenous leukaemia	364 (65.5)	339 (62.9)
Acute lymphocytic leukaemia	57 (10.3)	50 (9.3)
Non-Hodgkin's lymphoma	58 (10.4)	62 (11.5)
Other¶	77 (13.8)	88 (16.3)
Neutrophil count <100 per mm^3—no. (%)	400 (71.9)	406 (75.3)

* The 1095 patients in the modified intention-to-treat population, in which the primary efficacy analysis was conducted, received at least one complete dose of study therapy (i.e. active drug plus placebo) and had persistent fever and neutropenia. Among the 1123 patients who underwent randomization, 12 did not receive any study drug, 15 did not have documented fever or neutropenia at study entry, and 1 did not receive a full dose of study drug. In all, 17 patients were excluded from the caspofungin group (9 because they did not receive study drug), and 11 were excluded from the liposomal amphotericin B group (3 because they did not receive study drug).
† Race was determined by the individual site investigator.
‡ Some of these patients had received chemotherapy for relapse of acute leukaemia.
§ Antifungal prophylaxis before enrolment was used at the discretion of the investigator. Fluconazole was the most commonly used agent.
¶ This category included chronic myelogenous leukaemia, multiple myeloma, Hodgkin's lymphoma, solid tumours, and the myelodysplastic syndrome.
Source: Walsh et al. (2004).

Despite the far superior toxicity profile of liposomal amphotericin compared with the parent compound, this drug continues to cause significant problems, usually related to renal toxicity. This is seen increasingly, as more patients who have already been multiply treated and whose renal function is suboptimal to start with are put through yet more rounds of cytotoxic and nephrotoxic therapy. Whilst even a trial of this size recruited only 27 baseline fungal infections to each group, prompting much

Table 3.4 Results of the safety analyses

Variable	Caspofungin (*n* = 564)	Liposomal amphotericin B (*n* = 547)	Difference (95% CI)* percentage points	*P* value
	percentage of patients			
Nephrotoxicity†	2.6	11.5	–8.9 (–12.0 to –5.9)	<0.001
Infusion-related event‡	35.1	51.6	–16.4 (–22.2 to –0.7)	<0.001
Discontinuation of study therapy because of a drug-related adverse event	5.0	8.0	–3.1 (–6.0 to –0.02)	0.04
Any drug-related adverse event§	54.4	69.3	–14.9 (–20.5 to –9.2)	<0.001
Most commonly reported drug-related adverse events¶				
Clinical (any)	47.0	59.6	–12.6 (–18.4 to –6.8)	<0.001
Fever	17.0	19.4	–2.4 (–6.9 to 2.2)	
Chills	13.8	24.7	–10.9 (–15.5 to –6.2)	
Rash	6.2	5.3	0.9 (–1.8 to 3.6)	
Headache	4.3	5.7	–1.4 (–4.0 to 1.1)	
Hypokalaemia	3.7	4.2	–0.5 (–2.8 to 1.8)	
Nausea	3.5	11.3	–7.8 (–10.9 to –4.7)	
Vomiting	3.5	8.6	–5.0 (–7.8 to –2.2)	
Dyspnoea	2.0	4.2	–2.3 (–4.3 to –0.2)	
Flushing	1.8	4.2	–2.4 (–4.4 to –0.4)	
Laboratory (any)	22.5	32.0	–9.5 (–14.7 to –4.3)	<0.001
Increase in alanine aminotransferase	8.7	8.9	–0.1 (–3.5 to 3.2)	
Increase in aspartate aminotransferase	7.0	7.6	–0.6 (–3.7 to 2.4)	
Increase in alkaline phosphatase	7.0	12.0	–5.1 (–8.5 to –1.6)	
Decrease in potassium	7.3	11.8	–4.5 (–7.9 to –1.0)	
Increase in total bilirubin	3.0	5.2	–2.1 (–4.5 to 0.2)	
Increase in direct bilirubin	2.6	5.2	–2.6 (–5.3 to 0.2)	
Decrease in magnesium	2.3	2.6	–0.3 (–2.2 to 1.6)	
Increase in blood urea nitrogen	1.9	3.1	–1.2 (–3.9 to 1.5)	
Increase in creatinine	1.2	5.5	–4.3 (–6.4 to –2.1)	

* CI, confidence interval. Negative values indicate a smaller proportion of patients in the caspofungin group.
† Nephrotoxicity (defined as a doubling of the serum creatinine level or, if the creatinine level was elevated at enrolment, an increase of at least 1 mg per decilitre [88 μmol per litre]) was assessed in 547 patients in the caspofungin group and 522 in the liposomal amphotericin B group who had a creatinine clearance above 30 ml per minute.
‡ The most frequently reported infusion-related events were fever, chills, headache, nausea, and vomiting.
§ Events categorized as possibly, probably, or definitely related to study therapy were considered drug-related.
¶ The events listed are those with an incidence of at least 2% in at least one treatment group. For laboratory drug-related adverse events, only the results of tests performed on more than 100 patients are shown.
Source: Walsh *et al.* (2004).

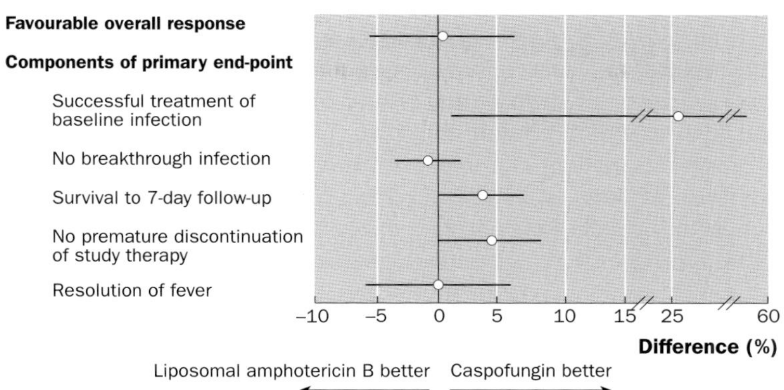

Fig. 3.5 Differences between the treatment groups in the rate of overall response (adjusted) and individual components of the primary end-point (observed), with 95.2 and 95% confidence intervals, respectively. Source: Walsh *et al.* (2004).

discussion about exactly how far the results can be interpreted, two features stand out clearly: caspofungin is at least as effective as liposomal amphotericin as an antifungal agent, and is certainly less toxic. As long as its price is comparable to that of liposomal amphotericin, there seems little reason now not to consider this agent – with very little significant toxicity and potential for drug interaction – as the drug of choice for the empirical therapy of neutropenic fever.

Conclusion

This chapter was specifically put together to allow physicians to get a feel for the rapidly changing field of antifungal therapy. I make no apologies for not discussing papers relating to animal work, the disposition of drugs, molecular mechanisms of action, or other equally important aspects of these drugs and their action. This is because clinicians need to know first and foremost when and how to use them; this requires clinical rather than theoretical information. Unlike the situation as little as 3 years ago, we now have choices for invasive fungal infection in terms not only of route of administration and pharmacodynamics but also of drug interaction and side effect profile. Two drugs have got to market ahead of the others and have emerged as particularly promising, namely voriconazole (developed from the very successful triazole family of agents) and caspofungin (representing a completely new class of agent with a new target of action: the echinocandins). Several messages come through loud and clear: caspofungin seems as effective as liposomal amphotericin for both *Candida* and *Aspergillus* infection, and voriconazole has an exceedingly broad spectrum of action and gets into the CNS probably better than any other drug except

5-flucytosine, which unfortunately cannot and must not be used as single-agent therapy. Decisions concerning which of these new agents to use in specific situations continue to need some degree of subtlety, however: caspofungin is not active against all fungal pathogens (although data concerning *Candida* would suggest that, for now at least, it seems particularly predictably active), and voriconazole has a very significant drug interaction profile in areas of medicine (intensive care, haematological oncology) that are already infamous for their polypharmacy.

Clarity, therefore, emerges out of several papers in this chapter, namely those basing their results and conclusions on randomized trials. We now know that an amphotericin B/5-fluorocytosine combination remains the gold standard for *Cryptococcus* meningitis, that caspofungin is an effective treatment for infections with most if not all strains of *Candida*, that itraconazole is effective despite its toxicity and drug interaction profile for the prophylaxis of high-risk patients, and that caspofungin seems as effective as liposomal amphotericin for the empirical treatment of neutropenic fever and is less toxic.

There remains, however, much confusion and uncertainty despite these trials. Why? Because despite the enormous effort invested in the development of these new drugs with superior clinical efficacy and toxicity profiles, no drug seems to be the magic bullet. This is not for reasons of spectrum of activity or of pharmacodynamics, but for reasons of one aspect of the biology of these infections which remains poorly understood. The fact remains that, even if, for the sake of argument, these drugs really did kill all fungi stone dead at no toxicity cost to the host, none of us would be any the wiser as to whether highly significant differences in mortality would emerge—and this surely must be the only end-point when treating life-threatening disease. In this context, the Walsh trial reminds us that 'efficacy', as judged by the end-points defined in that study, remains below 40% in both treatment arms. Is this because the drugs just do not work (sometimes)? Is it because they do work—but that this is of no relevance to the outcome in over half the patients? I also find it difficult to understand the concept of 'breakthrough infection' in treated patients, unless the drug does not work. And if does not work, why not? Even the simple question of whether this might be due to lack of tissue penetration or lack of susceptibility of that particular strain for that particular drug remains unanswered. If that were not bad enough, the current (appalling) quality of diagnostic technology as applied to invasive fungal infection other than candidaemia injects enormous noise into any large study, most, if not all, of which have to include 'possible' and 'probable' diagnostic categories to satisfy the hunger for large numbers and European Organisation for Research Trials in Cancer (EORTC) stringencies. Klastersky's insightful commentary |6| prompted by Walsh's paper is certainly worth reading, and contains more of the same concerns.

What of the other papers I chose? They simply represent the fascinating balance between the truly useful information which flows from one-off cases – in this context voriconazole's undoubted ability to penetrate the CNS – and the awful mess we will end up in if we succumb to combining antifungal agents without the context of properly designed studies. I quote in evidence the rigour of Brouwer's paper, and another in this chapter which is quite the contrary. The pressure to save life will, however, see much more combination therapy. Time will tell whether this is the way to go, and surely combination trials must follow. Far more interesting is the possibility of using adjuvant biological response modifiers, such as GM-CSF, which is why I included Bethell's paper. A trial here would be expensive and I doubt that the sort of sums involved could be generated from those companies manufacturing such niche products.

The other papers discussed are included simply to illustrate the constantly evolving nature of the field. I suspect that trials will also flow from such new compounds, assuming that they make it that far.

References

1. Denning D. Echinocandin antifungal drugs. *Lancet* 2003: **362**: 1142–51.

2. Kirkpatrick WR, Perea S, Coco BJ, Patterson TF. Efficacy of caspofungin alone and in combination with voriconazole in a guinea pig model of invasive aspergillos. *Antimicrob Agents Chemother* 2002; **46**(8): 2564–8.

3. Serrano M del C, Valverde-Conde A, Chávez-Caballero M, Bernal S, Claro RM, Peman J, Ramírez M, Martín Mazuelos E. *In vitro* activity of voriconazole, itraconazole, caspofungin, anidulafungin (VER002, LY303366) and amphotericin B against Aspergillus spp. *Diagn Microbiol Infect Dis* 2003; **45**: 131–5.

4. Ellis M, Watson R, McNabb A, Lukic M, Nork M. Massive intracerebral aspergillosis responding to combination high dose liposomal amphotericin B and cytokine therapy without surgery. *J Med Microbiol* 2002; **51**: 70–5.

5. Stevens DA. Azoles in the management of systemic fungal infections. *Infect Dis Clin Pract* 2004; **12**: 81–92.

6. Klastersky J. Antifungal therapy in patients with fever and neutropenia—more rational and less empirical? *N Engl J Med* 2004; **351**: 1445–7.

Part II

Emerging problems and solutions to antibiotic-resistant bacteria

4

Methicillin-resistant *Staphylococcus aureus*

NEIL WIGGLESWORTH, MARK WILCOX

Introduction

Methicillin-resistant *Staphylococcus aureus* (MRSA) is an endemic hospital pathogen that continues to consume excessive healthcare resources and cause morbidity and mortality. Ten studies have been selected to highlight current areas of research in order to further the understanding and control of MRSA. The startling emergence of community-acquired MRSA infection has stimulated much research to understand the epidemiology of this new significant threat |1,2|. Two recent reports succeed considerably in this respect. Vandenesch *et al.* report that the gene coding for Panton–Valentine leucotoxin is a stable genetic marker found in all the 117 community-acquired (CA) MRSA strains examined. Their data imply that CA-MRSA strains have evolved as successful community-based pathogens, and that they have spread to distinct geographical locations. A detailed molecular investigation by Mongkolrattanothai and colleagues of *S. aureus* isolates causing severe community-acquired infection in four children concludes that it is likely that these and other CA-MRSA strains emerged as a result of the mobile chromosomal cassette encoding methicillin resistance (SCC*mec* type IV) have been acquired by methicillin-susceptible *S. aureus* (MSSA) strains. A study from The Netherlands (misleadingly titled as the isolates did not originate there) found a surprisingly high prevalence of MRSA isolates with reduced susceptibility to glycopeptides, highlighting the need for microbiology laboratories to use methods capable of detecting this trait.

Patients with nasal carriage of *S. aureus* have an increased risk of *S. aureus* surgical site infections. Topical mupirocin is effective in some but not all patients in eliminating nasal *S. aureus* carriage. Two studies examine the effectiveness of perioperative prophylaxis including mupirocin application to prevent surgical site infections. Contrasting results were obtained in these, and the findings are discussed in the context of the effect of choice of prophylaxis regimen and study design on outcome. Although evidence associating fluoroquinolone exposure with MRSA infection has been published, this has largely been of low quality |3,4|. The study by Weber *et al.* is a well-designed epidemiological study specifically designed to investigate whether there is a differential effect on the acquisition of either MRSA or MSSA associated with the use of fluoroquinolones. Lucet and colleagues have attempted to define whether risk factors can be used to identify which patients should be screened for MRSA in the intensive care unit (ICU) setting.

Adding to the now considerable body of evidence of the adverse effect on patient outcome of delay in initiating effective antibiotic therapy, Lodise *et al.* have produced further support. They found that appropriate treatment in *S. aureus* bacteraemia was associated with decreased mortality and morbidity. MRSA infection was the most significant predictor of delayed appropriate treatment. The study by Wunderink *et al.* is a potentially important advance in the treatment of nosocomial pneumonia. Using a retrospective analysis on two combined large patient cohorts, they have produced evidence of superior outcome in terms of both clinical cure and mortality for patients with MRSA pneumonia treated with linezolid compared with vancomycin.

Lastly, the findings of an impressive systematic review by Cooper and colleagues of the evidence for the effectiveness of patient isolation to control MRSA spread are discussed. The review emphasizes that current practice is based on weak evidence. Mathematical modelling has been used to predict whether patient isolation can be an effective control measure.

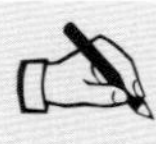

Linezolid versus vancomycin: analysis of two double-blind studies of patients with methicillin-resistant *Staphylococcus aureus* nosocomial pneumonia

Wunderink RG, Rello J, Cammarata SK, Croos-Dabrera RV, Kollef MH. *Chest* 2003; **124**: 1789–97

BACKGROUND. Current treatment options for MRSA pneumonia are limited and are generally associated with suboptimal outcome. This is a retrospective data analysis of two prospective, randomized, multicentre, multinational, double-blind studies, each of identical design, comparing vancomycin and linezolid (with or without aztreonam) for the treatment of hospital-acquired pneumonia. The aim was to determine the effect of baseline variables and treatment on outcome in patients with nosocomial pneumonia particularly due to MRSA. A total of 1019 patients with suspected Gram-positive nosocomial pneumonia, including 339 patients with documented *S. aureus* pneumonia and 160 patients with documented MRSA pneumonia (MRSA subset), were examined. Clinical cure rates for linezolid versus vancomycin were 59.0 versus 35.5% for the MRSA subset (*P* <0.01). Logistic regression analysis confirmed that the difference favouring linezolid remained significant after adjusting for baseline variables (odds ratio [OR] 3.3; 95% confidence interval [CI] 1.3–8.3; *P* = 0.01). Kaplan–Meier survival rates for linezolid versus vancomycin were 80.0 versus 63.5 for the MRSA subset (*P* = 0.03). Logistic regression analysis confirmed that the increased survival associated with linezolid therapy remained significant after adjusting for baseline variables (OR 2.2; 95% CI 1.0–4.8; *P* = 0.05).

INTERPRETATION. In this retrospective analysis, initial treatment of nosocomial MRSA pneumonia with linezolid compared with vancomycin was associated with significantly superior outcome both in terms of survival and clinical cure.

Comment

This analysis is open to potential criticism because of its retrospective nature and the use of data from two studies. However, because of the number of subjects examined, it dwarfs other studies of antibiotic efficacy in nosocomial staphylococcal, particularly MRSA, pneumonia. Interestingly, in an earlier important study Gonzales and colleagues found a significant difference in mortality in bacteraemic patients with MSSA pneumonia treated with vancomycin as opposed to cloxacillin (47 versus 0%; *P* <0.01) |5|. These results were also derived retrospectively as a subanalysis and from a total of 27 patients, i.e. less than a quarter of the number of MRSA cases in the present study. In the present study the two patient cohorts can reasonably be considered to be similar, given that they were selected via common inclusion and exclusion criteria.

Importantly, the results of the study by Wunderink *et al.* provide evidence for superior outcome in linezolid-treated as opposed to vancomycin-treated patients with an infection associated with poor outcome. Several factors known to be associated with reduced mortality in critically ill patients, such as low APACHE II and younger age, were confirmed here. Such findings lend credence to the results showing superior clinical cure and survival rates in linezolid recipients with MRSA, including after adjustment for the effects of baseline risk factors associated with poor outcome. The superior outcome associated with linezolid therapy probably centres around improved pharmacokinetics compared with vancomycin, which penetrates lung tissue to yield concentrations approximately equivalent to only 15% of plasma levels |6,7|.

The challenge now is how to identify patients who could benefit from linezolid therapy, i.e. those with MRSA pneumonia. Previous antibiotic therapy, diabetes, recent surgery and old age are all known risk factors for MRSA sepsis. Factors associated with MRSA carriage in a multivariate analysis of ICU patients in a study reviewed in this chapter were older than 60 years, prolonged hospital stay in transferred patients, a history of hospitalization or surgery, and the presence of open skin lesions in directly admitted cases (see Lucet *et al.* in this chapter). However, most ICU patients have one or more of such risk factors. Rapid diagnostic methods coupled with the use of invasive techniques to establish the pathogens causing pneumonia are required to permit early identification of MRSA pneumonia cases. A recent retrospective analysis of the same cohort of patients, but focusing on patients with MRSA ventilator-associated pneumonia (VAP), similarly found that linezolid was associated with better outcome compared with vancomycin |8|.

Table 4.1 Results of logistic regression analysis of factors associated with clinical cure in patients with *S. aureus* and MRSA nosocomial pneumonia*

Predictors	OR (95% CI)	*P* value
S. aureus pneumonia (*n* = 272)		
Linezolid therapy	1.6 (0.9–2.7)	0.090
APACHE II score ≤20	2.2 (1.0–4.6)	0.046†
Single-lobe pneumonia	2.0 (1.2–3.5)	0.014†
Absence of VAP	2.5 (1.4–4.6)	0.003†
Absence of cardiac comorbidities	2.1 (1.1–4.1)	0.034†
Absence of oncologic comorbidities	4.4 (1.4–13.5)	0.011†
Absence of renal comorbidities	13.5 (3.0–62.5)	<0.001†
MRSA pneumonia (*n* = 123)		
Linezolid therapy	3.3 (1.3–8.3)	0.011†
Single-lobe pneumonia	3.7 (1.5–9.5)	0.006†
Absence of VAP	2.9 (1.1–7.5)	0.028†
Absence of oncologic comorbidities	21.7 (3.7–125.0)	<0.001†
Absence of renal comorbidities	16.4 (3.2–83.3)	<0.001†
Absence of hepatic comorbidities	4.2 (0.6–31.3)	0.154

* Data from patients with clinical outcomes assessed as indeterminate or missing were excluded.
† Significant at 0.05 level.
VAP, ventilator-acquired pneumonia.
Source: Wunderink *et al.* (2003).

Use of perioperative mupirocin to prevent methicillin-resistant *Staphylococcus aureus* (MRSA) orthopaedic surgical site infections

Wilcox MH, Hall J, Pike H, *et al.* *J Hosp Infect* 2003; **54**: 196–201

BACKGROUND. There is limited evidence that peri-operative prophylaxis aimed at reducing nasal carriage of *S. aureus* may reduce the incidence of MRSA surgical site infections (SSIs). This was a controlled before-and-after study on patients from four orthopaedic wards, undergoing orthopaedic surgery with insertion of metal prostheses and/or fixation. Patients were given peri-operative prophylaxis with nasal mupirocin for 5 days, and a shower or bath with 2% (v/v) triclosan before surgery (PPNMT). After introduction of PPNMT there was a significant reduction in the incidence of MRSA SSIs from 23 per 1000 operations in the 6 months beforehand (period A) to 3.3 (*P* <0.001) and 4 per 1000 operations (*P* <0.001) in subsequent consecutive 6-month periods (periods B and C, respectively). Eleven MRSA SSI cases occurred during periods B and C, but only one of these had actually received PPNMT; 10 occurred after acute, as opposed to elective, surgery (*P* <0.001). Nasal MRSA carriage decreased from 38% before PPNMT to 23% immediately after, and 20, 7, 10 and 8% (*P* <0.001) at 6-monthly intervals after intervention. Conversely, the prevalence of nasal MRSA carriage in a control elderly medicine ward did not

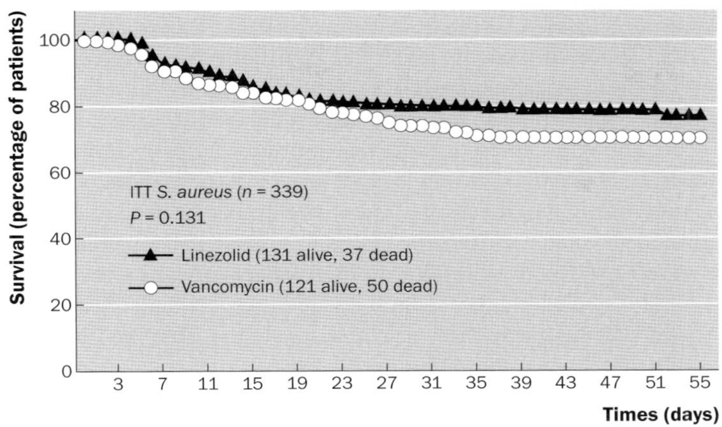

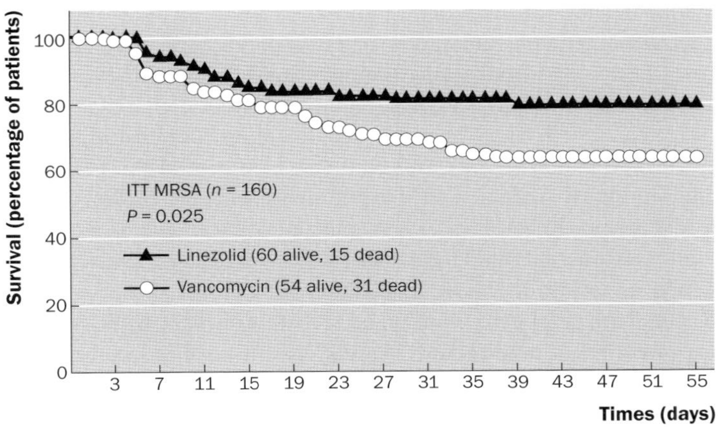

Fig. 4.1 Kaplan–Meier survival curves for uncensored data on patients with *S. aureus* (top) and MRSA (bottom) nosocomial pneumonia treated with either linezolid or vancomycin. Source: Wunderink *et al.* (2003).

alter. Vancomycin usage declined by 23%. There was no increase in low-level mupirocin resistance in *S. aureus* isolates associated with the introduction of PPNMT or during 2 years of follow-up; no isolates with high-level mupirocin resistance were found.

INTERPRETATION. PPNMT can reduce the incidence of MRSA SSIs after orthopaedic surgery, probably by reducing nasal MRSA carriage in the endemic setting. Use of short-duration PPNMT prophylaxis was not associated with the development of mupirocin resistance.

Comment

Several studies have now highlighted the potential use of nasal mupirocin prophylaxis to prevent SSIs, notably in patients undergoing cardiothoracic surgery |**9,10**|, and possibly upper gastrointestinal surgery |**11**|. However, a placebo-controlled study of nasal mupirocin prophylaxis in patients undergoing orthopaedic prosthetic implant surgery found a reduction in *S. aureus* nasal carriage but no effect on SSI incidence |**12**|. Perl *et al.* also recently failed to show an overall benefit in terms of reduction in an SSI incidence study using empirical mupirocin prophylaxis in general surgical patients, although a significant reduction in SSIs was seen in those patients who were nasal *S. aureus* carriers |**13**|. However, the duration of peri-operative mupirocin prophylaxis appeared to be relatively short (not stated in the report) and topical antiseptics were not used. Furthermore, there was a relatively low baseline incidence of staphylococcal SSIs, and it is possible that the randomized study design meant that the opportunity to reduce nasal *S. aureus* carriage in study patients was limited compared with that seen using a cohort or crossover type of approach (such as in the present study).

Wilcox *et al.* initiated a controlled before-and-after study after an increasing incidence of MRSA SSIs in patients undergoing orthopaedic surgery. The hypothesis was that cohort use of PPNMT would reduce the prevalence of nasal MRSA carriage and thus in turn the incidence of MRSA SSI. Despite only modest compliance with the prophylaxis protocol, particularly in patients undergoing acute as opposed to elective surgery, there was a marked reduction in the incidence of MRSA SSIs. Also, there was a highly significant reduction in the prevalence of nasal MRSA carriage (decreased from 38% before PPNMT to 23% immediately after, and 20, 7, 10 and 8 at 6-monthly intervals after PPNMT; $P < 0.001$). Conversely, the prevalence of nasal MRSA carriage in a control elderly medicine ward did not decrease during the study period. The main risk of the widespread use of mupirocin-based prophylaxis, namely the promotion of mupirocin resistance, was not realized in the 2-year follow-up period. This probably reflects the use of only short-term mupirocin administration in individual patients. Perl *et al.* similarly did not experience the emergence of mupirocin resistance despite (short-term) use in almost 2000 patients during a study lasting more than 3 years; they recovered only four mupirocin-resistant isolates, three of which were obtained from patients who were not treated with mupirocin |**13**|.

SSIs cause a marked prolongation of hospital stay |**14**|, and the authors estimated a potential saving of 520 orthopaedic bed days per annum by using PPNMT secondary to preventing approximately 51 orthopaedic MRSA SSIs each year. Further evidence of the effectiveness of the protocol was the 23% reduction in the use of vancomycin in the orthopaedic wards studied. Such savings are likely to more than offset the increased acquisition cost for mupirocin and triclosan. The value of mupirocin-based prophylaxis is clearly likely to be maximal in MRSA-endemic settings.

Community-acquired methicillin-resistant *Staphylococcus aureus* carrying Panton–Valentine leukocidin genes: worldwide emergence

Vandenesch F, Naimi T, Enright MC, *et al*. *Emerg Infect Dis* 2003; **9**: 978–84

BACKGROUND. CA-MRSA has been reported worldwide. This study aimed to investigate the degree of genetic similarity among 117 CA-MRSA isolates from the US, France, Switzerland, Australia, New Zealand, and Western Samoa. Polymerase chain reaction (PCR) for 24 virulence factors and the methicillin-resistance determinant, pulsed-field gel electrophoresis and multilocus sequence typing (MLST) were performed. All the CA-MRSA strains shared a SCC*mec* type IV cassette and possessed a Panton–Valentine leukocidin (PVL) locus. However, the distribution of other toxin genes was linked to the geographical origin of strains. Pulsed field gel electrophoresis (PFGE) and MLST analysis indicated distinct genetic backgrounds associated with each of these origins. Within each continent, the genetic background of CA-MRSA strains did not correspond to that of the hospital-acquired MRSA.

INTERPRETATION. The PVL locus appears to be a stable genetic marker in CA-MRSA strains, and thus explains the frequency of primary skin infections and occasionally necrotizing pneumonia associated with these strains. The data imply that CA-MRSA strains have evolved as successful community-based pathogens.

Comment

These results should be read in conjunction with the findings of Mongkolrattanothai *et al.* in this chapter. Only two genes (SCC*mec* type IV cassette and the PVL locus) were shared by the 117 CA-MRSA isolates examined. However, the genetic background of CA-MRSA was different in each of the three continents. Also, MLST and PFGE analysis showed that, within a continent, the genetic background of CA-MRSA strains did not match that of the local hospital-acquired (HA) MRSA strains. This implies that CA-MRSA did not emerge from local HA-MRSA. The main difference between CA-MRSA strains was predominantly restricted to the accessory gene regulator (*agr*), which is the central regulatory system that controls gene expression for a large set of virulence factors.

Hence, dissemination of a single CA-MRSA clone appears not to have occurred around the world. Instead, it is likely that there has been simultaneous co-evolution of CA-MRSA organisms in different locations. It has been suggested that isolates of the New York/Japanese pandemic MRSA clone may be predisposed to become vancomycin-resistant because of mutations in the *agr* gene |**15**|. Notably, Howe *et al.* have recently reported that reduced susceptibility to vancomycin has also emerged in many successful epidemic MRSA lineages |**16**|. Thus, a pattern of spread of both antibiotic-resistant and CA-MRSA that is specific to distinct geographical locations continues to emerge.

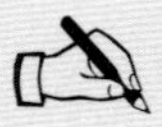

High percentage of methicillin-resistant *Staphylococcus aureus* isolates with reduced susceptibility to glycopeptides in The Netherlands

Van Griethuysen A, Van 't Veen A, Buiting A, *et al. J Clin Microbiol* 2003; **41**: 2487–91

BACKGROUND. The epidemiology and significance of *S. aureus* isolates with reduced susceptibility to glycopeptides remain contentious issues. During *in vitro* antimicrobial susceptibility testing of 107 MSSA and 250 MRSA strains, the authors unexpectedly found that 19 (7.6%) of MRSA isolates had apparently reduced glycopeptide susceptibility, as determined by E-test using a large inoculum (no. 2 McFarland standard) and extended incubation time (48 h) on brain–heart infusion agar. Further testing by population analysis profile–area under the curve analysis confirmed that 15 of these isolates were heterogeneously resistant to glycopeptides (hGISA). The MIC_{50} and MIC_{90} for MSSA isolates according to the E-test with the large inoculum were 3 and 4 mg/l, respectively, for both teicoplanin and vancomycin; corresponding values for MRSA isolates were 3 and 8 mg/l for teicoplanin and 3 and 4 mg/l for vancomycin.

INTERPRETATION. This first report of hGISA isolates collected (but not originating) in The Netherlands showed a surprisingly high prevalence and emphasizes the need to examine specifically for such strains to determine their epidemiology accurately.

Comment

The abstract and title of this study is misleading as most if not all the hGISA MRSA isolates that were detected actually originated outside The Netherlands. The collection of MRSA isolates used in this study, assembled in The Netherlands between 1989 and 1998, predominantly comprised isolates from patients hospitalized in other countries, given the low prevalence of MRSA in The Netherlands. Hence, the countries of origin of the patients (details available for 12 of the 15 hGISA isolates) were Turkey and Italy (three each), France and Greece (two each), and Germany and Ivory Coast (one each) (Table 4.2). What is not clear is how the particular isolates were selected to be part of the isolate collection in the first place, and this is a surprising omission by these authors. Without this information it is impossible to gauge the precise significance of the startlingly high prevalence of glycopeptide intermediately resistant *S. aureus* (GISA) strains that were detected.

Microdilution susceptibility testing methods are able to detect *S. aureus* isolates with reduced susceptibilities to vancomycin, but cannot detect heteroresistance [17]. Indeed, none of the isolates detected in the present study were correctly classified as (h)GISA by the broth microdilution method. Conversely, the E-test with a large inoculum (no. 2 McFarland standard), a longer incubation time (48 h) and the use of rich BHI medium was the only method that correctly identified Mu3, a hetero-resistant isolate first reported by Hiramatsu *et al.* [18,19]. The false-positive GISA rate as determined by E-test for MRSA isolates was 1.6%, which is very similar to

Table 4.2 Origins and results of testing of 19 MRSA isolates found to have reduced glycopeptide susceptibility by E-test criteria

Isolate	Yr of isolation	Country of origin	Isolate source	MIC (μg/ml) with E-test system		Vancomycin MIC (μg/ml) by broth microdilution	PAP-AUC ratio*	Interpretation for hGISA†
				Vancomycin	Teicoplanin			
1	1990	Turkey	–‡	6	12	1	1.09	+
2	1991	France	–	8	12	1	1.12	+
3	1992	Turkey	–	8	8	1	0.99	+
4	1992	Turkey	–	4	24	1	1.03	+
5	1994	India	Perineum	6	12	0.5	0.82	–
6	1994	France	Burn wound	8	16	1	1.16	+
7	1994	Italy	Pus	4	12	2	1.05	+
8	1994	–	Nares	8	16	2	1.07	+
9	1994	South Africa	Nares	4	24	2	0.84	–
10	1994	Greece	Skin	3	12	1	1.13	+
11	1994	Italy	Wound	4	12	1	1.04	+
12	1994	France	Pus	3	12	0.5	0.78	–
13	1995	Germany	Perineum	8	12	2	1.28	+
14	1995	Greece	Pus	6	12	1	1.06	+
15	1998	Argentina	Wound	2	12	1	0.88	–
16	1998	Ivory Coast	Perineum	12	16	4	1.23	+
17	1998	–	Pus	6	12	0.5	1.00	+
18	1998	Italy	Nares	16	96	2	0.97	+
19	1998	–	–	12	16	1	0.93	+

* PAP-AUC ratio criteria for vancomycin resistance are defined in the text.
† Interpretation of PAP-AUC ratio +, hGISA; –, glycopeptide-sensitive *S. aureus*.
‡ –, unknown.
Source: Van Griethuysen *et al*. (2003).

that reported (2.1%) |**20**|. Walsh *et al.* also found that the E-test method with a large inoculum is a reliable and sensitive screening method for the detection of glycopeptide resistance, including heteroresistance |**20**|. In the same study, the population analysis profile–area under the curve (PAP-AUC) ratio proved to be a reliable method for the confirmation of E-test results. However, PAP-AUC testing is more difficult to perform than the E-test. These results therefore offer a practicable way for non-specialist laboratories to determine the prevalence of reduced glycopeptide susceptibility in MRSA.

Severe *Staphylococcus aureus* infections caused by clonally related community-acquired methicillin-susceptible and methicillin-resistant isolates

Mongkolrattanothai K, Boyle S, Kahana MD, Daum RS. *Clin Infect Dis* 2003; **37**: 1050–8

BACKGROUND. There is increasing concern about the emergence of CA-MRSA. This was a retrospective analysis of the genetic relatedness of five CA *S. aureus* isolates obtained from four consecutive paediatric patients presenting with sepsis syndrome and severe pneumonia during a 3-week period in 2000. Two of the children were infected with MSSA and two were infected with MRSA. The PFGE profiles for the two CA-MRSA isolates were identical to each other, as were the patterns for the three CA-MSSA isolates. A two-band difference reflecting the presence of a staphylococcal cassette chromosome mec (SCC*mec* type IV) element distinguished the CA-MRSA isolates from the CA-MSSA isolates.

INTERPRETATION. An insertion or, less likely, a deletion of the SCC*mec* type IV element occurred in a highly virulent *S. aureus* strain. These data increase the evidence that CA-MRSA infections may be caused by isolates closely related to MSSA isolates.

Comment

This group recently described a novel SCC*mec* type, type IV, that is smaller in size than SCC*mec* types I–III and, like SCC*mec* type I, lacks resistance determinants other than *mecA* |**21**|. SCC*mec* type IV has been found in most CA-MRSA isolates reported to date, and therefore CA-MRSA isolates are usually resistant only to β-lactams. This detailed molecular analysis of *S. aureus* MSSA and MRSA isolates recovered from four paediatric cases of severe CA-MRSA infection aimed to provide clues about the origin of strains that contain SCC*mec* type IV. The striking interpretation of these molecular studies is that the common virulent CA-MRSA strain that was recovered from these children appears to have evolved from a virulent MSSA strain that acquired SCC*mec* type IV. Thus, the only observed difference in the PFGE DNA profile of the CA-MRSA and CA-MSSA isolates recovered from the children was the presence of an SCC*mec* element in a fragment of the CA-MRSA isolates, as demonstrated by Southern blot hybridization. Furthermore, MLST, which targets seven relatively conserved genes, also could not distinguish between a pair of MRSA/

MSSA strains from these paediatric cases. Notably, the CA-MRSA strain identified in these paediatric cases is indistinguishable (by DNA fingerprinting and by sequencing of rare toxin genes) from a known sequenced virulent CA-MRSA strain |22|.

There are two potential explanations for this observation. It is possible that SCC*mec* type IV was lost from a CA-MRSA isolate to yield the MSSA strain. Alternatively, SCC*mec* IV may have inserted into a CA-MSSA isolate, thereby creating a CA-MRSA strain. Spontaneous loss of methicillin resistance *in vitro* has been described previously, usually secondary to deletion of SCC*mec* |23–25|. However, these instances have been characterized by a simultaneous deletion of the plasmid encoding the structural β-lactamase gene and its regulatory elements. Hence, the resulting MSSA strains are susceptible to penicillin. The MSSA strains in the present report produced β-lactamase and were penicillin-resistant. The authors therefore believe that the most likely explanation for these strains is the acquisition of SCC*mec* type IV by MSSA to yield CA-MRSA.

This report adds to the growing understanding of the emergence of MRSA clones. The diversity in the lineages of MRSA isolates indicates that horizontal transfer of SCC*mec* into MSSA recipient backgrounds has probably occurred relatively frequently |21,26,27|. Just how frequently this occurs and the conditions that favour such genetic transfer are unknown. Intriguingly, there is some evidence that there may be a barrier to efficient transfer of *mecA* into MSSA strains |28|, although the nature of this and its significance remain to be elucidated.

Fluoroquinolones and the risk for methicillin-resistant *Staphylococcus aureus* in hospitalized patients

Weber SG, Gold HS, Hooper DC, Karchmer AW, Carmeli Y. *Emerging Infect Dis* 2003; **9**: 1415–22

BACKGROUND. Previous studies have implicated fluoroquinolone use as predisposing patients to colonization and/or infection with MRSA. However, these studies were not designed specifically to elicit this outcome. The authors here describe parallel case–control studies that examine the risk of both MRSA and MSSA acquisition following exposure to both ciprofloxacin and levofloxacin. Patients with nosocomially acquired MRSA ($n = 222$) or MSSA ($n = 163$) were compared with 343 concurrent controls. Univariate analysis identified exposure to both ciprofloxacin and levofloxacin as being associated with MRSA, but not with MSSA acquisition (OR 5.4; $P < 0.0001$ and OR 2.2; $P < 0.003$, respectively). After logistic regression analysis (Table 4.3) including potential confounders, both agents remained significantly associated with subsequent isolation of MRSA but not MSSA (ciprofloxacin OR 3.4; $P < 0.0001$; levofloxacin OR 2.5; $P < 0.005$). The authors also compared the two agents with each other but found no significant difference in their effect on MRSA or MSSA acquisition.

INTERPRETATION. In hospital patients the administration of fluoroquinolones may significantly increase the risk of nosocomial MRSA acquisition. The choice of antimicrobial agents may need to take account of this specific and unwanted effect.

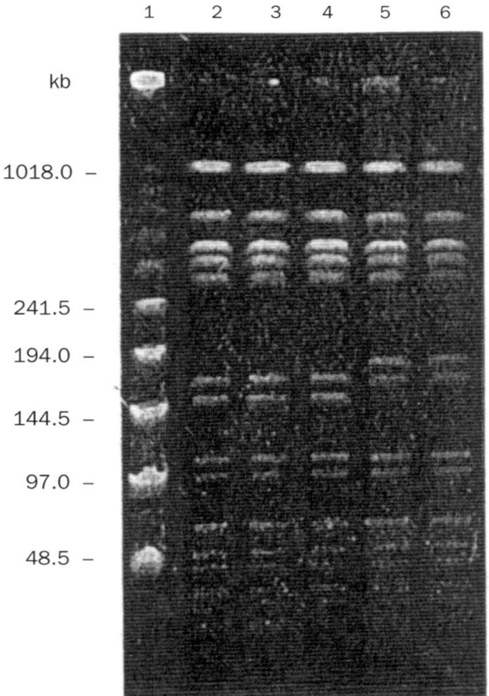

Fig. 4.2 PFGE of *Sma*I-digested genomic DNA of *S. aureus* isolates recovered from four children. *Lane 1,* Molecular weight marker D 2476; *lane 2,* MSSA isolate 2352 recovered from child 2A; *lane 3,* MSSA isolate 2353 recovered from child 1A; *lane 4,* MSSA isolate 2354 recovered from child 2A; *lane 5,* MRSA isolate 2355 recovered from child 1B; *lane 6,* MRSA isolate 2356 recovered from child 2B. All five isolates have an identical PFGE pattern, except for a two-band difference reflecting the presence of staphylococcal cassette chromosome *mec* in the community-acquired MRSA isolates (lanes 5 and 6). Source: Mongkolrattanothai *et al.* (2003).

Comment

This rigorously designed epidemiological study is the first to specifically investigate whether there is a differential effect on the acquisition of either MRSA or MSSA associated with the use of fluoroquinolones. Earlier studies have implicated antimicrobials in general and specific classes (including fluoroquinolones), in particular in the promotion of antibiotic resistance in both hospital and community patients. The authors suggest that this effect of fluoroquinolones may be irrespective of their antibacterial action. *In vitro* studies have demonstrated that exposure of *S. aureus* to subinhibitory levels of fluoroquinolones results in increased expression of adherence factors, thus promoting colonization. This increase in the ability to colonize patients combined with the susceptibility of most MSSA isolates to fluoroquinolones may explain the differential promotion of MRSA acquisition in this study (i.e. colonization by *S. aureus* is promoted but the majority of MSSA strains are eliminated by fluoroquinolones, leaving only MRSA strains).

Interestingly, the authors also identified a (non-significant) tendency towards a protective effect of ciprofloxacin in MSSA acquisition. This study is further evidence that the prevention of MRSA colonization and infection depends on a variety of factors and that it may be possible to target strategies such as reducing antimicrobial use more effectively to concentrate on agents with a proven propensity to increase microbial acquisition.

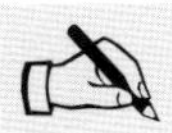

Outcomes analysis of delayed antibiotic treatment for hospital-acquired *Staphylococcus aureus* bacteraemia

Lodise TP, McKinnon PS, Swiderski L, Rybak MJ. *Clin infect Dis* 2003; **36**; 1418–23

BACKGROUND. Delayed treatment with an appropriate antimicrobial agent may increase mortality and morbidity. However, this phenomenon has not been extensively investigated in *S. aureus* bacteraemia (SAB). This is a retrospective

Table 4.3 Results of multivariable analysis

Risk	MRSA cases		MSSA cases	
	OR (95% CI)	**P value**	**OR (95% CI)**	**P value**
Primary covariates				
Levofloxacin	3.38 (1.94–5.90)	<0.001	0.69 (0.34–1.40)	0.30
Ciprofloxacin	2.48 (1.32–4.67)	0.005	0.47 (0.21–1.02)	0.06
Other covariates				
Lung disease	3.94 (2.43–6.40)	<0.001	2.33 (1.43–3.81)	<0.001
Renal disease	*		1.98 (1.03–3.80)	0.04
Penicillin	*		1.78 (0.93–3.39)	0.08
Metronidazole	1.92 (1.10–3.37)	0.02	1.29 (0.65–2.56)	0.46
ICU stay	5.33 (3.28–8.68)	<0.001	4.60 (2.90–7.30)	<0.001
Emergent admission	1.74 (1.09–2.78)	0.02	1.90 (1.17–3.08)	0.01
Admission service				
Medical	*		–	–
Obstetrical	*		0.29 (0.08–1.05)	0.06
Surgical	*		1.82 (1.12–2.97)	0.02

* All results adjusted for time at risk. Only variables significant (*P* ≤0.05) on univariate anlysis were included in final models. Several variables (indicated with an asterisk) met criteria for inclusion in the MSSA (methicillin-susceptible *Staphylococcus aureus*), but not the MRSA (methicillin-resistant *Staphylococus aureus*) model. OR, odds ratio; CI, confidence interval; ICU, intensive care unit.
Source: Weber *et al.* (2003).

analysis of all eligible cases of hospital-acquired (defined as occurring after >2 days of hospitalization) SAB over a 2-year period (n = 167). The authors used classification and regression tree analysis to identify the breakpoint in time after identification of S. aureus in blood cultures that corresponds to delayed treatment. Appropriate treatment instigated up to this point (44.75 h) was considered 'early' and thereafter 'delayed'. Infection-related mortality (IRM) and length of stay after bacteraemia were compared using multivariate analysis and were found to be significantly greater in the delayed treatment group (OR of IRM with delayed treatment 3.8; 95% CI 1.3–11.0; P = 0.01; mean length of stay 20.2 days for delayed versus 14.3 days for early treatment; P = 0.05). The effect of delayed treatment on mortality was significantly greater in more severely ill patients (APACHE II score >15.5) and patients in whom the source of infection was considered high-risk (i.e. associated with mortality greater than 10%). After logistic regression analysis involving clinical and treatment data, MRSA infection was the most significant predictor of delayed treatment (OR 8.3; 95% CI 2.6–16.8).

INTERPRETATION. Failure to initiate appropriate treatment in SAB may lead to increased mortality and morbidity. Poor outcome associated with delayed treatment is compounded by other patient risk factors, such as APACHE II score and those with a source of infection considered to have a high risk of bacteraemia. MRSA infection was the most significant predictor of delayed appropriate treatment.

Comment

This study supports the growing body of evidence that delayed antimicrobial treatment with an effective agent may lead to poor patient outcomes |**29–31**|. In this case, failure to treat SAB optimally within the first 2 days after identification increases the specific risk of IRM (rather than mortality in general, for which the evidence is less strong), and increases length of stay for survivors, and presumably the risk of further iatrogenic complications. The contribution of high MRSA prevalence (62% of patients with SAB in this study) is considerable and suggests that, in situations where MRSA is endemic, empirical treatment of SAB without glycopeptides or other agents with action against MRSA presents an unacceptable risk of delaying effective treatment initiation, with ensuing poor outcome.

Two outcomes from this study are striking. Firstly it should be possible, using locally defined risk factor data, to identify patients at high risk of IRM secondary to SAB, and those whose SAB may be caused by MRSA. In doing so, it should be possible to target appropriate empirical therapy without a wholesale move to glycopeptide use. Secondly, the proportion of SAB caused by MRSA in this study is very high and the results may not be generalizable to situations where this proportion is lower. More studies in settings where MRSA, as a proportion of SAB, is less prevalent may be needed to support the findings of this study. In settings with such a low prevalence of MRSA the accuracy of establishing that there is a MRSA risk becomes even more important.

Randomized clinical trial of pre-operative intranasal mupirocin to reduce surgical-site infection after digestive surgery

Suzuki Y, Kamigaki T, Fujino Y, Tominaga M, Ku Y, Kuroda Y. *Br J Surg* 2003; **90**; 1072–5

BACKGROUND. Use of nasal mupirocin to prevent Gram-positive infections has been reported in cardiothoracic surgery, orthopaedic surgery and renal patients with vascular devices *in situ*. This study examines the use of nasal mupirocin in complex digestive surgery, where MRSA infection is potentially a serious adverse outcome. A prospective randomized controlled trial of pre-operative nasal mupirocin versus no treatment was carried out in 395 patients (193 treated, 202 controls). Peri-operatively, both groups were otherwise managed identically according to local standard procedures. There were no significant differences in the groups with regard to demographics, comorbidities or types of procedure performed. Of 50 SSIs (28 in the mupirocin group and 22 in the control group), nine were caused solely by Gram-positive organisms; there was no significant difference between the groups. The authors also documented other infectious complications in the patients studied and noted a statistically significant reduction in post-operative pneumonias in the mupirocin group (0 versus 5 in the control group; *P* = 0.028). In all of the patients in whom pneumonias were identified, sputum culture yielded *S. aureus* (*n* = 4 MRSA).

INTERPRETATION. No reduction in SSIs in patients undergoing complex digestive surgery was found with the use of pre-operative nasal mupirocin. An unexpected reduction in post-operative pneumonias was identified in the mupirocin treatment group.

Comment

Comment on this study should be considered together with that for the report by Wilcox *et al.* in this chapter. Suzuki and colleagues' study highlights the issue of selecting the most appropriate infection prevention strategies for the population in question. Infections in the study population in this case were mainly caused by Gram-negative bacteria; thus, the finding of little benefit from pre-operative nasal mupirocin is unsurprising. The use of nasal mupirocin in the prevention of serious Gram-positive infections is still an area of debate, and concerns are being raised about the possible promotion of mupirocin resistance amongst Gram-positive bacteria (no data are given regarding this in the present study).

The unexpected significant reduction in the incidence of post-operative pneumonia in the treatment group is interesting and merits further study. However, this result must be interpreted with caution as it was not an aim of the study to examine this outcome, and other characteristics of the subjects and/or the study design may have confounded the results.

It is surprising that the authors refer to the use of a pre-operative ritual that has been shown to increase the risk of SSIs, namely pre-operative shaving |**32**|. In addition, the cases received mupirocin for 3 days pre-operatively in total. This may not be the optimum regimen. Wilcox *et al.* used nasal mupirocin from 1 day before to 4 days after surgery, plus topical washing with triclosan. The days immediately following surgery are a high-risk period, given the presence of the fresh skin wound. Thus, as discussed elsewhere, the design of this study means that patients may still have been exposed to nosocomial pathogens in the post-operative period, and were not receiving prophylaxis at this time.

Prevalence and risk factors for carriage of methicillin-resistant *Staphylococcus aureus* at admission to the intensive care unit

Lucet JC, Chevret S, Durand-Zaleski I, Chastang C, Regnier B; Multicenter Study Group. *Arch Intern Med* 2003; **163**: 181–8

BACKGROUND. A significant proportion of patients admitted to the ICU will be colonized or infected with MRSA, particularly where MRSA is endemic. In a multicentre study in 14 ICUs, prevalence and risk factors for MRSA in patients admitted to the ICU were examined prospectively. There was also an attempt to devise a cost-effective predictive score to identify those patients at high risk of MRSA colonization/infection, to allow targeting of screening and isolation precautions accordingly. All admissions to the ICUs for 6 months were screened using nasal, intact skin and clinical swabs. The overall MRSA prevalence at admission was 6.9% (range for ICUs, 3.7–20%). Using multivariate analysis, the identified risk factors were different for patients admitted directly to the ICU (history of hospitalization or surgery and presence of open skin lesions) than for patients transferred from other departments (age >60 years and prolonged hospital stay). Fitting these risk factors to a predictive score enabled the authors to identify the proportion of cases who would have been screened and the MRSA detection rate depending on the number of risk factors present (Table 4.4).

INTERPRETATION. The authors concluded that only universal screening was sensitive enough to identify carriers. A cost–benefit analysis of screening and precautionary isolation compared with effects of excess MRSA infections is claimed to demonstrate a net benefit from universal screening. However, the authors when arriving at this conclusion have made a number of important assumptions.

Comment

The debate on the most appropriate screening strategies for the detection of MRSA continues but there is perhaps general agreement that screening may be of most value in high-risk populations. This large multicentre study highlights the consistently high level of MRSA introductions into ICU populations. Although risk factors were identified, these were not universally present and a screening policy based on the presence of one or more of these factors would fail to identify a proportion of MRSA carriers.

The cost–benefit analysis is both based on and makes a number of assumptions that would have to be borne out by further study. The first of these is the likelihood that each undetected case of MRSA will transmit the organism to between one and three other patients; this is based on a report of an outbreak in a neonatal unit |33|, and it is hard to see how this can be generalized to adult ICUs with endemic MRSA. It also remains unknown whether, in this setting, a policy of universal contact precautions is as effective as screening and selective precautions in preventing MRSA clinical infections. Such a study is currently in progress |34|. Finally, the data suggest that any of the suggested screening strategies described would result in a net cost–benefit, although the authors appear to reject this finding in their analysis, concluding that only universal screening or screening on the basis of one identified risk factor are cost effective (Fig. 4.3).

Systematic review of isolation policies in the hospital management of methicillin-resistant *Staphylococcus aureus*: a review of the literature with epidemiological and economic modelling

Cooper BS, Stone SP, Kibbler CC, *et al. Health Technol Assess* 2003; **7**(39): 1–194

BACKGROUND. Isolation of patients colonized or infected with MRSA remains central to recommendations for limiting the spread of the bacterium, particularly

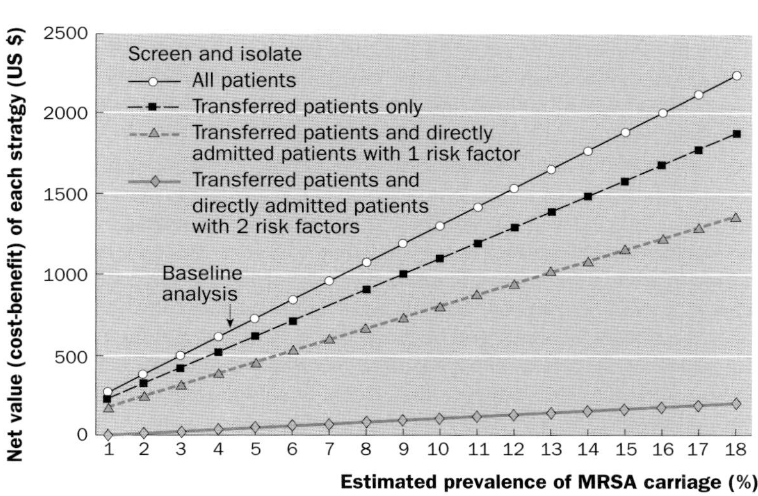

Fig. 4.3 Threshold for MRSA carriage on ICU admission making the strategy beneficial, according to screening and preventive isolation precautions among different populations. Source: Lucet *et al.* (2003).

Table 4.4 Yield of various screening strategies for detecting carriage of MRSA at ICU admission

No. of risk factors	Sensitivity	Positive predictive value	Patients screened
Transferred patients			
≥0	100.0% (58/53)	7.1% (53/744)	100.0% (744/744)
≥1	86.8% (46/53)	8.8% (46/524)	70.4% (524/744)
2	43.4% (23/53)	19.7% (23/117)	15.7% (117/744)
Directly admitted patients			
≥0	100.0% (43/43)	3.0% (43/1443)	100.0% (1443/1443)
≥1	88.4% (38/43)	4.2% (38/900)	62.6% (902/1441)
≥2	55.8% (24/43)	8.7% (24/277)	19.2% (277/1441)
≥3	18.6% (8/43)	15.4% (8/52)	3.6% (52/1441)

Source: Lucet *et al.* (2003).

to susceptible individuals, and is widely practised in hospitals. There has been significant debate regarding the evidence base for this approach, and this review seeks to clarify the current state of our knowledge. Of the more than 4000 papers retrieved, the authors found that 254 were specific enough to the questions being asked and 46 of these were deemed to be of a standard worthy of data extraction. The strategies identified included isolation wards, nurse cohorting and single-room isolation on general wards. The methodological quality of the studies reviewed was largely poor, with many unplanned and/or multiple interventions and many sources of potential bias and confounding. Studies were mainly interrupted time series before-and-after studies, and a significant proportion of them were retrospective without the comparison(s) being fixed before data extraction. Meta-analysis was not deemed appropriate because of the heterogeneous nature of the study designs and populations (including single wards/units, whole hospitals and multiple hospitals). The main conclusions were mixed, with evidence both for and against the use of the isolation strategies identified. The authors concluded that there was some evidence that concerted interventions that include an element of intervention can reduce MRSA prevalence even in the endemic situation. No conclusions could be drawn about the cost-effectiveness of the strategies employed because of the lack of any robust economic analysis in the published literature. The transmission dynamics of MRSA in the endemic situation were modelled, as were the effects of a dedicated isolation facility on endemic MRSA, allowing for variations in transmissibility and levels of carrier detection. This modelling suggests that, in many scenarios, the number of cases introduced into a hospital will overwhelm a fixed capacity for isolation. Given an adequate capacity for isolation, the authors showed that it may be possible to reduce endemic levels of MRSA over perhaps 10 years; however, these reductions are dependent on available resources, both for screening and isolation. It was not possible to model the economic impact of these requirements in great detail because of the paucity or simplistic nature of the available economic data.

INTERPRETATION. The existing evidence for isolation in the control of MRSA is generally of poor methodological quality. There is considerable bias and confounding, and many plausible alternative explanations for reported reductions in MRSA. There is no evidence that current strategies should be abandoned, but further methodologically sound research in this area is urgently required. Modelling suggests that to control endemic MRSA using isolation would require large isolation facilities with scalable capacity.

Comment

This is a comprehensive, systematic and extensive review of isolation as a strategy in controlling MRSA. The authors have highlighted the paucity of well-designed prospective studies that support current practice in this area. Of the numerous reports studied, only eight could be considered to present strong evidence, lacking in systematic bias. These eight studies presented conflicting evidence for the efficacy of isolation, the authors concluding that sufficient evidence exists that intensive measures including isolation *may* be effective, and that there is no evidence that such measures are ineffective and should be abandoned.

The recommendations of the review team—that well-designed prospective studies focusing on planned interventions with systematic evaluation and adjustment for confounders—must be taken seriously and should be a priority for research funding bodies and researchers. The most serious drawback of the recommendations provided is the focus on isolation wards as the potential way forward. This may be a possibility, but a number of potential problems lie in wait, not least the quality of care available to patients from multiple specialities placed on a mixed-function isolation ward.

The modelling presented is very detailed and includes patient admission and re-admission patterns as well as the dynamics of MRSA with and without a range of isolation facilities available. The models also suggest that such strategies could be cost-effective in the longer term, although large initial investment would be necessary. Such modelling holds out the possibility of reducing MRSA using adequately resourced isolation facilities, ideally introduced before endemic levels have become established. However, in most developed countries MRSA is already endemic in many hospital settings. It remains to be seen whether any healthcare system has the resources to test these model scenarios in real life.

Conclusion

The prevalent threat of MRSA means that effective control strategies are urgently required. As we struggle to control nosocomial MRSA, community-acquired MRSA infection represents a significant new challenge. The description of community-acquired MRSA strains that probably originated as MSSA strains and that have subsequently acquired a mobile chromosomal cassette, requires further investigation to understand how and why this occurs. Importantly, we need to know what we can do to limit the emergence and spread of such strains. Unfortunately, a large systematic review of the evidence for the effectiveness of patient isolation to control MRSA spread reveals that current practice is based on weak evidence.

Peri-operative prophylaxis strategies, ideally avoiding systemic antibiotics, are an attractive goal. Accumulating data indicate that topical mupirocin-based prophylaxis warrants detailed study to determine when and where this may be effective. It is likely also that increasing attempts will be made to limit MRSA selection in high-risk settings by using low-risk antibiotics in preference to cephalosporins and possibly fluoroquinolones. Rotational antimicrobial prescribing may be a way forward here. Therapeutic alternatives to glycopeptides are urgently required, given the intense use of this class of antimicrobials, and the increasing evidence of the emergence of resistance. Linezolid is a significant addition to the anti-MRSA formulary, and indeed may be a more efficacious choice in some infections, particularly where glycopeptide drug penetration is suboptimal.

References

1. Outbreaks of community-associated methicillin-resistant *Staphylococcus aureus* skin infections—Los Angeles County, California. MMWR 2002–2003 02/07/2003; **52**: 88. Available at: http://www.cdc.gov/mmwr/PDF/wk/mm5205.pdf.

2. Dufour P, Gillet Y, Bes M, Lina G, Vandenesch F, Floret D, Etienne J, Richet H. Community acquired methicillin-resistant *Staphylococcus aureus* infections in France: emergence of a single clone that produces Panton–Valntine leukocidin. *Clin Infect Dis* 2002; **35**: 819–24.

3. Isaacs RD, Kunke PJ, Cohen RL, Smith JW. Ciprofloxacin resistance in epidemic methicillin-resistant *Staphylococcus aureus*. *Lancet* 1988; **ii**: 843.

4. Manhold C, von Rolbicki U, Brase R, Timm J, von Pritzbuer E, Heimesaat M, Kljucar S. Outbreaks of *Staphylococcus aureus* infections during treatment of late onset pneumonia with ciprofloxacin in a prospective, randomized study. *Intensive Care Med* 1998; **24**: 1327–30.

5. Gonzalez C, Rubio M, Romero-Vivas J, Gonzalez M, Picazo JJ. Bacteremic pneumonia due to *Staphylococcus aureus*: a comparison of disease caused by methicillin-resistant and methicillin-susceptible organisms. *Clin Infect Dis* 1999; **29**: 1171–7.

6. Lamer C, de Beco V, Soler P, Calvat S, Fagon JY, Dombret MC, Farinotti R, Chastre J, Gibert C. Analysis of vancomycin entry into pulmonary lining fluid by bronchoalveolar lavage in critically ill patients. *Antimicrob Agents Chemother* 1993; **37**: 281–6.

7. Honeybourne D, Tobin C, Jevons G, Andrews J, Wise R. Intrapulmonary penetration of linezolid. *J Antimicrob Chemother* 2003; **51**: 1431–4.

8. Kollef MH, Rello J, Cammarata SK, Croos-Dabrera RV, Wunderink RG. Clinical cure and survival in Gram-positive ventilator-associated pneumonia: retrospective analysis of two

double-blind studies comparing linezolid with vancomycin. *Intensive Care Med* 2004; **30**: 388–94.

9. Kluytmans JA, Mouton JW, VandenBergh MF, Manders MJ, Maat AP, Wagenvoort JH, Michel MF, Verbrugh HA. Reduction of surgical-site infections in cardiothoracic surgery by elimination of nasal carriage of Staphylococcus aureus. *Infect Control Hosp Epidemiol* 1996; **17**: 780–5.

10. Cimochowski GE, Harostock MD, Brown R, Bernardi M, Alonzo N, Coyle K. Intranasal mupirocin reduces sternal wound infection after open heart surgery in diabetics and nondiabetics. *Ann Thorac Surg* 2001; **71**: 1572–8.

11. Yano M, Doki Y, Inoue M, Tsujinaka T, Shiozaki H, Monden M. Preoperative intranasal mupirocin ointment significantly reduces postoperative infection with Staphylococcus aureus in patients undergoing upper gastrointestinal surgery. *Surg Today* 2000; **30**: 16–21.

12. Kalmeijer MD, Coertjens H, Kluytmans JAJ, Van Nieuwland-Bollen E, Bogaers-Hofman D, De Baere GAJ. Perioperative eradication of nasal carriage of Staphylococcus aureus by mupirocin nasal ointment as prevention of surgical site infections in orthopedic surgery. In: *Abstracts of the 39th Interscience Conference on Antimicrobial Agents and Chemotherapy, September 1999*. Washington, DC: American Society for Microbiology; Abstract 514: p 591.

13. Perl TM, Cullen JJ, Wenzel RP, Zimmerman MB, Pfaller MA, Sheppard D, Twombley J, French PP, Herwaldt LA; Mupirocin And The Risk Of Staphylococcus Aureus Study Team. Intranasal mupirocin to prevent postoperative Staphylococcus aureus infections. *N Engl J Med* 2002; **346**: 1871–7.

14. Coello R, Glenister H, Fereres J, Bartlett C, Leigh D, Sedgwick J, Cooke EM. The cost of infection in surgical patients: a case–control study. *J Hosp Infect* 1993; **25**: 239–50.

15. Sakoulas G, Eliopoulos GM, Moellering RC Jr, Wennersten C, Venkataraman L, Novick RP, Gold HS. Accessory gene regulator (agr) locus in geographically diverse Staphylococcus aureus isolates with reduced susceptibility to vancomycin. *Antimicrob Agents Chemother* 2002; **46**: 1492–502.

16. Howe RA, Monk A, Wootton M, Walsh TR, Enright MC. Vancomycin susceptibility within methicillin-resistant Staphylococcus aureus lineages. *Emerg Infect Dis* 2004; **10**: 855–7.

17. Trakulsomboon S, Danchaivijitr S, Rongrungruang Y, Dhiraputra C, Susaemgrat W, Ito T, Hiramatsu K. First report of methicillin resistant Staphylococcus aureus with reduced susceptibility to vancomycin in Thailand. *J Clin Microbiol* 2001; **39**: 591–5.

18. Hiramatsu K, Hanaki H, Ino T, Yabuta K, Oguri T, Tenover FC. Methicillin-resistant Staphylococcus aureus clinical strain with reduced vancomycin susceptibility. *J Antimicrob Chemother* 1997; **40**: 135–6.

19. Wootton M, Howe RA, Hillman R, Walsh TR, Bennett PM, MacGowan AP. A modified population analysis profile (PAP) method to detect hetero-resistance to vancomycin in Staphylococcus aureus in a UK hospital. *J Antimicrob Chemother* 2001; **47**: 399–403.

20. Walsh T R, Bolmstrom A, Qwarnstrom A, Ho P, Wootton M, Howe RA, MacGowan AP, Diekema D. Evaluation of current methods for detection of staphylococci with reduced susceptibility to glycopeptides. *J Clin Microbiol* 2001; **39**: 2439–44.

21. Daum RS, Ito T, Hiramatsu K, Hussain F, Mongkolrattanothai K, Jamklang M, Boyle-Vavra S. A novel methicillin-resistance cassette in community-acquired methicillin-resistant Staphylococcus aureus isolates of diverse genetic backgrounds. *J Infect Dis* 2002; **186**: 1344–7.

22. Baba T, Takeuchi F, Kuroda M, Yuzawa H, Aoki K, Oguchi A, Nagai Y, Iwama N, Asano K, Naimi T, Kuroda H, Cui L, Yamamoto K, Hiramatsu K. Genome and virulence determinants of high virulence community-acquired MRSA. *Lancet* 2002; **359**: 1819–27.

23. Al Salihy SM, James AM. Loss of methicillin-resistance from resistant strains of Staphylococcus aureus. *Lancet* 1972; **ii**: 331–2.

24. Wada A, Katayama Y, Hiramatsu K, Yokota T. Southern hybridization analysis of the mecA deletion from methicillin-resistant Staphylococcus aureus. *Biochem Biophys Res Commun* 1991; **176**: 1319–25.

25. Hiramatsu K, Suzuki E, Takayama H, Katayama Y, Yokota T. Role of penicillinase plasmids in the stability of the mecA gene in methicillin resistant Staphylococcus aureus. *Antimicrob Agents Chemother* 1990; **34**: 600–4.

26. Hiramatsu K, Kondo N, Ito T. Genetic basis for molecular epidemiology of MRSA. *J Infect Chemother* 1996; **2**: 117–29.

27. Enright MC, Robinson DA, Randle G, Feil EJ, Grundmann H, Spratt BG. The evolutionary history of methicillin-resistant Staphylococcus aureus (MRSA). *Proc Natl Acad Sci USA* 2002; **99**: 7687–92.

28. Katayama Y, Zhang HZ, Hong D, Chambers HF. Jumping the barrier to beta-lactam resistance in Staphylococcus aureus. *J Bacteriol* 2003; **185**: 5465–72.

29. Kollef MH, Sherman G, Ward S, Fraser VJ. Inadequate antimicrobial treatment of infections: a risk factor for hospital mortality among critically ill patients. *Chest* 1999; **115**: 462–74.

30. Kollef MH, Ward S. The influence of mini-BAL cultures on patient outcomes: implications for the antibiotic management of ventilator-associated pneumonia. *Chest* 1998; **113**: 412–20.

31. Ibrahim EH, Sherman G, Ward S, Fraser VJ, Kollef MH. The influence of inadequate antimicrobial treatment of bloodstream infections on patient outcomes in the ICU setting. *Chest* 2000; **118**: 146–55.

32. Mangram AJ, Horan TC, Pearson ML, Silver LC, Jarvis WR. Guideline for prevention of surgical site infection. Centers for Disease Control and Prevention (CDC) Hospital Infection Control Practices Advisory Committee. *Am J Infect Control* 1999; **27**: 97–132.

33. Jernigan JA, Titus MG, Gröschel DH, Getchell-White S, Farr BM. Effectiveness of contact isolation during a hospital outbreak of methicillin-resistant Staphylococcus aureus. *Am J Epidemiol* 1996; **143**: 496–504.

34. Marshall C, Wesselingh S, McDonald M, Spelman D. Control of endemic MRSA—what is the evidence? A personal view. *J Hosp Infect* 2004; **56**: 253–68.

5

Enterococci

ALAN JOHNSON

Introduction

Enterococci are part of the normal microbial flora of the human intestinal tract. They were regarded for a long time as minor opportunistic pathogens causing occasional cases of endocarditis or urinary tract infection (UTI). However, since the late 1980s enterococci have been increasingly recognized as important nosocomial pathogens, affecting particularly cancer patients who are neutropenic or have underlying haematological malignancies, patients in intensive care units (ICUs) or renal units, and recipients of transplanted organs. Moreover, the treatment of enterococcal infections is often problematic because of the intrinsic resistance of enterococci to cephalosporins, low levels of other β-lactams and aminoglycosides, and their well-documented ability to develop resistance to most other classes of antimicrobial agents, including glycopeptides, often by acquisition of genes encoding resistance. Recently the ability of enterococci to exchange genetic material has achieved new prominence with the finding that genes encoding resistance to vancomycin appear to have passed from vancomycin-resistant enterococci (VRE) to *Staphylococcus aureus*, resulting in clinical isolates of the latter species with high-level resistance |**1–3**|.

Clinical, epidemiological and microbiological aspects of infections caused by enterococci, including strains resistant to glycopeptides

As a result of the prominent role that enterococci now play as nosocomial pathogens, a considerable body of work has been undertaken with a view to increasing our understanding of the clinical and epidemiological aspects of enterococcal infections. The therapeutic efficacy and safety of new therapeutic drugs has also been the subject of investigation. While some studies have investigated enterococci *per se*, a large number have focused more specifically on strains resistant to glycopeptides, which are particularly widespread in hospitals in the US. The underlying rationale for these studies is that a fuller understanding of the epidemiology of enterococcal infections may lead to improved strategies for reducing their incidence and clinical impact. It is hoped that the papers discussed below will give the reader a flavour of the type of work currently being undertaken in many centres around the world.

Risk factors for infective endocarditis in patients with enterococcal bacteremia: a case–control study

Anderson DJ, Murdoch DR, Sexton DJ, *et al. Infection* 2004; **32**: 72–7

BACKGROUND. Although enterococci cause both hospital-acquired bacteraemia and endocarditis, nosocomial bacteraemia was not believed to present a serious risk of development of endocarditis. This perception stemmed from studies performed from the 1960s through to the 1980s which indicated that enterococcal endocarditis was primarily a disease of older Caucasian men, and was generally community-acquired. In many of these studies, however, the case definitions of endocarditis used do not meet current criteria, and in addition many were uncontrolled. This study evaluated the relationship between enterococcal bacteraemia and endocarditis by comparing the clinical and demographic characteristics of patients with enterococcal endocarditis with those of patients with enterococcal bacteraemia but without endocarditis, over an 8-year period.

INTERPRETATION. Between 1992 and 1999, 41 patients with 'possible' or 'definite' enterococcal endocarditis were diagnosed by application of the modified Duke criteria |4|, and their clinical, microbiological and demographic data were collected from relevant hospital records. The same data were additionally collected for 84 control patients without endocarditis randomly chosen from among the 455 patients who had two or more blood cultures that yielded enterococci over the same period. By univariate and multivariable analyses, the presence of a prosthetic valve and infection with *Enterococcus faecalis* were significantly associated with endocarditis, while age, gender, race, polymicrobial infection and community-acquired infection were not (Table 5.1). Thirty-nine per cent of the cases of enterococcal endocarditis were nosocomial in origin.

Table 5.1 Univariate analyses for patients with enterococcal endocarditis versus patients with enterococcal bacteraemia without endocarditis

	Patients with enterococcal bacteraemia (*n* = 84)	Patients with enterococcal endocarditis (*n* = 41)	*P* value
Median age (range)	56 (18–88)	65 (29–88)	0.12
Male gender	40 (48%)	21 (51%)	0.71
Race			0.99
Caucasian	47 (56%)	25 (61%)	
African–American	31 (37%)	14 (34%)	
Other races	6 (7%)	2 (5%)	
Prosthetic valve present	1 (1%)	10 (24%)	<0.001
Infection with *E. faecalis*	58 (69%)	34 (89%)	0.02

Source: Anderson *et al.* (2004).

Comment

The authors rightly point out that enterococcal endocarditis can no longer be regarded as primarily a community-acquired disease of Caucasian men. Interestingly, Fernández-Guerrero *et al.*, in a recent paper, also concluded that there is a significant risk of endocarditis in patients with nosocomial bacteraemia due to *E. faecalis* and that patients with underlying valvulopathy are particularly prone to infection |5|. The differences between the findings of earlier studies and the present ones may reflect a number of factors, including the looser criteria for diagnosing endocarditis used in earlier studies. However, the findings may well also reflect the increasing rate of nosocomial bacteraemia due to enterococci. From the standpoint of the clinician, the take-home message is that the occurrence of enterococcal bacteraemia (particularly if it involves *E. faecalis*) in a patient with an abnormal or prosthetic heart valve should raise suspicion of endocarditis.

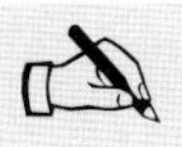

Molecular epidemiology of *Enterococcus faecalis* in liver transplant patients at University Hospital Groningen

Waar K, Willems RJ, Slooff MJ, Harmsen HJ, Degener JE. *J Hosp Infect* 2003; **55**: 53–60

BACKGROUND. *E. faecalis* is an important cause of infection in liver transplant patients. It was originally thought that such infections were endogenous, arising from the patient's own enterococcal flora. However, studies of nosocomial enterococcal infections have also indicated that enterococci are capable of spreading between patients. To investigate the epidemiology of enterococcal infections in their liver unit, Waar *et al.* undertook prospective surveillance in which patients were screened (stool and throat cultures) weekly for carriage of *E. faecalis*. In addition, all clinical and surveillance isolates of *E. faecalis* were typed using the DNA fingerprinting method, amplified fragment length polymorphism (AFLP).

INTERPRETATION. A total of 133 *E. faecalis* isolates were cultured from the faeces and throats (95 isolates) or clinical sites (35 isolates) of 43 liver transplant patients. Among these 133 isolates, 15 different AFLP types (designated A–O) could be identified, of which nine comprised isolates from more than one patient (Fig. 5.1). For five of these, the patients from whom the identical isolates were obtained were linked epidemiologically, being on the same wards at the same time. The isolates belonging to one particular AFLP type (type K) showed a high degree of epidemic potential, being isolated from 23 liver transplant patients during 15 months. Antimicrobial susceptibility testing did not reveal any multiresistant isolates.

Comment

This study, which combined epidemiological monitoring of patients in a liver transplant unit with microbiological surveillance and typing of isolates by AFLP, indicated that transmission of *E. faecalis* occurred frequently in the unit. Nine of the AFLP types comprised isolates from multiple patients, one particular type having spread

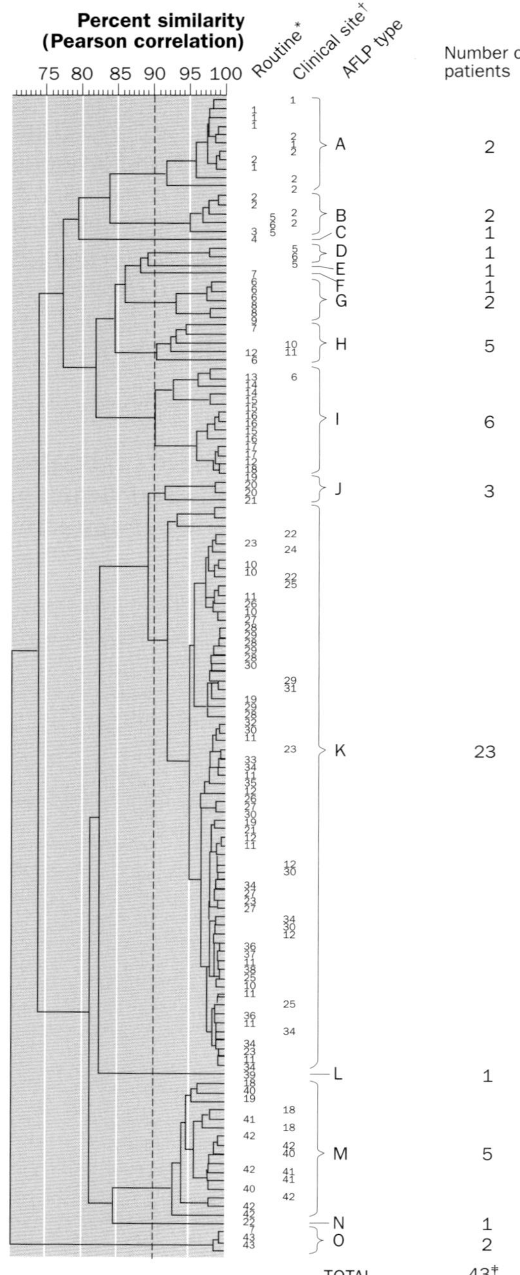

Fig. 5.1 Dendrogram of 133 *E. faecalis* isolates recovered from 43 liver transplant patients. Percentages on the horizontal axis indicate percentage similarities (Pearson product–moment correlation coefficient). A–O, different AFLP types with a similarity of >90%. Patients are numbered 1–43; numbers behind the branches in the dendrogram indicate the patient from which the *E. faecalis* was isolated and the source (routine or clinical isolate). *Routine surveillance isolates from faeces or throat; † includes wound (10), bile (10), ascites (8), sputum (5), blood (1) and intravascular catheter (1); ‡ five patients had two different isolates and four patients had three different isolates. Source: Waar *et al.* (2003).

widely. Interestingly, 25% of the isolates belonging to the 'epidemic' types were obtained from clinical sites rather than carriage sites, compared with 43% of non-epidemic isolates. Thus, although the epidemic strains have a greater potential to spread between patients, they do not appear to be more pathogenic. Of particular note was the fact that resistance to amoxicillin and vancomycin were not seen in any isolates during the study period. Thus, selection of antibiotic-resistant strains by antibiotic use in the unit did not seem to be an important factor in determining the spread of *E. faecalis*. With regard to possible mechanisms of inter-patient spread, the authors comment that type K isolates appeared able to adhere to the surfaces of biomaterials, and harboured the *esp* gene, which encodes an enterococcal surface protein (ESP) that is thought by some to mediate such adherence. However, this is a controversial area, as another article reviewed later in the chapter (Kristich *et al.*, 2004) highlights data indicating that ESP does not play such a role.

Role of environmental contamination as a risk factor for acquisition of vancomycin-resistant enterococci in patients treated in a medical intensive care unit

Martinez JA, Ruthazer R, Hansjosten K, Barefoot L, Snydman DR. *Arch Intern Med* 2003; **163**: 1905–12

BACKGROUND. Previous studies have identified several risk factors for acquisition of VRE in the ICU, including proximity to another case, exposure to a nurse caring for another case, enteral feeding, and the use of vancomycin, cephalosporins or other antibiotics. However, the role of contaminated environmental surfaces has not been well delineated. Martinez *et al.* undertook a retrospective case–control study of patients admitted to the medical ICU of a tertiary-care university medical centre during a 9-month period. Thirty patients who acquired VRE (cases) were each matched with two randomly selected control subjects who did not acquire VRE and had been in the ICU for at least the same number of days.

INTERPRETATION. During the 9-month study period, patients were screened microbiologically (rectal swab) for VRE on admission to the ICU, and weekly thereafter. An environmental survey was also undertaken, in which numerous surfaces in rooms of the ICU where patients with VRE had been located were sampled after the patients had been discharged and the rooms had been subjected to routine cleaning. Univariate analysis indicated that cases were more likely to have been in the hospital for longer than 7 days before ICU admission, to have occupied a particular room with surfaces that remained contaminated with VRE after cleaning, to have had a central venous catheter, to have received vancomycin, cephalosporins or quinolones before ICU admission, or to have received vancomycin or metronidazole after ICU admission. Multivariate logistic regression analysis showed that a hospital stay of longer than 1 week before ICU admission, receipt of vancomycin before or after ICU admission, use of quinolones before ICU admission, and placement in a particular room with contaminated surfaces were independent risk factors for VRE acquisition (Table 5.2).

Table 5.2 Multivariable conditional logistic regression model explaining the acquisition of VRE

Variable	OR (95% CI)	P value
Hospitalization longer than 1 week before ICU admission	18.5 (1.1–301.0)	0.04
Administration of vancomycin before or during ICU admission	6.3 (1.2–34.0)	0.03
Administration of quinolones before or during ICU admission	14.8 (1.2–180.0)	0.04
Location in a high-risk ICU room	81.7 (2.2–3092.0)	0.02

OR, odds ratio; CI, confidence interval.
Source: Martinez *et al.* (2003).

Comment

Despite numerous studies of factors related to VRE acquisition having been published during the last decade, some questions remain unanswered or controversial. In particular, although it is well documented that VRE can contaminate the surfaces and equipment of hospital rooms and remain viable for several days, it has not been clearly proven that such environmental contamination contributes to the acquisition of VRE by patients. In this study, in addition to well-documented risk factors, such as prolonged hospital stay and receipt of antibiotics, the location of patients in a specific room was an independent risk factor for VRE acquisition. The room in question appeared not to have any particular characteristic that would have made it more likely to be occupied by specific types of patient, and during an environmental survey items were found still to be contaminated with VRE despite the room having undergone routine cleaning. This epidemiological link between placement of patients in a contaminated room and VRE acquisition constitutes new evidence supporting the putative role of environmental contamination in VRE transmission. The finding that the room remained contaminated after routine cleaning underscores the need for better cleaning in the hospital environment if VRE and other nosocomial pathogens are to be controlled.

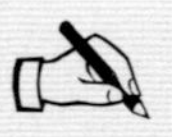

Active surveillance reduces the incidence of vancomycin-resistant enterococcal bacteremia

Price CS, Paule S, Noskin GA, Peterson LR. *Clin Infect Dis* 2003; **37**: 921–8

BACKGROUND. Although it is well recognized that infection control measures are important in containing the spread of VRE in the hospital setting, assessing the efficacy of intervention strategies can be problematic. There is some evidence that the occurrence of VRE can be reduced through routine surveillance for the colonization of high-risk patients and the subsequent isolation of patients found to be colonized or infected. To investigate this further, Price *et al.* undertook a 6-year retrospective analysis of the prevalence of bacteraemia due to VRE in two

neighbouring hospitals with similar demographics, one of which (hospital A) did not routinely screen patients for VRE colonization, while the other (hospital B) actively screened high-risk patients.

INTERPRETATION. The analysis was backdated to when VRE were first isolated from blood cultures at each hospital. The two hospitals were similar with regard to numbers of beds, admissions per year and surgical procedures per year. Both undertook solid-organ transplants and the mean number of defined daily doses of vancomycin per 1000 patient-days per year (hospital A, 70.3 [range 64–81]; hospital B, 65.5 [range 49–72]) were not significantly different ($P = 0.34$). The rate of VRE bacteraemia in hospital A (17.1 per 100 000 patient-days) was 2.1-fold higher than that at hospital B (8.2 per 100 000 patient-days). Typing of VRE by pulsed-field gel electrophoresis (PFGE) showed that most hospital A isolates were clonally related, with four clones responsible for infection in >75% of patients, while in hospital B the four commonest clones accounted for 37%.

Comment

Although some studies have shown a correlation between vancomycin usage and VRE infection rates, differences in vancomycin usage did not account for the different rates of VRE bacteraemia at these two hospitals. While it is possible that the use of other antimicrobials, such as cephalosporins, could have affected the rates of VRE bacteraemia, this would not explain the difference in the clonality of the VRE populations in the two hospitals. Another consideration is that VRE emerged in the two hospitals at different times (the first VRE bacteraemias occurred in hospitals A and B in November 1990 and July 1992, respectively); hence, the time courses over which the rates of VRE infection were compared were not identical. However, despite these limitations of the study design, the data appear quite compelling and indicate that routine screening of patients at risk of VRE, followed by isolation of those found to be colonized, is associated with lower rates of VRE bacteraemia and a more poly-clonal VRE population in the hospital, reflecting less horizontal strain transmission. The results of this study support a growing body of literature that shows the benefit of hospital infection-control programmes that use routine active screening and patient isolation to reduce the spread of resistant bacteria in hospitals.

Prospective, randomized study comparing quinupristin–dalfopristin with linezolid in the treatment of vancomycin-resistant *Enterococcus faecium* infections

Raad I, Hachem R, Hanna H, *et al*. *J Antimicrob Chemother* 2004; **53**: 646–9

BACKGROUND. In the past, options for the antibiotic management of infections caused by vancomycin-resistant *Enterococcus faecium* (VREF) were often minimal or, on occasions, non-existent, because of the high level of multiresistance shown by many isolates. However, this situation has radically changed within the last 4 years

following the licensing of two novel antimicrobial agents, the streptogramin quinupristin–dalfopristin and the oxazolidinone linezolid. Quinupristin–dalfopristin is active against *E. faecium*, including strains resistant to glycopeptides, but lacks activity against *E. faecalis*, while linezolid is active against both species. Although trials had been undertaken to independently evaluate the clinical efficacy and safety of quinupristin–dalfopristin and linezolid in the treatment of VREF infections, the two agents had not previously been compared directly. This report describes a prospective, randomized study of the comparative efficacy and safety of these two drugs in cancer patients with infections caused by VREF.

INTERPRETATION. Forty adult (age >18 years) cancer patients with VREF infection were randomized to receive either quinupristin–dalfopristin (7.5 mg/kg every 8 h) or linezolid (600 mg every 12 h), and were followed up for 30 days after treatment had been discontinued. The characteristics of the two patient groups, including age, sex, underlying malignancy, frequency and duration of neutropenia, site of infection and duration of treatment, were broadly comparable, apart from more of the patients receiving quinupristin–dalfopristin being critically ill and having concurrent pneumonia. The patients receiving quinupristin–dalfopristin and linezolid had comparable clinical and microbiological responses (Table 5.3). Thirty-three per cent of the patients who received quinupristin–dalfopristin had myalgias and/or arthralgias, whereas these symptoms were not reported by any of those who received linezolid. In contrast, drug-related thrombocytopenia occurred in 11% of patients who received linezolid, but was not observed in the quinupristin–dalfopristin group.

Comment

This study indicates that quinupristin–dalfopristin and linezolid appear to have comparable efficacy in the treatment of VREF infections in cancer patients with haematological malignancy. It should be stressed, however, that because of the lack of activity of quinupristin–dalfopristin against *E. faecalis*, it is essential that clinicians ensure that enterococci implicated in infections are fully identified to species level before treatment is started. In this regard, the reader is directed to the article immediately following (Winston *et al.*, 2004), which addresses issues relating to the identification of enterococci. Another consideration is that quinupristin–dalfopristin can only be given by the intravenous route, while linezolid is available as both intravenous and oral formulations, allowing a change from intravenous to oral adminis-

Table 5.3 Outcome associated with linezolid and quinupristin–dalfopristin

Outcome	Linezolid (*n* = 19)	Quinupristin–dalfopristin (*n* = 21)	*P* value
Clinical response (at end of therapy), *n* (%)	11 (58)	9 (43)	0.6
Microbiological response, *n* (%)	17 (90)	15 (71)	0.3
Death caused by infection, *n* (%)	3 (16)	2 (10)	0.7
Relapse, *n* (%)	4 (21)	2 (10)	0.4

Source: Raad *et al.* (2004).

tration, which may simplify patient management. The study confirmed previous findings that quinupristin–dalfopristin treatment is associated with a relatively high frequency of myalgias/arthralgias, a side effect not associated with linezolid administration. However, the occurrence of thrombocytopenia in patients receiving linezolid (also reported previously) might limit the choice of this agent, particularly in patients with underlying haematological malignancy.

API 20 Strep identification system may incorrectly speciate enterococci with low level resistance to vancomycin

Winston LG, Pang S, Haller BL Wong M, Chambers HF, Perdreau-Remington F.
Diagn Microbiol Infect Dis 2004; **48**: 287–8.

BACKGROUND. As described above, the activity of quinupristin–dalfopristin against *E. faecium* but not *E. faecalis* means that accurate identification of enterococci is an essential pre-requisite for the use of this agent. Identification of enterococci is also essential for understanding the epidemiology of VRE infection, as vancomycin-resistant *E. faecium* and *E. faecalis* are important nosocomial pathogens, while other *Enterococcus* species, such as *E. casseliflavus* and *E. gallinarum*, which exhibit intrinsic low-level resistance to vancomycin, show limited patient-to-patient transmission and cause little morbidity. Traditional biochemical testing methods for identifying enterococci are time- and labour-intensive, and laboratories may use the API 20 Strep system, a commercial identification system with 20 biochemical tests designed for the identification of *Streptococcus* and *Enterococcus* species. In this paper Winson *et al.* report their experience that the API 20 Strep system incorrectly speciated enterococci with low levels of resistance to vancomycin.

INTERPRETATION. Following the introduction of active surveillance for VRE among patients admitted to the ICU, the API 20 Strep system was used to speciate suspected enterococcal isolates (catalase-negative Gram-positive cocci in pairs or chains with α or γ haemolysis). Of 119 VRE identified as *E. faecium*, 46 had low vancomycin minimum inhibitory concentrations (MICs) (16–32 mg/l) and unique PFGE patterns, and contrasted with isolates with high vancomycin MICs ($\geq$256 mg/l), many of which had PFGE patterns that showed they were related to a genotype endemic in the hospital over the previous 4 years. The microbiology laboratory subsequently re-identified the 46 low-MIC isolates by applying their usual protocol, which comprised using the POS ID Type 2 panel on the MicroScan WalkAway and also assessing motility and pigment production by conventional methods. The 46 isolates were identified by the clinical microbiology laboratory as follows: 41 *E. gallinarum*, four *E. faecium* and one *E. faecalis*. Four isolates (two *E. faecium*, one *E. faecalis*, one *E. gallinarum*) required conventional tube biochemical tests to make a final identification.

Comment

In summary, the API 20 Strep system misidentified 42 of 46 enterococcal isolates with low-level vancomycin resistance, primarily *E. gallinarum*, as *E. faecium*. The abbreviated identification protocol adopted for the purpose of active surveillance did not include motility assessment, which would probably have revealed the problem sooner. The authors highlight that they initially believed the API 20 Strep system was performing well as in each case it indicated an excellent match for a specific enterococcal species. The authors recommend that additional tests should be used in addition to the commercial API 20 Strep system for the speciation of enterococci with low-level vancomycin resistance. This is particularly of importance if quinupristin–dalfopristin is being considered as a treatment option.

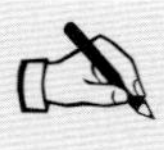

Occurrence of co-colonization or co-infection with vancomycin-resistant enterococci and methicillin-resistant *Staphylococcus aureus* in a medical intensive care unit

Warren DK, Nitin A, Hill C, Fraser VJ, Kollef MH. *Infect Control Hosp Epidemiol* 2004; **25**: 99–104

BACKGROUND. Three isolates of methicillin-resistant *S. aureus* (MRSA) resistant to vancomycin have been reported from Michigan, Pennsylvania and New York, respectively |1–3|. In each case, the resistance was encoded by *vanA*, the gene for glycopeptide resistance found in enterococci. In the first two cases there was microbiological evidence for co-colonization of the patient with MRSA and glycopeptide-resistant *E. faecalis*, the indication being that the glycopeptide-resistant staphylococci acquired their resistance by gene transfer from the resistant enterococcus. At the time of writing, only preliminary data are available from the third case. Nonetheless, co-colonization of patients with VRE and MRSA appears to be a potential risk factor for the emergence of glycopeptide resistance in MRSA. Recently, Warren *et al.* reported a study of the occurrence of such co-colonization or co-infection among adult patients in an ICU in a teaching hospital in the southern US.

INTERPRETATION. Eight hundred and seventy-eight consecutive patients treated in the ICU for at least 48 h, who had had at least one microbiological culture performed, were evaluated. Of these, 402 (45.8%) did not have evidence of colonization or infection with either VRE or MRSA, 355 (40.4%) were colonized or infected with VRE, 38 (4.3%) were colonized or infected with MRSA, and 83 (9.5%) had co-colonization or co-infection with both organisms. Multiple logistic regression analysis demonstrated that increasing age, hospitalization during the preceding 6 months and admission to a long-term-care facility were independently associated with colonization or infection with VRE and with co-colonization/infection with VRE and MRSA.

Comment

The recent emergence of vancomycin-resistant MRSA due to inter-species transfer of the *vanA* gene complex from VRE suggests that patients harbouring both VRE and MRSA are at risk of having their infecting or colonizing strain of MRSA acquire resistance to glycopeptides. Although only three cases of infection with vancomycin-resistant MRSA have been reported to date, in two of the cases susceptibility testing using automated systems (Microscan and Vitek) failed to detect the vancomycin resistance initially. This raises the possibility that other strains of vancomycin-resistant MRSA may already have emerged without having been detected. The finding in this study, that nearly 10% of patients in a medical ICU were co-colonized or co-infected with VRE and MRSA, supports the need for aggressive infection control measures in the ICU.

Dogs should be included in surveillance programs for vancomycin-resistant enterococci

Herrero IA, Fernandez-Garayzabal JF, Moreno MA, Dominguez L. *J Clin Microbiol* 2004; **42**: 1384–5

BACKGROUND. Enterococci are part of the commensal gut flora of both humans and animals. The observation made in the early 1990s by Bates and colleagues that the intestinal flora of farm animals may include enterococci resistant to vancomycin |6| raised the possibility that VRE in farm animals might spread to humans either directly or via the food chain. This in turn has led investigators to question whether companion animals might serve as a reservoir of VRE. To investigate this possibility, Herrero et al. screened dogs treated at an animal hospital for intestinal carriage of VRE.

INTERPRETATION. Eighty-seven dogs from households in different neighbourhoods of Madrid, which were treated at an animal hospital between 1998 and 2003, were randomly selected for microbiological examination. Faeces were investigated for the presence of VRE using selective medium containing vancomycin (8 mg/l) and isolates were identified to species level. Fifteen dogs (13%) yielded vancomycin-resistant isolates (MIC >128 mg/l), comprising eleven *E. faecium* and four *E. gallinarum*, all of which contained the *vanA* gene when tested by a polymerase chain reaction (PCR) method. All the vancomycin-resistant isolates were multiresistant, being resistant to four or more agents.

Comment

Although there have been previous reports of the isolation of VRE from dogs |7,8| most documented the presence of VRE in animals living on farms, where such strains are known to occur in other farm animals. This report differs in that the population of dogs investigated lived in an urban area, and the majority did not have any known contact with farm animals. Moreover, none had clinical records of treatment with vancomycin. It is therefore of interest to note the presence of VRE in the apparent absence of obvious selection pressure for this resistance trait. The major issues that this study raises are the possibility that the VRE might spread from the colonized dogs to their owners and that they may emerge as important nosocomial pathogens in veterinary medicine. With regard to the former, previous reports have indicated direct transmission of VRE from farm animals to humans |9,10|. At present, however, there are no data to indicate whether such concerns are valid for dogs, and further microbiological surveillance, focusing not only on dogs but also on their owners, will need to be undertaken if these potential problems are to be addressed. A further point is that similar surveillance of carriage of VRE in pets needs to be undertaken in other regions and countries, as the rates of carriage in other regions may differ from that seen in Madrid.

Studies of the pathogenicity of enterococci

The historical perception that enterococci were primarily commensal organisms inhabiting the intestinal tract and caused only occasional opportunistic infections meant that little attention was paid to their pathogenic potential. It was only with the realization that enterococci have become an important cause of nosocomial infection that researchers have started to investigate the means by which they might cause disease. A number of putative virulence determinants have been identified, including gelatinase, cytolysin, collagen-binding protein, endocarditis antigen, capsule, hyaluronidase, the *fsr* quorum-sensing system, aggregation substance (AS) and ESP. At present much work is being undertaken to define the importance (or otherwise) of these various factors, either by looking for their presence in isolates of enterococci from various clinical or environmental settings, or by assessing their impact on the virulence of enterococci in experimental systems, such as animal models of infection or appropriate cell culture systems.

Survey for virulence determinants among *Enterococcus faecalis* isolated from different sources

Creti R, Imperi M, Bertuccini L, *et al. J Med Microbiol* 2004; **53**: 13–20

BACKGROUND. In an attempt to determine the importance of a range of putative virulence factors, Creti *et al.* undertook a survey to determine their presence or absence in 74 isolates of *E. faecalis* from invasive (26) and non-invasive (32) hospital infections, the environment (six) and the faeces or throats of healthy individuals (ten). The PCR was used to determine the presence or absence of genes encoding collagen-binding protein (*ace*), endocarditis antigen (*efaA*), haemolysin activator (*cylA*), gelatinase (*gelE*), AS (*asa1* and *asa373*), ESP (*esp*) and two novel putative surface antigens (*EF0591* and *EF3314*), and phenotypic assays were used to test for the production of gelatinase, haemolysin and AS.

INTERPRETATION. The general finding was that isolates from endocarditis, biliary stents and the environment tended to possess fewer genes encoding putative virulence factors than isolates from other sources, with isolates from UTIs possessing the highest number (Fig. 5.2). With regard to the prevalence of specific factors, the *ace* and *efaA* genes were found in all isolates, with the next commonest being *gelE*, which was present in 74.3% of isolates. *Esp* and *cylA* were not detected in endocarditis isolates (Table 5.4). Interestingly, for each of the three factors for which evidence of phenotypic expression was sought (gelatinase, haemolysin

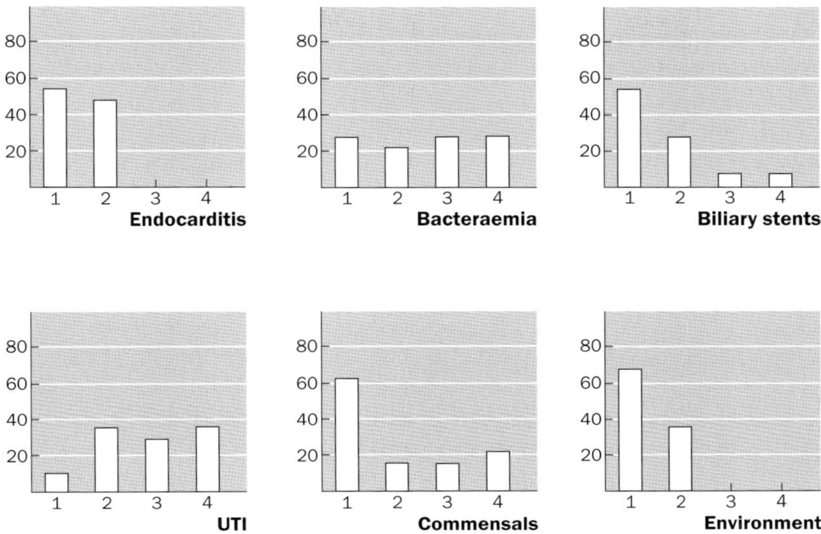

Fig. 5.2 Incidence of single or multiple virulence determinants possessed by *E. faecalis* isolates. The *x* axis shows the number of factors and the *y* axis shows the percentage of strains that possess a certain number of factors. Source: Creti *et al.* (2004).

Table 5.4 Incidence (%) of virulence factors among *E. faecalis* isolates from different types of infection

Type of infection	*esp*	*cylA*	*asa1*	*asa373*	*gelE*
Invasive					
Endocarditis	0	0	44	0	100
Bacteraemia	73	36	55	18	73
Other	33	33	67	50	83
Non-invasive					
Biliary stents	50	0	50	8	67
UTIs	67	42	67	8	91
Other	50	38	100	13	63

Source: Creti *et al.* (2004).

and AS), the presence of the gene did not correlate with expression. Among 55 isolates with the *gelE* gene, only 19 (35%) expressed the gene, while 65% of *cylA*-positive isolates expressed haemolysin and 66% of isolates containing *asa1* and/or *asa373* produced AS.

Comment

This study highlights the difficulty of determining the role (if any) that each of the putative virulence factors found in enterococci plays in the pathogenesis of enterococcal infection. A major problem is that while the genes for these determinants may be present in individual isolates, it is clear that they may or may not be expressed. A full understanding of this phenomenon will require a knowledge of the environmental factors that influence gene expression both *in vivo* and *in vitro*. In addition, it should be remembered that studies of this kind, which focus specifically on the presence or absence of potential virulence factors in the bacterium, fail to take into account relevant host factors that have a major influence on disease progression, such as valve disease in patients at increased risk of enterococcal endocarditis (see paper by Anderson *et al.*, above).

Enterococcal aggregation substance and binding substance are not major contributors to urinary tract colonization by *Enterococcus faecalis* in a mouse model of ascending unobstructed urinary tract infection

Johnson JR, Clabots C, Hirt H, Waters C, Dunny G. *Infect Immun* 2004; **72**: 2445–8

BACKGROUND. AS is a plasmid-encoded enterococcal surface protein that interacts with enterococcal binding substance (EBS), its cognate receptor on other enterococci, to form bacterial clumps called mating complexes. AS appears to be epidemiologically associated with UTIs, increases enterococcal adherence to cultured renal tubular cells, and protects *E. faecalis* from killing by polymorphonuclear leukocytes, and it has therefore been postulated that it may have a role in the pathogenesis of UTIs. Johnson *et al.* investigated this by comparing the ability of isogenic *E. faecalis* strains that differed in their expression of AS and EBS to produce UTIs in experimentally infected mice.

INTERPRETATION. Four derivatives of *E. faecalis* strain OG1SSp were studied; two of them expressed plasmid-encoded AS and EBS (one inducibly, one constitutively) and two did not do so. Female CBA/J and Swiss Webster mice were inoculated perurethrally and colonization was assessed by quantitative sampling of urine, bladder and kidneys 24 h, 48 h or 5 days after inoculation. There was no evidence that production of AS and EBS enhanced the ability of *E. faecalis* strain OG1SSp to colonize the murine urinary tract, when compared with the two derivatives lacking these factors, as the proportion of inoculated mice showing evidence of infection was similar in the two groups.

Comment

The findings reported fail to support the hypothesis that AS and EBS are urovirulence factors for *E. faecalis*. This was an unexpected finding, given the epidemiological association of the production of AS and EBS with UTI. The authors speculated that for the strain in which expression of AS was inducible there may have been insufficient expression, while for the strain with constitutive expression plasmid loss may have occurred. However, the frequency of plasmid loss *in vivo* in these experiments was similar to that observed during non-selective *in vitro* growth, suggesting that the expression of AS *in vivo* did not provide selective pressure for the maintenance of the plasmid. This is further, albeit indirect, evidence against a major role for AS in the pathogenesis of UTIs. To date, ESP is the only seemingly confirmed urovirulence factor in enterococci. However, the role that ESP plays in enhancing infection is associated only with infections of the bladder, not the kidney. Given that in the experiments reported here kidney infections were noted despite the bacteria being inoculated into the lower urinary tract, it seems reasonable to postulate that additional urovirulence factors in *E. faecalis* that promote ascending infection in the urinary tract remain to be identified.

Esp-independent biofilm formation by *Enterococcus faecalis*

Kristich CJ, Li Y-H, Cvitkovitch DG, Dunny GM. *J Bacteriol* 2004; **186**: 154–63

BACKGROUND. Bacteria growing on the surfaces of indwelling medical devices exist in complex microbial communities, known as biofilms, which are typically encased in an extracellular polymeric matrix. Biofilm formation has been associated with chronic infection, due in part to poor penetration of antimicrobial agents. *E. faecalis* is often isolated from biofilms and clinical isolates have been shown to be capable of biofilm formation *in vitro*. To investigate the molecular basis of biofilm formation by *E. faecalis*, Kristich *et al.* examined the ability of *E. faecalis*, including some genetically manipulated strains lacking the putative virulence factor ESP, to form biofilms on glass rods inserted into a chemostat fermenter and on the surface of microtitre plates.

INTERPRETATION. Scanning electron microscopy showed that the growth of genetically manipulated strains of *E. faecalis* lacking ESP on glass rods in the chemostat progressed through the stages associated with biofilm formation, namely initial attachment of individual cells, microcolony formation and the development of a typical complex architecture (Fig. 5.3). Analysis of enterococcal biofilms produced on microtitre plates containing different media indicated that some environmental conditions allowed both biofilm formation and persistence, while others allowed initial formation of biofilms that subsequently showed a decrease in bacterial cell density. In addition, it was found that *E. faecalis* that had been genetically manipulated to produce the secreted metalloprotease GelE showed enhanced biofilm formation.

Comment

Infection of indwelling medical devices, such as prostheses and catheters, is an important clinical problem. Often, such infections appear refractory to treatment with antimicrobial agents, and clinical resolution may require removal of the infected device. Bacterial biofilm formation is now known to be a central component of the pathogenesis of such infections and is the subject of much current research. In this

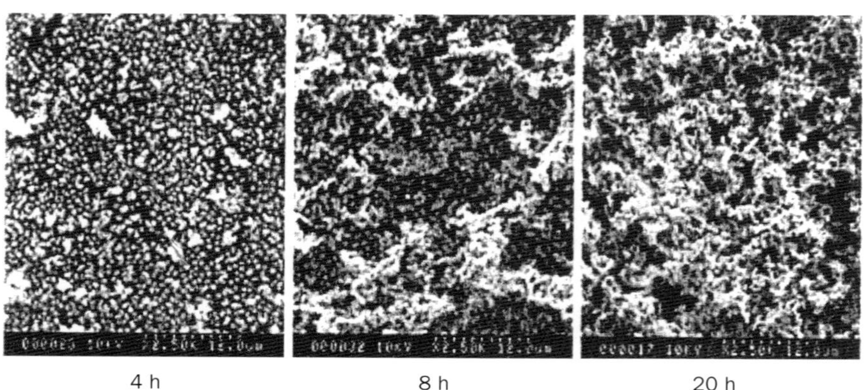

Fig. 5.3 Analysis by scanning electron microscopy of biofilm development by *E. faecalis* in the chemostat-based biofilm fermenter. Glass rods carrying biofilms were removed from the fermenter and processed for scanning electron microscopy at the times indicated. Source: Kristich *et al.* (2004).

paper, Kristich *et al.* report that the putative enterococcal virulence determinant ESP is not required for biofilm formation to occur, a finding that is consistent with a recent report by Sandoe *et al.* |**11**|, who evaluated 70 bloodstream isolates of *E. faecalis* using a microtitre plate assay and found no association between the presence of *esp* and biofilm-forming ability. In contrast, Toledo-Arana *et al.* recently reported a significant correlation between the presence of *esp* and the capacity of *E. faecalis* to form biofilms in a microtitre assay, and suggested that ESP is involved in biofilm formation by this organism |**12**|. However, these workers also noted that two *esp*-deficient mutants retained the ability to produce biofilms, although other such mutants lost this ability. Moreover, genetic complementation studies revealed that ESP expression in an *E. faecalis esp*-deficient strain restored the ability to produce biofilms *in vitro*. Thus, there are conflicting data on the role, if any, that ESP plays in biofilm production. In addition, the finding that the secreted metalloprotease GelE appears to enhance biofilm formation by *E. faecalis* opens a further avenue of investigation. Clearly, further work is required for this scientifically perplexing and clinically important problem to be fully resolved.

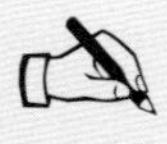

Translocation of *Enterococcus faecalis* strains across a monolayer of polarized human enterocyte-like T84 cells

Zeng J, Teng F, Weinstock GM, Murray BE. *J Clin Microbiol* 2004; **42**: 1149–54

BACKGROUND. It is well recognized that some patients with enterococcal bacteraemia lack a readily identifiable primary focus of infection. From studies of mice experimentally infected with enterococci, it is now thought that this may reflect direct seeding of the bloodstream by intestinal enterococci that migrate across the gut lining, passing through columnar epithelial cells within cytoplasmic vacuoles, by an incompletely understood process termed 'translocation'. In the present study, a human colon carcinoma cell line, T84, that forms a polarized columnar epithelial monolayer with tight or occluding intercellular junctions was used to mimic the translocation of enterococci across intestinal epithelial cells. The strains of *E. faecalis* studied in this model included nine clinical isolates from different sources, five faecal isolates, two well-characterized laboratory strains (OG1RF and JH2-2) and two mutants of OG1RF with disruptions in the *epa* gene cluster, which encodes the synthesis of a major antigenic polysaccharide needed for virulence and resistance to killing by polymorphonuclear leukocytes.

INTERPRETATION. Strain OG1RF and eight clinical isolates (two endocarditis, one urine, five faecal) showed translocation in this assay, while six other clinical isolates (three endocarditis, three urine) and strain JH2-2 did not (Fig. 5.4). One *epa* mutant (TX5179) was unable to translocate, while another (TX5180), with an *epa* disruption further downstream, showed a moderate decrease in translocation, indicating that the *epa* gene cluster is important for translocation. This was confirmed by complementation of TX5179 with *epa* genes, which restored its translocation ability. These findings demonstrate that strains of *E. faecalis* differ in their ability to undergo intestinal translocation, and that the *epa* gene product may influence this process.

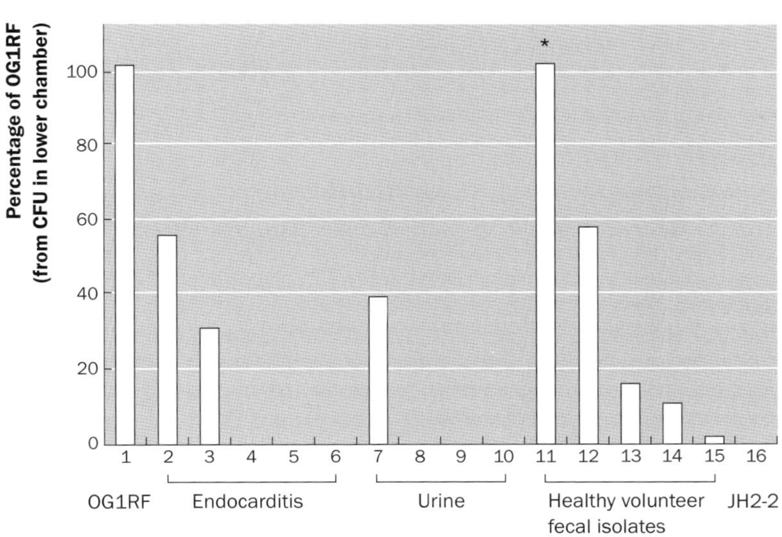

Fig. 5.4 Translocation of *E. faecalis* strains across a T84 monolayer, expressed as the percentage of concurrently determined results for OG1RF. Results are shown for three combined experiments. For six human isolates and JH2-2, no bacteria were recovered in the lower chamber. Levels of recovery of the other eight isolates ranged from 2 to 267%. *, 267%. Source: Zeng *et al.* (2004).

Comment

At present, the mechanisms involved in the translocation of enterococci across the gut mucosa are incompletely understood. This report demonstrates that the human colon carcinoma cell line T84, which can be cultured *in vitro* as a tall columnar epithelial monolayer with tight intercellular junctions, showing phenotypic similarity to colonic crypt cells, can be used to investigate the translocation of enterococci across intestinal epithelial cells. Using this model, it is apparent that clinical isolates of enterococci show considerable variation in their ability to translocate across columnar gut epithelial cells. Related to this was the observation that each of five faecal isolates underwent translocation, as opposed to only three of nine clinical isolates, suggesting the possibility that translocation ability may be a common feature of organisms recently derived from faeces. Although the numbers are too small to allow firm conclusions to be drawn at this stage, this concept merits further investigation. Of particular interest was the finding that the ability to undergo translocation was reduced or lost in two strains with mutations in the *epa* gene cluster. The fact that there was a difference between the level of translocation seen with the two mutants suggests that other, as yet undefined, differences exist between these mutants. Further characterization of these mutants and of the *epa* gene cluster will be helpful in understanding these differences. Continued research using this model will hopefully lead to a fuller understanding of the pathogenesis of enterococcal bacteraemia resulting from intestinal translocation, and the development of strategies (vaccination, for example?) for preventing such infections.

Conclusion

Over the last few decades, enterococci appear to have evolved from being primarily intestinal commensals, causing only occasional opportunistic infections, to being a major cause of nosocomial infections. Our interest in, and knowledge of, this bacterial genus has broadly evolved in parallel. With regard to the clinical importance of enterococci, our understanding of their role in certain diseases, such as endocarditis, is becoming clearer. In addition, numerous investigations of the epidemiology of nosocomial enterococcal infections, particularly those associated with strains resistant to glycopeptides, have identified a number of risk factors. However, the challenge of using this information effectively to reduce the clinical and economic burden imposed by enterococci clearly remains, as evidenced by the continuing (and, in many hospitals, increasing) prevalence of enterococcal infections. Although new drugs (such as quinupristin–dalfopristin and linezolid) that are active against enterococci, including glycopeptide-resistant strains, have been developed, issues such as the emergence of resistance and potential toxicity mean that they are not the final solution.

In addition to clinically orientated studies of enterococci, much basic work on their potential mechanisms of pathogenicity have been undertaken in recent years.

Although progress in understanding the pathogenesis of enterococcal infections is being made, a number of such studies have produced conflicting findings. This may be due to a number of factors, such as differences in methods and in the biological properties of the strains of enterococci being studied in different laboratories. Nonetheless, it is to be hoped that continuing work in this area, particularly work making use of the revolution in molecular biology that is currently under way, will result in significant advances in our understanding of this fascinating group of organisms. The ultimate goal is that such advances will be translated into practical interventions, such as vaccines and improved diagnostic tests, that will enable us to counter the continuing threat posed by this important group of nosocomial pathogens.

References

1. Chang S, Sievert DM, Hageman JC, Boulton ML, Tenover FC, Downes FP, Shah S, Rudrik JT, Pupp GR, Brown WJ, Cardo D, Fridkin SK; Vancomycin-Resistant *Staphylococcus aureus* Investigative Team. Infection with vancomycin-resistant *Staphylococcus aureus* containing the *vanA* resistance gene. *N Engl J Med* 2003; **348**: 342–7.

2. Tenover FC, Weigel LM, Appelbaum PC, McDougal LK, Chaitram J, McAllister S, Clark N, Killgore G, O'Hara CM, Jevitt L, Patel JB, Bozdogan B. Vancomycin-resistant *Staphylococcus aureus* isolate from a patient in Pennsylvania. *Antimicrob Agents Chemother* 2004: **48**: 275–80.

3. Centers for Disease Control and Prevention. Brief report: Vancomycin-resistant *Staphylococcus aureus*. New York: *Morbid Mortal Wkly Rep* 2004; **53**: 322–3.

4. Li JS, Sexton DJ, Mick N, Nettles R, Fowler VG, Ryan T, Bashore T, Corey GR. Proposed modifications to the Duke criteria for the diagnosis of infective endocarditis. *Clin Infect Dis* 2000; **30**: 633–8.

5. Fernández-Guerrero ML, Herrero L, Bellver M, Gadea I, Roblas RF, de Górgolas M. Nosocomial enterococcal endocarditis: a serious hazard for hospitalized patients with enterococcal bacteraemia. *J Intern Med* 2002; **252**: 510–15.

6. Bates J, Jordens JZ, Griffiths DT. Farm animals as a putative reservoir for vancomycin-resistant enterococcal infection in man. *J Antimicrob Chemother* 1994; **34**: 507–16.

7. Van Belkum A, van den Braak N, Thomassen R, Verbrugh H, Endtz H. Vancomycin-resistance enterococci in cats and dogs. *Lancet* 1996; **348**: 1038–9.

8. Devriese LA, Cruz Colque JI, De Herdt P, Haesebrouck F. Identification and composition of the tonsillar and anal enterococcal and streptococcal flora of dogs and cats. *J Appl Bacteriol* 1992; **73**: 421–5.

9. Simonsen GS, Haaheim H, Dahl KH, Kruse H, Lovseth A, Olsvik O, Sundsfjord A. Transmission of VanA-type vancomycin-resistant enterococci and *vanA* resistance elements

between chicken and humans at avoparcin-exposed farms. *Microb Drug Res* 1998; **4**: 313–18.

10. Stobberingh E, van den Bogaard A, London N, Driessen C, Top J, Willems R. Enterococci with glycopeptide resistance in turkeys, turkey farmers, turkey slaughterers, and (sub)urban residents in the south of The Netherlands: evidence of transmission of vancomycin resistance from animals to humans? *Antimicrob Agents Chemother* 1999; **43**: 2215–21.

11. Sandoe J, Witherden AIR, Cove JH, Heritage J, Wilcox MH. Correlation between enterococcal biofilm formation in vitro and medical-device-related infection potential in vivo. *J Med Microbiol* 2003; **52**: 547–50.

12. Toledo-Arana A, Valle J, Solano C, Arrizubieta MJ, Cucarella C, Lamata M, Amorena B, Leiva J, Penades JR, Lasa L. The enterococcal surface protein, Esp, is involved in *Enterococcus faecalis* biofilm formation. *App Environ Microbiol* 2001; **67**: 4538–45.

6

Pneumococcal vaccination

DAVID McINTOSH

Introduction

To become familiar with the three generations of pneumococcal vaccines, it is important to review the immunological basis upon which they are believed to function. The 23-valent pneumococcal polysaccharide 'grandparent' vaccine contains T-cell-independent antigens capable only of inducing a restricted immunoglobulin G (IgG) response with poor immunological memory [1]. The 7-valent pneumococcal conjugate 'parent' vaccine acts by T-cell-dependent mechanisms to induce T-helper cells to stimulate polysaccharide-specific B cells to maturation. These become either antibody-producing plasma cells or memory cells. While there is a degree of cross-reactivity between pneumococcal serotypes within serogroups, essentially a 7-valent vaccine can be relied upon to cover for the seven serotypes included, a 9-valent vaccine to cover the nine serotypes, etc. Pneumococcal conjugates will be the dominant pneumococcal vaccines for the time being. The next generation will be protein vaccines, but their mechanism of action is as yet barely understood.

The structure of this chapter is based loosely around this pedigree and, while not dismissing the 23-valent pneumococcal polysaccharide vaccine out of hand, it is becoming apparent that its usefulness is limited (Jackson *et al.*). This vaccine is becoming an integral part of the retirement and superannuation package, and is often combined with influenza vaccination. However, the 7-valent pneumococcal conjugate vaccine may supplant its use in adults, not only when administered directly but also when administered to infants and young children via herd immunity (Whitney *et al.*). Recent evidence suggests that the conjugate vaccines may even have a role in preventing viral pneumonia (Klugman *et al.*).

Exploring the theme of indirect immunization further, at the individual rather than at the population level, both haematopoietic stem cell recipients and newborn babies stand to benefit from pneumococcal vaccination of the donor and the mother respectively (Molrine *et al.*, Richter *et al.*). While the former should become the standard of care, the latter awaits further ethical consideration. The role of either 23-valent pneumococcal polysaccharide vaccine or 7-valent pneumococcal conjugate vaccine in other transplant situations, such as renal transplantation, remains to be defined, with immune responses competing against more powerful immunosuppressive therapy (Kumar *et al.*). Information on the role of such therapies and the optimal vaccination regimes are two of the huge gaps in pneumococcal research (Nachman *et al.*).

A major area of debate surrounds the role of pneumococcal conjugate vaccines in mucosal infections such as otitis media and the potential for serotype replacement disease, both local and systemic (Fireman *et al.*, Dagan *et al.*). For the time being the overwhelming benefits of reduction in invasive pneumococcal disease and the impressive reductions in antibiotic resistance outweigh these risks. In any case, there will be newer and perhaps more generic pneumococcal vaccines in the future to address such issues (Dagan *et al.*, McCool *et al.*).

Finally, two papers are included as much for their remarkable methodologies as for their important results. A group-randomized approach to Phase III trial design was adopted successfully in a study of pneumococcal vaccination in North American indigenous populations (O'Brien *et al.*), while direct inoculation of human volunteers with *Streptococcus pneumoniae* constituted the design of a Phase I trial (McCool *et al.*).

23-valent pneumococcal polysaccharide vaccine

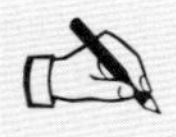

Effectiveness of pneumococcal polysaccharide vaccine in older adults

Jackson LA, Neuzil KM, Yu O, *et al.*, for the Vaccine Safety Datalink. *N Engl J Med* 2003; **348**: 1747–55

BACKGROUND. 23-valent pneumococcal polysaccharide vaccine is recommended and used widely but its efficacy/effectiveness in preventing pneumococcal infection has been called into question. It is already known to have low immunogenicity in infants and young children but its role in adults, especially the elderly, is uncertain. This retrospective study examined its effectiveness in preventing pneumococcal bacteraemia and all-cause pneumonia in those ≥65 years of age. Of the 47 365 cohort members, 1428 were hospitalized with community-acquired pneumonia, 3061 were managed as outpatients with pneumonia and 61 had pneumococcal bacteraemia. Whilst the vaccine was associated with a significant reduction in the risk of pneumococcal bacteraemia (multivariate-adjusted hazard ratio 0.56; 95% confidence interval [CI] 0.33–0.93; point effectiveness 44%), this was not the case for pneumonia.

INTERPRETATION. While an aetiological agent is not sought in most cases of pneumonia, *Streptococcus pneumoniae* is assumed to cause around 30% of cases |2|. In failing to demonstrate effectiveness against pneumonia at the population level, it is still possible that it has a degree of efficacy at the level of the individual. The results are at variance with another retrospective study which did show a reduction in the risk of hospitalization for pneumonia (and influenza), of 0.57 |3|. The vaccine is useful in preventing invasive pneumococcal disease, but newer approaches such as the use of pneumococcal conjugate vaccines may produce greater overall benefit for the elderly.

Comment

Retrospective studies have limitations and possible confounding factors. The results of a large-scale prospective study of 23-valent pneumococcal polysaccharide vaccine in 152765 healthy military recruits were presented at the fourth International Symposium on Pneumococci and Pneumococcal Disease (ISPPD) held in Helsinki from 9 to 12 May 2004 by K. Russell and colleagues. The vaccine did not result in a decrease in all-cause pneumonia. Nor was a protective effect noted for either preventing community-acquired pneumonia or diminishing its severity in a Catalonia study reported at the same meeting by Ochoa Gondar and colleagues. There will be cost-effectiveness implications for newer vaccine approaches, but for the present the elderly are not going to be denied this vaccine and there may be renewed impetus for identifying the causative agents in adult (and paediatric) pneumonias.

Indirect immunization

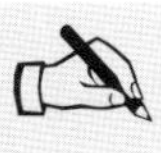

Donor immunization with pneumococcal conjugate vaccine and early protective antibody responses following allogeneic hematopoietic cell transplantation

Molrine DC, Antin JH, Guinan EC, *et al. Blood* 2003; **101**: 831–6

BACKGROUND. Ninety-six patients at least 2 years of age with haematological malignancy were randomized to receive allogeneic non-T cell-depleted haematopoietic cell transplantation with or without pre-vaccination of the donor with 7-valent pneumococcal conjugate vaccine (7–10 days in advance). All patients received the vaccine at 3, 6 and 12 months after transplantation, and serotype-specific antibody concentrations were determined by enzyme-linked immunosorbent assay (ELISA) after each dose. Sixty-five patients (68%) could be evaluated. Transplantation patients in the immunized donor group had higher geometric mean antibody concentrations to all seven vaccine serotypes after one and two doses of vaccine compared with patients whose donors were unimmunized. The differences were statistically significant after one dose for serotypes 6B, 9V, 18C, 19F and 23F ($P <0.05$) and after two doses for serotypes 6B, 14, 19F and 23F ($P <0.03$). After the third dose, both groups had more than 60% of patients with antibody concentrations regarded as being protective (≥ 0.5 µg/ml) to all seven serotypes. In the second part of this study, the antibody levels of all patients immunized with 7-valent pneumococcal conjugate vaccine were compared with those of historical patients immunized with 23-valent pneumococcal polysaccharide vaccine. The geometric mean concentrations of antibody to the seven serotypes included in both vaccines were significantly higher for patients who received a three-dose series of 7-valent pneumococcal conjugate vaccine at 3, 6 and 12 months compared with those of patients who received an initial dose of 23-valent pneumococcal polysaccharide vaccine at 12 months.

INTERPRETATION. Donor immunization enables haematopoietic cell transplant recipients to respond early to their own immunization. Given that antibody responses to 23-valent pneumococcal polysaccharide vaccine are weak and unlikely to be protective during the time of greatest disease risk |4|, immunization with 7-valent pneumococcal conjugate vaccine should be considered as an alternative. Furthermore, should the donor agree to pre-vaccination, the transplant recipient may receive even greater protection.

Comment

The recipient of haematopoietic cell transplantation is likely to be investigated for infection at the slightest sign of fever, especially that associated with neutropenia. The vaccination approach suggested above has the potential to decrease the number of febrile episodes and the need for antibiotics. Conventionally, the donor would be expected to be immune to hepatitis B virus and to be screened for other blood-borne pathogens. Now there is the expectation that the donor should be 'primed' in order for the transplanted cells to be optimized. This approach needs to be investigated for a wider range of malignancies and transplant situations.

Immunization of female mice with glycoconjugates protects their offspring against encapsulated bacteria

Richter MY, Jakobsen H, Birgisdottir A, *et al*. *Infect Immun* 2004; **71**: 187–95

BACKGROUND. Vaccination strategies are needed that confer protective immunity very early in life. Infants born with high circulating antibodies due to active immunization of their mother may be passively protected during the time required for them to mount an immune response of their own to vaccination. Adult female mice were immunized with native pneumococcal polysaccharide of serotypes 1, 6B and 19F or with polysaccharide conjugated to tetanus protein (6B and 19F being adjuvanted). Not only did the conjugated vaccine elicit much higher specific antibodies in the mothers than did native polysaccharide, but also these antibodies were transmitted to the offspring at up to 322% of the maternal levels by 3 weeks. Furthermore, the offspring of mothers immunized with conjugate were protected against a lethal challenge with *Streptococcus pneumoniae* while the other offspring were not.

INTERPRETATION. Protection was demonstrated not only for infant pneumococcal lung infection but also for lethal blood infection. As expected, there was a decline in the antibody levels in the mice over time – this would need to be extrapolated to humans to determine the optimal time for infant immunization. Nevertheless, the murine model is suitable for studying maternal immunization despite probable differences from humans, such as the proportion and concentration of antibody subclasses transferred, the invasiveness of different pneumococcal serotypes, and the immune responses.

Comment

For organisms that are capable of causing infection early in infancy, such as group B streptococcus, respiratory syncytial virus and *S. pneumoniae*, the infant immune system may not be capable of mounting a response to vaccination. Furthermore, there is a risk of hyporesponsiveness to subsequent doses. While maternal immunization may be a realistic option for conferring early protection, the ethical, legal and logistical issues are formidable, and there is a risk of interference with responses to vaccines administered in infancy unless the timing is optimized.

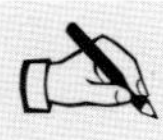

Decline in invasive pneumococcal disease after the introduction of protein-polysaccharide conjugate vaccine

Whitney CG, Farley MM, Hadler J, *et al.*, for the Active Bacterial Core Surveillance of the Emerging Infections Program Network. *N Engl J Med* 2003; **348**: 1737–46

BACKGROUND. Population-based data from the Active Bacterial Core Surveillance of the Centers for Disease Control and Prevention in the US were evaluated to determine the effectiveness of 7-valent pneumococcal conjugate vaccine in preventing invasive pneumococcal disease since its licensing in early 2000. Trends were assessed in seven geographical areas with continuous participation in the scheme from 1998 to 2001, covering a population of 16 million. As expected, there was an overall large decline in invasive pneumococcal disease in the target age group, infants and young children less than 2 years of age (188 cases per 100 000 to 59 cases per 100 000, a 69% decrease; $P < 0.001$) (Fig. 6.1). For vaccine serotypes this decrease was 78% while for vaccine-related serotypes the decrease was 50%. What was unexpected were significant decreases in the rates of invasive pneumococcal disease in adults: 32% for adults 20–39 years of age ($P < 0.001$), 8% for those 40–64 years of age ($P = 0.03$) and 18% for those 65 years of age and older ($P < 0.001$).

INTERPRETATION. In that the decreases in rates in adults were mainly in serotypes covered by 7-valent pneumococcal conjugate vaccine, it is likely that the effect was due to decreased transmission from infants and young children rather than the use of 23-valent pneumococcal polysaccharide vaccine.

Comment

To cover the period up to 2003, Whitney and colleagues at the fourth ISPPD have updated the data. For infants and children less than 2 years of age the overall reductions in invasive pneumococcal disease are between 77 and 83%, while for vaccine and vaccine-related serotypes the reductions are 96 and 35% respectively. However, there has been a statistically significant increase in disease due to non-vaccine serotypes, although small in overall numbers. What is remarkable is the sustained and further reduction in overall adult invasive pneumococcal disease: 41% for those 20–39 years of age, 20% for those aged 40–64 years, and 31% for those 65 years of age and older. These reductions are coupled with large decreases in antibiotic resistance.

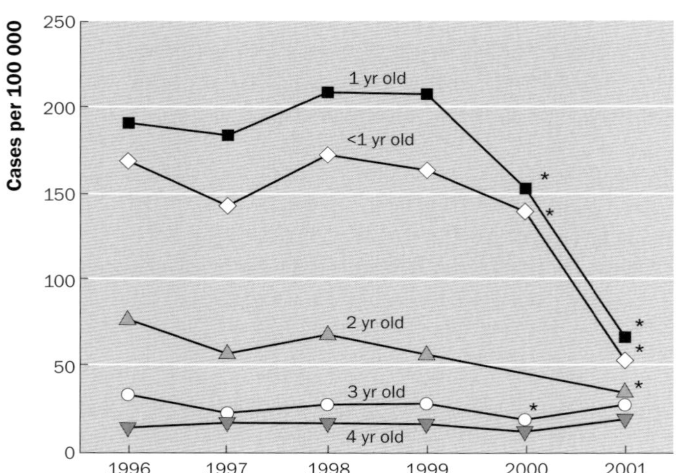

Fig. 6.1 Rates of invasive pneumococcal disease among children under 5 years of age, according to age and year. Data are from the US Active Bacterial Core Surveillance from 1996 to 2001. *, *P* <0.05 for comparisons of the rate in 2000 or 2001 with the combined rate for 1998 and 1999 (the 1996 and 1997 rates do not include data from New York State). Source: Whitney *et al.* (2003).

Licensure and assays

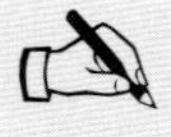

Serological criteria for evaluation and licensure of new pneumococcal conjugate vaccine formulations for use in infants

Jódar L, Carlone G, Dagan R, *et al. Vaccine* 2003; **21**: 3265–72

BACKGROUND. The lack of a definitive serological correlate of protection and the multiplicity of antigens present in pneumococcal conjugate vaccines (at present count 7+) are barriers to the licensure of such vaccines. The only currently licensed pneumococcal conjugate vaccine has been subject to a large pivotal efficacy trial |5| but the clinical efficacy of most of the individual serotypes represented is not established. It would aid the licensure of new vaccines, for example in determining non-inferiority, if there were agreement about the immunological correlates of protection. The World Health Organization sponsored a consultation to consider the assessment of antibody responses, persistence of antibodies, priming/memory and functionality.

INTERPRETATION. Inferences for protection against bacteraemia and meningitis can be made from the serological results of the efficacy trial |5|, although this is more difficult for pneumonia and otitis media. Inferiority for rarer serotypes in a vaccine may be counterbalanced by at least covering for more serotypes, assuming that a common aggregate threshold for all serotypes would be relatively close to thresholds for individual serotypes. Immunological memory can be measured by evidence of boosting; that is, an augmented immune response to either 23-valent pneumococcal polysaccharide vaccine or pneumococcal conjugate vaccine. In addition, it can be implied by a response that is dominated by IgG and by increased antibody avidity. The immunological issues to be considered in the licensure of pneumococcal conjugate vaccines are summarized in Table 6.1.

Comment

While 7-valent pneumococcal conjugate vaccine covers a high proportion of serotypes in both developed and developing countries, vaccines covering more serotypes are desirable. However, the logistics of conducting vast efficacy trials for licensing purposes argue for basing efficacy on surrogate markers. For determining non-inferiority, some would argue that an absolute IgG level by ELISA of 0.35 μg/ml should be the benchmark while others would argue for a lower level of 0.2 μg/ml, provided an inhibition step is performed. There are pneumococcal conjugate vaccines under development with more serotypes and different protein carriers, and a consensus will have to be reached in order for licensing authorities to be assured of the ability of the vaccine to prevent disease. In fact, guidance protocols have been formulated by a multinational group |6| and are available at http://www.vaccine. uab.edu. The reference laboratory in the UK has noted discrepancies between assays based on the 23-valent polysaccharide antigen and those that are serotype-specific |7|.

Table 6.1 Proposed end-points for licensure of pneumococcal conjugate vaccine based on serological criteria

Measurement	Interpretation
IgG by ELISA 4 weeks after three-dose priming series	Optimal for registration
Single pooled threshold antibody concentration	Derived from efficacy
Percentage of non-responders	Determination of non-inferiority
Single primary end-point	Sufficient for registration
Age-matched opsonophagocytic assay	Functionality of antibody
Antibody concentrations after boosting	Evidence of memory
Avidity of antibodies	Evidence of memory

Source: Jódar *et al.* (2003).

At-risk situations

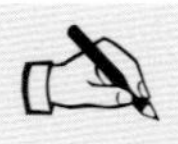

Safety and immunogenicity of a heptavalent pneumococcal conjugate vaccine in infants with human immunodeficiency virus type 1 infection

Nachman S, Kim S, King J, *et al.*, for the Pediatric AIDS Clinical Trials Group Study 292 Team. *Pediatrics* 2003; **112**: 66–73

BACKGROUND. Given the poor immunogenicity of 23-valent pneumococcal polysaccharide vaccine in those with HIV infection |8| and in the context of the efficacy results described above, it is important to document both safety and immunogenicity in patients with HIV infection. Infants with HIV infection were randomized to receive three doses of 7-valent pneumococcal conjugate vaccine or placebo at 2-month intervals, starting at between 56 and 180 days of age, with a booster dose at 15 months of age. Thirty infants with HIV infection received vaccine and 15 received placebo. In the light of what is said in the section 'Licensure and assays' (see above), the two composite primary end-points were prespecified for assessing immunogenicity: an epidemiological criterion of a 4-fold increase in IgG from pre-immunization levels for all vaccine serotypes after the primary series, and the scientific criterion of a 4-fold increase for three or more of the vaccine serotypes. Immunogenicity was further measured by means of geometric mean concentrations of antibody, mean fold changes and rates of achieving type-specific antibody levels of both 0.5 μg/ml and 0.15 μg/ml.

INTERPRETATION. Five severe acute reactions were experienced by four subjects (three in the vaccine arm of the study), although all resolved within 48 h. For all serological end-points 22 of 24 subjects receiving vaccine achieved levels satisfying the criteria. For all vaccine serotypes, geometric mean concentrations and mean fold rises were statistically significantly higher in the vaccine arm; more than 95% of vaccine recipients achieved antibody levels of 0.15 μg/ml and at least 80% achieved 0.5 μg/ml after the primary series. After the booster dose, booster rates as measured by 4-fold increases ranged from 30 to 70% depending on serotype.

Comment

The composite primary serological end-points avoid inflating the false-positive rates associated with testing for immunogenicity against individual serotypes. The 7-valent pneumococcal conjugate vaccine was found to be immunogenic in infants with HIV infection. Further studies are required to assess the longevity of these immune responses, to ascertain the optimum schedule, to examine the effect of different forms of antiretroviral therapy on safety and immunogenicity, and to evaluate the role of 23-valent pneumococcal polysaccharide vaccine. In relation to the last point, it is important to remember that non-specific antibodies have been shown to interfere with the standardized ELISA for pneumococcal polysaccharide capsular antibodies in HIV-infected adults and that it is necessary to remove non-specific antibodies by means of absorption with heterologous pneumococcal polysaccharide, such as 22F |9|. Finally, it is important to note that patients with HIV infection or AIDS have an odds ratio of 8.4 (95% CI 3.5–20.3) for recurrent invasive pneumococcal disease |**10**|.

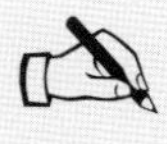

Efficacy and safety of seven-valent conjugate pneumococcal vaccine in American Indian children: group randomised trial

O'Brien KL, Moulton LH, Reid R, *et al. Lancet* 2003; **362**: 355–61

BACKGROUND. People of the Navajo and White Mountain Apache tribes of the south-western US suffer high rates of invasive pneumococcal disease: up to 1820 per 100 000 in White Mountain Apache infants and children less than 2 years of age |11|. A group-randomized approach was used to assess the safety and efficacy of 7-valent pneumococcal conjugate vaccine in these populations. The study design was unusual in that there were 38 randomization units, these being clusters of existing, well-defined communities; within each unit for every infant or child that participated a similar vaccine or a similar control was administered.

INTERPRETATION. Around 80% of the infants and children in the target population were assessed, with a final enrolment of 8292. By per-protocol analysis for vaccine serotypes, the efficacy for those less than 2 years of age was 81.7%, while in the intention-to-treat analysis the efficacy was 86.4%. For infants enrolled by 7 months of age these efficacies were 76.8 and 82.6% respectively. There was no significant increase in non-vaccine serotype invasive pneumococcal disease and there was no pattern of increased adverse events in infants and children receiving the vaccine.

Comment

Whilst having some limitations, such as maintaining the masking throughout the trial, a reduction in the effective sample size and the mixing of intervention and control populations, this study was designed to serve as a pivotal trial for vaccine licensure and serves as a model for future trials, especially in populations divisible into distinct units. By contrast, 23-valent pneumococcal polysaccharide vaccine was tested for its effectiveness in preventing invasive pneumococcal disease in Navajo adults and was found to be inadequate in prevention |**12**|.

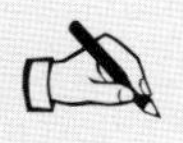

Randomized, double-blind, controlled trial of pneumococcal vaccination in renal transplant recipients

Kumar D, Rotstein C, Miyata G, Arlen D, Humar A. *J Infect Dis* 2003; **187**: 1639–45

BACKGROUND. Immunosuppression is likely to impair the immune response not only to infection but also to vaccination. At the same time as restoring renal function, renal transplantation ameliorates the systemic effects of renal failure but exacerbates susceptibility to infection by encapsulated organisms such as *Streptococcus pneumoniae* |13|. In order to compare the quantitative and functional antibody production arising from 23-valent pneumococcal polysaccharide vaccine as opposed to 7-valent pneumococcal conjugate vaccine, 60 adult Canadian renal transplant patients who had not received pneumococcal vaccination within the preceding 5 years participated in a double-blind, randomized, controlled study. Patients were administered a single dose of vaccine and immune responses were measured before vaccination and then at 8 weeks.

INTERPRETATION. By ELISA, the overall response rates to each individual serotype were poor in both groups: 13–40% for the 23-valent pneumococcal polysaccharide group and 17–50% for the 7-valent pneumococcal conjugate vaccine group. Nor were the functional antibody responses, as measured by opsonophagocytic assay, different between the two groups (Table 6.2). The fold increase between baseline and 2 months was not significantly different between groups for all 7 serotypes.

Comment

While both vaccines exhibited some degree of immunogenicity, the authors applied a protective threshold of 1.0 μg/ml and it is not clear whether this would be protective in the clinical setting. Probably more than one dose of pneumococcal vaccine is required, including a combination of the two types of vaccine; for example, priming with the conjugate and boosting with the polysaccharide or multiple doses of conjugate.

Table 6.2 Titre of opsonophagocytic assay for serotype-specific functional antibody before and after vaccination with polysaccharide and conjugate vaccines in renal transplant patients. Data are geometric mean titres (range)

Serotype	Polysaccharide vaccine		Conjugate vaccine	
	Baseline	**8 weeks**	**Baseline**	**8 weeks**
4	49.6 (4–1024)	172.8 (32–1024)	45.3 (4–256)	207.9 (32–2048)
6B	70.2 (8–512)	198.6 (32–4096)	70.2 (8–2048)	294.1 (32–4096)
9V	14.3 (4–256)	78.8 (4–1024)	16.0 (4–128)	82.5 (4–8192)
14	70.2 (8–1024)	203.3 (4–2048)	111.4 (8–1024)	238.9 (4–4096)
18C	30.6 (4–1024)	86.4 (4–2048)	19.7 (4–512)	119.4 (4–2048)
19F	49.6 (8–256)	111.4 (16–1024)	58.4 (4–4096)	147.0 (8–2048)
23F	12.4 (4–128)	28.5 (4–512)	16.8 (4–1024)	64.0 (4–2048)

Source: Kumar *et al.* (2003).

Otitis media

Impact of the pneumococcal conjugate vaccine on otitis media

Fireman B, Black SB, Shinefield HR, Lee J, Lewis E. *Pediatr Infect Dis* J 2003; **22**: 10–16

BACKGROUND. In addition to studies on the efficacy of 7-valent pneumococcal conjugate vaccine in preventing invasive pneumococcal disease |5|, the vaccine has been studied for its ability to prevent non-invasive diseases, such as otitis media, many of which are deemed to be pneumococcal in origin.

INTERPRETATION. Starting at the first dose, 7-valent pneumococcal conjugate vaccine prevented 7% of otitis visits in the intention-to-treat analysis (95% CI 4.7–9.1%). However, three doses were required to sustain this decrease throughout the first year of life, the per-protocol efficacy after three doses reaching 7.8%. This translates into a reduction of 6.6% in episodes. Antibiotic prescriptions were reduced by 5.7% (95% CI 4.2–7.2%). Frequent episodes of otitis media were reduced by up to 26% while tube placements were reduced by 24% (95% CI 12–35%).

Comment

While clinicians in hospitals are likely to notice reductions in paediatric invasive pneumococcal disease after the introduction of 7-valent pneumococcal conjugate vaccine, it will be physicians in the community and specialists in otorhinolaryn gology that appreciate the decreases in otitis media. However, for parents the effect may be imperceptible, given the multiple causes of otitis media and the many pneumococcal serotypes that may be responsible. The knock-on effect will be decreased antibiotic prescribing and decreased antibiotic resistance. In what is certainly the largest depository of middle-ear fluid in Israel, which does not yet have a universal programme of infant pneumococcal vaccination, 477 (19%) of 2467 isolates from infants and young children with acute otitis media were shown to be non-vaccine serotypes (mainly 35B, 33F, 21 and 15B/C) |14|. This demonstrates the potential for non-vaccine strains, including antibiotic-resistant strains, to cause acute otitis media. Additionally, two of these serogroups (15 and 33) have been noted to be replacing vaccine serotypes as causes of invasive pneumococcal disease in the US |15|. Clonal analysis of pneumococcal isolates from the Finnish Otitis Media trial suggests that strains responsible for otitis media vary less in their potential to do so than do strains in their ability to cause invasive pneumococcal disease |16|. This gives further credence to the observation that replacement otitis media will occur after the intro-duction of conjugate pneumococcal vaccine |17|.

Newer pneumococcal vaccines

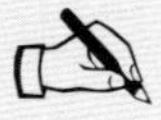

Effect of a nonavalent conjugate vaccine on carriage of antibiotic-resistant *Streptococcus pneumoniae* in day-care centers

Dagan R, Givon-Lavi N, Zamir O, Fraser D. *Pediatr Infect Dis J* 2003; **22**: 532–9

BACKGROUND. High rates of nasopharyngeal carriage tend to be found in day-care attendees, partly due to the age and partly due to the close proximity of these infants and children. Healthy day-care attendees in Israel aged between 12 and 35 months were randomized to receive either 9-valent pneumococcal conjugate vaccine (similar to the 7-valent vaccine but with the addition of globally important serotypes 1 and 5) or a conjugate meningococcal C vaccine. Nasopharyngeal cultures for *Streptococcus pneumoniae* were obtained prior to vaccination and frequently for 2 years after. The aim was to determine whether pneumococcal conjugate vaccine affected carriage, especially with regard to antibiotic-resistant strains.

INTERPRETATION. Most subjects were followed up for 18–24 months. Of the 3748 cultures obtained, 2450 (65%) were positive for *S. pneumoniae*, but of these nearly half were non-vaccine serotypes. However, the highest antibiotic resistance rates were found in serotypes 6B, 9V, 14, 19F and 23F (all covered by the existing pneumococcal conjugate vaccine), with 85% resistant to at least one antibiotic, 75% resistant to two or more antibiotics and 26% resistant to three or more antibiotics (penicillin, erythromycin, sulphamethoxazole/trimethoprim). The overall carriage rate of antibiotic-resistant *S. pneumoniae* was significantly reduced in the vaccinated compared with the control group. The significant reduction was observed only in serotypes included in the 9-valent pneumococcal conjugate vaccine plus serotype 6A, while there was a significant increase in carriage of serotypes not related to the vaccine (Table 6.3).

Table 6.3 Relative risks of nasopharyngeal carriage of pneumococcal serotypes in recipients of 9-valent pneumococcal conjugate vaccine versus control vaccine

Pneumococcal serotype	Relative risk	95% CI
6B, 9V, 14, 19F, 23F (vaccine)	0.63	0.54–0.73
1, 4, 5, 18C (vaccine)	0.30	0.14–0.67
6A (vaccine-related)	0.62	0.51–0.72
19A (vaccine-related)	1.01	0.70–1.45
Others (non-vaccine)	1.31	1.20–1.43

Source: Dagan *et al.* (2003).

Comment

The reduction in the serotypes most commonly associated with antibiotic resistance and the replacement with non-vaccine-related serotypes resulted in a large reduction in carriage of antibiotic-resistant *S. pneumoniae* among vaccinated day-care attendees. The global scale of the problem of antibiotic resistance is highlighted in an exposé in Emerging Infectious Diseases |**18**|. It appears that pneumococcal conjugate vaccines are going to have a major role not only in decreasing pneumococcal infection but also in decreasing antibiotic resistance (see also Whitney *et al.*, 2003, above). In a US study it was shown that non-susceptibility to penicillin is more common in pneumococcal strains related to 7-valent pneumococcal conjugate vaccine (45%) and potentially cross-reacting strains (51%) than in non-vaccine strains (8%) |**19**|. With monitoring and reporting in place, the importance of serotype replacement will become clearer.

As part of the same study in Israel, the younger siblings of day-care attendees provided monthly nasopharyngeal cultures |**20**|. There was a significant reduction in carriage of *S. pneumoniae* in not only the day-care attendees themselves but also the siblings of those attendees who had received the pneumococcal vaccine as opposed to those who had not (21% in vaccine siblings versus 34% in non-vaccine siblings; $P = 0.017$), although there were increases in non-vaccine serotypes in both attendees ($P <0.001$) and their siblings ($P = 0.15$). There were also significant decreases in the carriage of antibiotic-resistant *S. pneumoniae* in both the attendees and their siblings.

An 11-valent pneumococcal conjugate vaccine with a mixed carrier has also been under investigation by the same group and other groups |**21–23**|.

A trial of 9-valent pneumococcal conjugate vaccine in children with and those without HIV infection

Klugman KP, Madhi SA, Huebner RE, Kohberger R, Mbelle N, Pierce N, for the Vaccine Trialists Group. *N Engl J Med* 2003; **349**: 1341–8

BACKGROUND. The efficacy of 9-valent pneumococcal conjugate vaccine was evaluated in a randomized, double-blind trial in nearly 40 000 infants in Soweto, South Africa, half of whom received the vaccine and half placebo, administered at 6, 10 and 14 weeks. The incidence of vaccine-serotype-specific invasive pneumococcal disease was estimated to be 112 per 100 000 children. Follow-up continued until 15 children without HIV infection who were included in the per-protocol analysis met the primary end-point of invasive pneumococcal disease caused by a serotype included in the vaccine. The other primary end-point was an episode of radiologically confirmed pneumonia that occurred at least 14 days after the third dose in children without HIV infection who were included in the per-protocol analysis.

INTERPRETATION. For invasive pneumococcal disease in children without HIV, the serotype-specific per-protocol vaccine efficacy was 85% while for those with HIV the efficacy was 65%. In an update at the fourth ISPPD by Madhi *et al.*, corresponding figures were presented from the intention-to-treat perspective: 88% and 53.6% respectively. There were also reductions in disease caused by antibiotic-resistant strains. For pneumonia, the efficacy was 20% for HIV non-infected children. Based on the intention-to-treat analysis, the overall efficacies in preventing clinically diagnosed lower respiratory tract infection and hospitalized clinical pneumonia were 9.3% and 16.2%, respectively. Among HIV-infected children, these efficacies were 15.4% and 15%, while among HIV non-infected children the efficacies were 6.6% and 16.9%, respectively.

Comment

The 9-valent pneumococcal conjugate vaccine is effective in reducing invasive pneumococcal disease and pneumonia in infants and children with and without HIV infection, including infections caused by antibiotic-resistant strains. So far, the vaccine is not licensed. An unexpected effect was reported at the fourth ISPPD: a reduction not only in bacterial pneumonia but also a substantial reduction in hospitalization for viral pneumonia due to influenza A virus, parainfluenza virus and respiratory syncytial virus. This would add considerably to the benefits arising from widespread paediatric pneumococcal immunization.

Serum immunoglobulin G response to candidate vaccine antigens during experimental human pneumococcal colonization

McCool TL, Cate TR, Tuomanen EI, Adrian P, Mitchell TJ, Weiser JN. *Infect Immun* 2003; **71**: 5724–32

BACKGROUND. As an alternative to pneumococcal conjugate vaccine, which is based on pneumococcal polysaccharide, pneumococcal protein vaccines are under development. These could be based on the phosphorylcholine epitope of lipoteichoic acid, the choline-binding protein A (CbpA), pneumolysin, proteinase maturation protein, pneumococcal surface adhesin, pneumococcal surface protein A (PspA) or other recently identified surface proteins. CbpA is believed to be one of the pneumococcal virulence factors and binds to teichoic acid or lipoteichoic acid. PspA interferes with complement deposition and binds lactoferrin. Healthy uncolonized human volunteers were given an intranasal inoculum of either serotype 23F or 6B pneumococci. This was, in effect, a controlled vaccination. Six of the 14 inoculated with serotype 23F became colonized while six of the eight inoculated with 6B became colonized, the carrier state persisting for as long as 122 days. Sera from both the colonized and the uncolonized groups were used to measure specific antibody titres to the above proteins. By doing this it would be possible to ascertain the relative importance of particular immune responses. CbpA and PspA emerged as antigens of interest.

INTERPRETATION. Both CbpA and PspA were shown to be immunogenic during experimental human colonization with *Streptococcus pneumoniae*, eliciting serum IgG responses. By contrast there was no significant increase in antibodies to pneumococcal polysaccharide, at least for the two serotypes studied (23F and 6B). There was also strain-to-strain cross-reactivity, which was unexpected given the degree of sequence diversity represented by the genetic region tested.

Comment

The experiments were conducted in adults, not children. Although the adults were not colonized with *S. pneumoniae* at the time of inoculation, it is possible that they had been exposed to the organism earlier in life, thus altering the current immune response. It is also possible that mucosal antibody responses may not correlate with systemic responses. There have been concerns expressed about cross-reactivity between PspA and cardiac myosin, which may limit the potential of PspA to be developed into a vaccine. Given the global clonal spread of pneumococcal strains, generic vaccines such as pneumococcal proteins may become important in the future. In the meantime, this basic research paves the way for defining new correlates of protection.

Conclusion

Recent research into pneumococcal vaccines has revealed surprises and dilemmas. Of considerable surprise to young people would be the notion that, by being vaccinated themselves, they are preventing disease in their elders (Whitney *et al.*). Equally, the elderly would be entitled to a degree of scepticism regarding pneumococcal vaccination programmes targeted at their age group because of doubts over efficacy (Jackson *et al.*). A major dilemma lies in the very nature of *Streptococcus pneumoniae* and its 90 serotypes. Any hope of achieving successes such as those seen in the prevention of infections due to *Haemophilus influenzae* type b and *Neisseria meningitidis* Group C is tempered by the ubiquity and diversity of the pneumococcus.

New ways of achieving licensure are necessary either by agreeing on correlates of protection (Jödar *et al.*), by designing novel vaccine trials (O'Brien *et al.*) or both. Otherwise, the logistics of repeatedly conducting vast vaccine trials |5| will be prohibitive. In that a safety concern facing pneumococcal conjugate vaccines is that of serotype replacement (Dagan *et al.*, Kaplan *et al.*), it is important to maintain excellent infectious disease epidemiological surveillance and modelling to monitor the emergence of this phenomenon |**16,17**|.

How has pneumococcal vaccine altered clinical practice recently? In the US there is much less invasive pneumococcal disease (Whitney *et al.*, Kaplan *et al.*) and therefore fewer septic workups being performed. Where the 7-valent pneumococcal conjugate vaccine is used widely, a reduction in pneumococcal antibiotic resistance is to be expected (Whitney *et al.*), allowing a more rational choice of antibiotics. Where the vaccine is targeted towards at-risk groups, such as those receiving transplants (Molrine *et al.*, Kumar *et al.*) or those with HIV/AIDS (Nachman *et al.*) |**9,10**|, it provides an added defence against the effects of immunosuppression. I believe one area of intense research interest will be that of the safety, immunogenicity and efficacy of conjugate and other pneumococcal vaccines in those with HIV/AIDS. Another area of almost endless research possibilities is that of concomitant administration of vaccines and vaccine interactions. A third is obviously that of the immunological mechanism of action of protein vaccines (McCool *et al.*).

Finally, perhaps the most remarkable piece of evidence that has emerged recently is that of a bacterial vaccine, pneumococcal conjugate, preventing viral infection (Klugman *et al.*). The lethal synergism between influenza and *S. pneumoniae* has long been accepted dogma, but generally in this direction: preventing influenza prevents pneumococcal infection. Now it is necessary to study the immunological basis for the reverse process. Or is this an epidemiological epiphenomenon?

References

1. Eskola J. Immunogenicity of pneumococcal conjugate vaccines. *Pediatr Infect Dis J* 2000; 19: 388–93.

2. Ruiz-Gonzalez A, Falguera M, Nogues A, Rubio-Caballero M. Is *Streptococcus pneumoniae* the leading cause of pneumonia of unknown etiology? A microbiologic study of lung aspirates in consecutive patients with community-acquired pneumonia. *Am J Med* 1999; 106: 385–90.

3. Nichol KL, Baken L, Wuorenma J, Neslon A. The health and economic benefits associated with pneumococcal vaccination of elderly persons with chronic lung disease. *Arch Intern Med* 1999; 159: 2437–42.

4. Giebink GS, Warkentin PI, Ramsay NKC, Kersey JH. Titers of antibody to pneumococci in allogeneic bone marrow transplant recipients before and after vaccination with pneumococcal vaccine. *J Infect* 1986; 154: 590–6.

5. Black S, Shinefield H, Fireman B, Lewis EL, Ray P, Hansen JR, Elvin L, Ensor KM, Hackell J, Siber G, Malinoski F, Madore D, Chang IH, Kohberger R, Watson W, Austrian R, Edwards K, and the Northern California Kaiser Permanente Vaccine Study Center Group. Efficacy, safety and immunogenicity of heptavalent pneumococcal conjugate vaccine in children. *Pediatr Infect Dis J* 2000; 19: 187–95.

6. Wernette CM, Frasch CE, Madore D, Carlone G, Goldblatt D, Plikaytis B, Benjamin W, Quataert SA, Hildreth S, Sikkema DJ, Käyhty H, Jonsdottir I, Nahm MH. Enzyme-linked immunosorbent assay for quantitation of human antibodies to pneumococcal polysaccharides. *Clin Diagn Lab Immunol* 2003; 10: 514–19.

7. Balmer P, North J, Baxter D, Standford E, Melegaro A, Kaczmarski EB, Miller E, Borrow R. Measurement and interpretation of pneumococcal IgG levels for clinical management. *Clin Exp Immunol* 2003; 133: 364–9.

8. Rodriguez-Barradas MC, Alexandfaki I, Nazir T, Foltzer M, Mucher DM, Brown S, Thornby J. Response of human immunodeficiency virus-infected patients receiving

highly active antiretroviral therapy to vaccination with 23-valent pneumococcal polysaccharide vaccine. *Clin Infect Dis* 2003; 37: 438–47.

9. Feikin DR, Elie CM, Goet MB, Lennox JL, Carlone GM, Romero-Steiner S, Holder PF, O'Brien WA, Whitney CG, Butler JC, Breiman RF. Specificity of the antibody to the pneumococcal polysaccharide and conjugate vaccines in human immunodeficiency virus-infected adults. *Clin Diagn Lab Immunol* 2004; 11: 137–41.

10. King MD, Whitney CG, Parekh F, Farley MM, for the Active Bacterial Core Surveillance Team/Emerging Infections Program Network. Recurrent invasive pneumococcal disease: a population-based assessment. *Clin Infect Dis* 2003; 37: 1029–36.

11. Cortese MM, Wolff M, Almeido-Hill J, Reid R, Ketcham J, Santosham M, High incidence of invasive pneumococcal disease in the White Mountain Apache population. *Arch Intern Med* 1992; 152: 2277–82.

12. Benin AL, O'Brien KL, Watt JP, Reid R, Zell ER, Katz S, Donaldson C, Parkinson A, Schuchat A, Santosham M, Whitney CG. Effectiveness of the 23-valent polysaccharide vaccine against invasive pneumococcal disease in Navajo adults. *J Infect Dis* 2003; 188: 81–9.

13. Linneman CC Jr, First MR. Risk of pneumococcal infections in renal transplant patients. *JAMA* 1979; 241: 2619–21.

14. Porat N, Barkai G, Jacobs MR, Trefler R, Dagan R. Four antibiotic-resistant *Streptococcus pneumoniae* clones unrelated to the pneumococcal conjugate vaccine serotypes, including 2 new serotypes, causing acute otitis media in southern Israel. *J Infect Dis* 2004; 189: 385–92.

15. Kaplan SL, Mason EO Jr, Wald ER, Schutze GE, Bradley JS, Tan TQ, Hoffman JA, Givner LB, Yogev R, Barson WJ. Decrease in invasive pneumococcal infections in children among 8 children's hospitals in the United States after the introduction of the 7-valent pneumococcal conjugate vaccine. *Pediatrics* 2004; 113(3 Pt 1): 443–9.

16. Hanage WP, Auranen K, Syrjanen R, Herva E, Makela PH, Kilpi T, Spratt BG. Ability of pneumococcal serotypes and clones to cause acute otitis media: implications for the prevention of otitis media by conjugate vaccines. *Infect Immun* 2004; 72: 76–81.

17. McEllistrem MC, Adams J, Mason EO, Wald ER. Epidemiology of acute otitis media caused by *Streptococcus pneumoniae* before and after licensure of the 7-valent pneumococcal protein conjugate vaccine. *J Infect Dis* 2003; 188: 1679–84.

18. Albrich WC, Monnet DL, Harbarth S. Antibiotic selection pressure and resistance in *Streptococcus pneumoniae* and *Streptococcus pyogenes*. *Emerg Infect Dis* 2004; 10: 514–17.

19. Finkelstein JA, Huang SS, Daniel J, Rifas-Shiman SL, Kleinman K, Goldmann D, Pelton SI, DeMaria A, Platt R. Antibiotic-resistant *Streptococcus pneumoniae* in the heptavalent pneumococcal conjugate vaccine era: predictors of carriage in a multicommunity sample. *Pediatrics* 2003; 112: 862–9.

20. Givon-Lavi N, Fraser D, Dagan R. Vaccination of day-care center attendees reduces carriage of *Streptococcus pneumoniae* among their younger siblings. *Pediatr Infect Dis J* 2003; 22: 524–32.

21. Puumalainen T, Dagan R, Wuorimaa T, Zeta-Capeding R, Lucero M, Ollgren J, Käyhty H, Nohynek H. Greater antibody responses to an eleven valent mixed carrier diphtheria- or tetanus-conjugated pneumococcal vaccine in Filipino than in Finnish or Israeli infants. *Pediatr Infect Dis J* 2003; 22: 141–9.

22. Puumalainen T, Ekstrom N, Zeta-Capeding R, Loogren J, Jousimies K, Lucero M, Nohynek H, Käyhty H. Functional antibodies elicited by an 11-valent diphtheria-tetanus toxoid-conjugated pneumococcal vaccine. *J Infect Dis* 2003; **187**: 1704–8.

23. Dagan R, Käyhty H, Wuorimaa T, Yaich M, Bailleux F, Zamir O, Eskola J. Tolerability and immunogenicity of an eleven valent mixed carrier *Streptococcus pneumoniae* capsular polysaccharide–diphtheria toxoid or tetanus protein conjugate vaccine in Finnish and Israeli infants. *Pediatr Infect Dis J* 2004; **23**: 91–8.

7

Vancomycin resistance in *Staphylococcus aureus*

ROBIN HOWE

Introduction

The worldwide spread of methicillin-resistant *Staphylococcus aureus* (MRSA) during the 1980s and 1990s led to increasing reliance on the glycopeptides vancomycin and teicoplanin as the only agents displaying reliable activity against these strains. In 1988, high-level vancomycin resistance was first reported in enterococci (vancomycin-resistant enterococcus, [VRE]) [1] and throughout the 1990s it was feared that, with the increasing selective pressure due to high vancomycin use in hospitals and the increasing prevalence of both VRE and MRSA, vancomycin resistance would transfer from VRE into MRSA. In fact, when vancomycin resistance was first reported in a clinical strain of *S. aureus* in 1997 it had low-level resistance, due to a mechanism different from that seen in enterococci [2]. Such vancomycin-intermediate *S. aureus* (VISA) have subsequently been discovered in many countries around the world, although they remain rare [3]. Soon after the emergence of VISA, Hiramatsu described strains that are sensitive to vancomycin by conventional testing but have a subpopulation which can survive in the presence of higher vancomycin concentrations [4]. These so-called heterogeneous vancomycin-intermediate *S. aureus* (hVISA) appear to have a similar mechanism of resistance to VISA and have now been reported from all over the world, at rates varying from 0 to 20% of all MRSA [3].

Although VISA is rare, it seems clear that it is associated with a poor response to therapy with vancomycin. However, there remains considerable controversy regarding the clinical importance of hVISA and contradictory reports continue to be published (see below). Vancomycin resistance in hVISA/VISA is thought to be due to changes in cell wall metabolism that lead to a thickened cell wall with reduced cross-linking. However, the underlying genetic mechanisms that mediate these changes remain elusive and variability between strains suggests that there may be a number of mechanisms by which *S. aureus* can express a phenotype of low-level vancomycin resistance.

The most important recent development has been the emergence of high-level vancomycin resistance due to transfer of resistance from VRE. There have only been three strains isolated to date but experience with other forms of resistance suggests that vancomycin-resistant *Staphylococcus aureus* (VRSA) is likely to spread.

The field of vancomycin resistance in *S. aureus* has generated a number of acronyms, which has led to confusion in some situations. The acronyms used in this chapter are explained in Table 7.1; the terms GRSA, GISA and hGISA, used by some workers to refer to reduced susceptibility to glycopeptides, are equivalent to VRSA, VISA and hVISA, respectively. Where original authors have used alternative terms they have been changed to the equivalent term in the table in order to reduce confusion.

The emergence of VRSA

Vancomycin acts by inhibition of bacterial cell wall synthesis. It binds to the terminal D-ala-D-ala of the pentapeptide subunit of peptidoglycan and thereby inhibits cross-linking of the cell wall. The archetypal vancomycin resistance in enterococci is caused by a change of the D-ala-D-ala binding site to D-ala-D-lac, to which vancomycin cannot bind. The enzymes that mediate this change are encoded by a gene cassette (*vanA*) which is on transposon Tn1546. It was reported in 1992 that resistance could be transferred from *Enterococcus faecalis* to *S. aureus* in the laboratory and since then such transfer has been awaited in clinical practice. The initial report of the first VRSA was in 2002 and to date there have been three isolates, all from the USA. The following five papers describe clinical, microbiological and mechanistic studies on these strains.

Table 7.1 Acronyms used to denote different types of vancomycin resistance in *S. aureus*

Acronym	Expansion	Criteria
VRSA	Vancomycin-resistant *S. aureus*	Vancomycin MIC ≥32 mg/l
VISA	Vancomycin-intermediate *S. aureus*	NCCLS criteria • Vancomycin MIC 8–16 mg/l CDC criteria • Broth microdilution MIC 8–16 mg/l • E-test MIC ≥6 mg/l • Growth on commercial brain–heart infusion agar screen plates containing 6 mg/l vancomycin
SA-RVS	*S. aureus* with reduced susceptibility to vancomycin	Vancomycin MIC 4 mg/l
hVISA	Heterogeneous vancomycin-intermediate *S. aureus*	Vancomycin MIC ≤4 mg/l but a subpopulation of cells that can survive in the presence of ≥4 mg/l
VS-MRSA	Vancomycin-sensitive MRSA	Vancomycin MIC ≤4 mg/l

MIC, minimum inhibitory concentration; NCCLS, National Committee for Clinical Laboratory Standards.

Infection with vancomycin-resistant *Staphylococcus aureus* containing the vanA resistance gene

Chang S, Sievert DM, Hageman JC, *et al.*; Vancomycin-resistant *Staphylococcus aureus* Investigative Team. *N Engl J Med* 2003; **348**: 1342–7

BACKGROUND. In June 2002 the first clinical isolate of VRSA (minimum inhibitory concentration [MIC] >32 mg/l) was identified in Michigan. The patient was a 40-year-old female with diabetes mellitus and chronic renal failure for which she required haemodialysis. During the previous 6 months she had received a total of six and a half weeks of vancomycin therapy for recurrent foot ulcer infections and an MRSA infection of her arteriovenous dialysis graft. Dialysis was continued through temporary central catheters, but in June 2002 she presented with signs of an exit-site infection. The catheter was removed and, on culture, the tip grew VRSA (vancomycin MIC 1024 mg/l) and a vancomycin-resistant *E. faecalis* (VRE). VRSA was also grown from specimens from the plantar ulcers. The VRSA was sensitive to chloramphenicol, daptomycin, linezolid, minocycline, quinupristin–dalfopristin and trimethoprim–sulphamethoxazole. The patient was successfully treated with debridement and trimethoprim–sulphamethoxazole. Five hundred and forty-seven contacts from the community and three healthcare facilities were identified, and screening cultures were obtained from 371, of whom 110 (30%) were positive for *S. aureus* and 28 (8%) for MRSA; no VRSA was found. Use of the polymerase chain reaction (PCR) on the VRSA isolate revealed the presence of the *vanA* gene, and sequencing of this showed it to be identical to the *vanA* sequence from the patient's *E. faecalis* isolate. Pulsed-field gel electrophoresis (PFGE) of *Sma*I macrorestriction fragments showed that the initial VRSA isolate was indistinguishable from the vancomycin-sensitive MRSA grown from the patient's nose.

INTERPRETATION. This is the first report of a clinical isolate of *S. aureus* with high-level resistance to vancomycin mediated by the *vanA* gene from enterococci. The isolate remained susceptible to a number of other agents and was successfully treated with debridement and trimethoprim–sulphamethoxazole. Extensive screening of contacts did not reveal any evidence of spread of VRSA.

Comment

This report is important as it provides the first comprehensive evidence of the emergence of high-level vancomycin resistance in *S. aureus*. The *vanA* gene, which causes vancomycin resistance in VRE, is present in the VRSA and also in a vancomycin-resistant *E. faecalis* isolated from the patient. The implication is that the *vanA* gene has transferred from the VRE to MRSA *in vivo* to give rise to VRSA. It is encouraging that no spread of VRSA to contacts was demonstrated.

Genetic analysis of a high-level vancomycin-resistant isolate of *Staphylococcus aureus*

Weigel LM, Clewell DB, Gill SR, *et al. Science* 2003; **302**: 1569–71

BACKGROUND. A clinical isolate of *S. aureus* with high-level resistance to vancomycin (MIC 1024 mg/l) was isolated in June 2002 in Michigan, USA. The plasmid content of the VRSA, a vancomycin-sensitive MRSA and a vancomycin-resistant *E. faecalis* was analysed. The VRSA had single plasmid of 57.9 kb, the VS-MRSA had a single plasmid of ~47 kb, and the VRE had two plasmids (45 kb, 95 kb). Southern hybridization showed *vanA* on the VRE and VRSA plasmids but not on that of VS-MRSA. Filter-mating studies identified the VRSA plasmid as conjugative, and vancomycin resistance was transferred *in vitro* from the VRSA to the *S. aureus* COL strain. The prototype *vanA*-encoding element in enterococci, a 10.8-kb transposon, Tn1546, was localized to the VRSA plasmid and sequencing showed it to be complete without insertions or deletions, with 100% nucleotide identity with the prototype Tn1546. Additional elements on the VRSA plasmid encoded resistance to trimethoprim (*dfrA*), β-lactams (*blaZ*), aminoglycosides (*aacA-aphD*) and disinfectants (*qacC*). Genetic analyses suggest that the long-anticipated transfer of vancomycin resistance to a MRSA occurred *in vivo* by interspecies transfer of Tn1546 from a co-isolate of *E. faecalis*.

INTERPRETATION. The first clinical isolate of VRSA has the *vanA* gene on transposon Tn1546 localized to a 57.9 kb conjugative plasmid that also contains genes conferring resistance to multiple antimicrobial classes. The transposon appears to have transferred *in vivo* from a VRE that was also isolated from the patient. Filter-mating studies showed that the VRSA plasmid could transfer to another *S. aureus* strain and express vancomycin resistance.

Comment

The transfer of vancomycin resistance from enterococci to *S. aureus in vivo* has long been awaited and this study suggests that it has now occurred. In fact the authors attempted to reproduce the supposed transfer *in vitro* of resistance from the patient's VRE to the patient's own MRSA isolate but were unsuccessful. They suggest that the frequency of transfer may be low because the MRSA does not maintain the entero-coccal plasmid so that the establishment of resistance would require both the con-jugative transfer of the enterococcal plasmid and the excision and integration of the transposon into the resistance plasmid of the VS-MRSA. Alternatively, the trans-poson could be transferred by transduction. It is reassuring that the transfer of resist-ance from enterococci to *S. aureus* is difficult and this may explain why such an event has not been identified before now. However, the fact that the transposon integrated into a conjugative plasmid conferring multiple antimicrobial resistances and could transfer to an unrelated *S. aureus* strain gives us warning that such resistance is likely to spread.

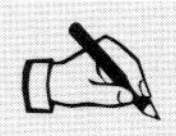

Vancomycin-resistant *Staphylococcus aureus* isolate from a patient in Pennsylvania

Tenover FC, Weigel LM, Appelbaum PC, *et al. Antimicrob Agents Chemother* 2004: **48**: 275–80

BACKGROUND. A VRSA was obtained from a patient in Pennsylvania, USA, in September 2002. Species identification was confirmed by standard biochemical tests and analysis of 16S ribosomal DNA, *gyrA* and *gyrB* sequences; all results were consistent with the *S. aureus* identification. The MICs of a variety of antimicrobial agents were determined by broth microdilution and macrodilution methods following NCCLS guidelines. The isolate was resistant to vancomycin (MIC 32 mg/l), aminoglycosides, β-lactams, fluoroquinolones, macrolides and tetracycline, but it was susceptible to linezolid, minocycline, quinupristin–dalfopristin, rifampicin, teicoplanin, and trimethoprim–sulphamethoxazole. The isolate, which was originally detected by using disc diffusion and a vancomycin agar screen plate, was vancomycin-susceptible by automated susceptibility testing methods. PFGE of *Sma*I-digested genomic DNA indicated that the isolate belonged to the USA100 lineage (also known as the New York/Japan clone), the most common staphylococcal PFGE type found in hospitals in the US. The VRSA isolate contained two plasmids of 120 and 4 kb and was positive for *mecA* and *vanA* by PCR amplification. The *vanA* sequence was identical to the *vanA* sequence present in Tn1546. A DNA probe for *vanA* hybridized to the 120 kb plasmid.

INTERPRETATION. The second VRSA isolate was obtained from a patient in Pennsylvania in 2002. The isolate contained the *vanA* gene on a 120 kb plasmid. The *vanA* sequence was identical to that in the transposon Tn1546. The isolate was resistant to vancomycin by broth microdilution (MIC 32 mg/l) but tested as sensitive by automated sensitivity testing methods. PFGE indicated that the VRSA belonged to the New York/Japan clone of MRSA, which is the commonest type found in US hospitals.

Comment

This paper reports the second isolate of VRSA mediated by transfer of the *vanA* gene from enterococci. The isolate in this case has a relatively modest MIC of 32 mg/l, which, the authors suggest, may be due to the level of expression of the *vanA* gene. PCR analysis suggests that sequences corresponding to the *vanR*, *vanS*, *vanX*, *vanY* and *vanH* elements of the *vanA* gene cassette on the transposon Tn1546 are present on a 120 kb plasmid. However, the 5′ end of the transposon may be truncated and there is additional DNA in two regions which may effect expression of the genes.

This paper also highlights potential difficulties in the laboratory identification of strains with this level of vancomycin resistance. Disk testing with a 30 μg vancomycin disc gave a small a small area of clearing within a zone of reduced growth that suggested resistance. However, automated sensitivity testing methods, such as the Microscan, Vitek, and Vitek2 systems, failed to identify resistance, as shown in

Table 7.2. Thus, it is recommended that if such methods are used an additional method should be employed to identify strains resistant to vancomycin.

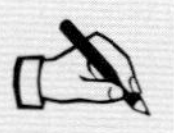

Vancomycin-resistant *Staphylococcus aureus* in the absence of vancomycin exposure

Whitener CJ, Park SY, Browne FA, *et al*. *Clin Infect Dis* 2004; **38**: 1049–55

BACKGROUND. This is a report of the world's second isolate of VRSA. A 70-year-old male with morbid obesity presented with an infected chronic heel ulcer and osteomyelitis. In the 3 years prior to hospital admission he had 63 courses of oral antimicrobials but, notably, no vancomycin since 1996. Numerous previous ulcer specimens had grown vancomycin-sensitive MRSA and VRE. Blood cultures from admission grew group B β-haemolytic streptococcus. Ulcer specimens grew a mixture of group B β-haemolytic streptococcus, *Pseudomonas aeruginosa*, *Stenotrophomonas maltophilia* and VRSA (vancomycin MIC 32 mg/l). The patient was treated with linezolid and piperacillin–tazobactam, plus trimethoprim–sulphamethoxazole. To assess VRSA transmission, a carriage study of 283 contacts and the patient's home environment was performed. Of the 262 contacts screened, 74 (28%) were positive for *S. aureus* and 21 (8%) for MRSA. No VRSA was isolated from contacts or from home environmental sampling.

INTERPRETATION. This second case of VRSA infection occurred in a patient who had received multiple courses of antimicrobials but notably no vancomycin in the previous 6 years. Screening of contacts and the home environment did not reveal any VRSA.

Comment

This paper gives further clinical information about the Pennsylvania VRSA. It is notable that the patient in this case had not been exposed to vancomycin for many years prior to isolation of VRSA. However, he had been documented to be positive for both MRSA and VRE in the previous year and had been exposed to multiple other antimicrobials. The *vanA* gene was localized on a 120 kb plasmid (see Tenover *et al.* above) which presumably carried resistance determinants for other antimicrobial

Table 7.2 Results of susceptibility testing of Pennsylvania VRSA isolate

S. aureus strain		MIC (mg/l) by method				
		Broth microdilution	E-test	Microscan	Vitek	Vitek2
VRSA	Uninduced	16–64	64	≤2–4	1–4	2
	Induced*	ND	ND	≤2–4	1–16	8

* Organisms were grown overnight on brain–heart infusion agar containing 6 mg/l vancomycin prior to testing. Uninduced strains were grown on sheep blood agar overnight. ND, not determined.
Source: adapted from Tenover *et al.* (2004).

classes, so that the use of non-glycopeptides may have selected for vancomycin resistance. The lack of transmission seen with the Michigan VRSA is mirrored in this case and might suggest that the expression of vancomycin resistance is associated with a loss of fitness compared with vancomycin-susceptible MRSA.

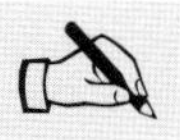

Vancomycin-resistant *Staphylococcus aureus*— New York, 2004

Centers for Disease Control and Prevention (CDC). *MMWR* 2004; **53**: 322–3

BACKGROUND. In March 2004 the third isolate of VRSA was isolated in New York from a urine sample from a resident of a long-term care facility. Initial susceptibility testing by Microscan gave a vancomycin MIC of 4 mg/l but an E-test gave an MIC of >256 mg/l. The reference broth microdilution using National Committee for Clinical Laboratory Standards (NCCLS) methods gave a vancomycin MIC of 64 mg/l. PCR analysis revealed the presence of the *vanA* gene. The isolate was susceptible to chloramphenicol, linezolid, minocycline, quinupristin–dalfopristin, rifampin and trimethoprim–sulphamethoxazole. The automated sensitivity testing methods Microscan and Vitek did not detect vancomycin resistance in this isolate.

INTERPRETATION. A third isolate of S. *aureus* with resistance to vancomycin mediated by the *vanA* gene has been isolated in New York. Although the isolate had an MIC of 64 mg/l when tested by a reference method, the automated susceptibility methods did not detect resistance.

Comment

This is only a preliminary report of the third VRSA isolate but highlights the difficulty of detecting resistance if automated susceptibility methods are used. It is suggested that a commercial screening plate with brain–heart infusion agar containing 6 mg/l vancomycin should be used in addition if automated susceptibility testing methods are routinely used.

Mechanism of resistance and epidemiology of VISA/hVISA

As noted above, vancomycin resistance in VISA/hVISA is not due to the same mechanism seen in enterococci. There are a number of characteristics that have been described in these strains, such as a thickened cell wall, reduced cross-linking of the peptidoglycan, increased glutamine-non-amidated muropeptides in the cell wall, increased production of some penicillin-binding proteins (PBPs), and decreased expression of PBP4. It has been suggested that the reduced cross-linking within a thickened cell wall results in increased free terminal D-ala-D-ala moieties in the outer layers of the cell wall. These can bind vancomycin and by stearic hindrance prevent penetration of vancomycin through the cell wall to potential binding sites at the cytoplasmic membrane, where vancomycin could exert its inhibitory effect. However, one of the problems in this area is that only a limited number of strains have been studied, and as more strains are investigated differences are being described. For example, strains have now been reported in which increased resistance to vancomycin is associated with increased rather than decreased cross-linking of peptidoglycan |5,6|.

One group in the US has suggested an association between *agr* type and vancomycin resistance. The accessory gene regulator (*agr*) locus in *S. aureus* is a quorum-sensing gene cluster that controls expression of a number of virulence factors. Polymorphisms within the *agr* locus define four types and a study of VISA from the US and Japan showed that all had the type II *agr* polymorphism |7|.

Over the last year, the mechanism of resistance has been studied in more strains from around the world and it has become clear that some of the characteristics of VISA/hVISA noted initially (such as *agr* type) may not be directly associated with vancomycin resistance but may rather reflect the strains in which resistance has emerged.

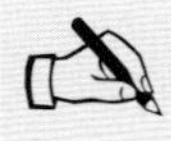

Cell wall thickening is a common feature of vancomycin resistance in *Staphylococcus aureus*

Cui L, Ma X, Sato K, *et al. J Clin Micro* 2003; **41**: 5–14

BACKGROUND. The authors have previously shown that a thickened cell wall is responsible for the vancomycin resistance of VISA strain Mu50. However, the mechanism of vancomycin resistance in other VISA strains has remained unclear. In this study, 16 clinical VISA strains from seven countries were subjected to serial daily passage in drug-free medium. After 10–84 days of passage in the non-selective medium, passage-derived strains with decreased MICs of vancomycin (MIC <4 mg/l) were obtained. However, all of the passage-derived strains except one (15 of 16) still possessed subpopulations that were resistant to vancomycin, as judged by population analysis, and vancomycin-resistant mutant strains were selected from the passage-derived strains by one-step vancomycin selection with a frequency of 4.25 × 10⁻⁶ to 1.64 × 10⁻³. The data indicate that vancomycin-resistant cells are frequently generated from the passage-derived strains even after vancomycin selective pressure is lifted. Cell wall thicknesses and MICs of glycopeptides (vancomycin and teicoplanin) and β-lactams (imipenem and oxacillin) were determined for a total of 48 strains, including 15 sets of three strains: the clinical VISA strain, the passage-derived strain, and the vancomycin-resistant mutant strain obtained from the passage-derived strain. No simple correlation between glycopeptide and β-lactam MICs was seen, while significant correlations between MICs of vancomycin and teicoplanin ($r = 0.679$; $P < 0.001$) and between MICs of imipenem and oxacillin ($r = 0.787$; $P < 0.001$) were recognized. Moreover, all of the VISA strains had significantly thickened cell walls, which became thinner with the loss of vancomycin resistance during drug-free passages and again became thick in the resistant mutant strains. The data show that cell wall thickness had a high correlation with the MICs of the two glycopeptides (correlation coefficients, 0.908 for vancomycin and 0.655 for teicoplanin) but not with those of the β-lactam antibiotics tested. These results, together with coupled changes in cell wall thickness and vancomycin MICs in 16 isogenic sets of strains, indicate that thickening of the cell wall is a common phenotype of clinical VISA strains and may be a phenotypic determinant for vancomycin resistance in S. *aureus*.

INTERPRETATION. Thickening of the bacterial cell wall is a common feature of VISA strains and the degree of thickening appears to correlate with the degree of resistance to vancomycin.

Comment

Initial reports of VISA strains described a thickened cell wall in the archetypal strain Mu50 |8|. The present study has investigated epidemiologically unrelated strains from Japan, USA, France, the UK, South Africa and Brazil and found that all VISAs had thickening of the cell wall. Passage in drug-free medium led to a decrease in vancomycin MIC and an associated decrease in cell wall thickness. Thus, this report confirms the suggestion that vancomycin resistance is associated with a thickened cell wall in VISA from geographically dispersed and epidemiologically unrelated strains.

Alterations of cell wall structure and metabolism accompany reduced susceptibility to vancomycin in an isogenic series of clinical isolates of *Staphylococcus aureus*

Sieradzki K, Tomasz A. *J Bacteriol* 2003; **185**: 7103–10

BACKGROUND. A series of isogenic MRSA isolates recovered from a bacteraemic patient were shown to acquire gradually increasing levels of resistance to vancomycin during chemotherapy with the drug. Sieradski and Tomasz compared properties of the earliest (parental) vancomycin-susceptible isolate, JH1 (MIC 1 μg/ml), to two late (progeny) isolates, JH9 and JH14 (vancomycin MIC 8 μg/ml). The resistant isolates produced abnormally thick cell walls and poorly separated cells when grown in antibiotic-free medium. Chemical analysis of the resistant isolates showed decreased cross-linkage of the peptidoglycan and drastically reduced levels of PBP4 as determined by the fluorographic assay. Resistant isolates showed reduced rates of cell wall turnover and autolysis. *In vitro* hydrolysis of resistant cell walls by autolytic extracts prepared from either susceptible or resistant strains was also slow, and this abnormality could be traced to a quantitative (or qualitative) change in the wall teichoic acid component of resistant isolates.

INTERPRETATION. Some change in the structure and/or metabolism of teichoic acids appears to be an important component of the mechanism of decreased susceptibility to vancomycin in S. *aureus*.

Comment

This study only examines a single isogenic set of strains and therefore the results may not be generalizable to all VISAs. Other workers have reported downregulation of PBP4 |9| and alterations in cell wall teichoic acid in VISA strains |10|. Since the PBP4 enzyme catalyses the cross-linking of peptidoglycan, downregulation could lead to the reduced cross-linking seen in most VISA/hVISA strains.

Accessory gene regulator group II polymorphism in methicillin-resistant *Staphylococcus aureus* is predictive of failure of vancomycin therapy

Moise-Broder PA, Sakoulas G, Eliopoulos GM, Schentag JJ, Forrest A, Moellering RC Jr. *Clin Infect Dis* 2004; **38**: 1700–5

BACKGROUND. The authors studied MRSA isolates to determine if the group II polymorphism at the accessory gene regulator (*agr*) locus demonstrated any relationship with the clinical efficacy of vancomycin. One hundred and twenty-two MRSA isolates from 87 patients treated with vancomycin were evaluated. Forty-five of 87 patients had no clinical or bacteriological response to vancomycin. Among the 36 clinically evaluable patients with the *agr* group II polymorphism, 31 had an infection that failed to respond to vancomycin, whereas only five had an infection that responded successfully to vancomycin. This finding is of interest in the light of our previous findings that glycopeptide-intermediately resistant *S. aureus* (VISA) and hVISA clinical isolates in the US and Japan are enriched for the *agr* group II polymorphism, and it suggests a possible intrinsic survival advantage of some *S. aureus* clones with this genetic marker under vancomycin selective pressure.

INTERPRETATION. MRSA with the accessory gene regulator group II polymorphism may possess a survival advantage under vancomycin selective pressure.

Comment

This group has previously studied a small collection of VISA from the US and Japan and found that all strains belonged to *agr* group II |7|. They have also suggested that *agr* group II strains may have an intrinsic advantage under vancomycin selective pressure |11|. In the present study they have found that patients infected with *agr* group II strains have a poor outcome when treated with vancomycin. The implication is that *agr* group II strains are in some way clinically resistant to vancomycin. The problem with this study is that it does not present any data regarding outcomes of therapy with other classes of antimicrobials. The poor outcome of *agr* group II strains may be due to the type of infection caused by these strains or increased virulence rather than resistance to vancomycin. It is already known that different *agr* groups are associated with different clinical scenarios: community MRSA usually belong to group III, exfoliatin-producing strains to group IV |12|, and most clinical isolates to group I |13|.

Staphylococcus aureus isolates with reduced susceptibility to glycopeptides belong to accessory gene regulator group I or II

Verdier I, Reverdy ME, Etienne J, Lina G, Bes M, Vandenesch F. *Antimicrob Agents Chemother* 2004; **48**: 1024–7

BACKGROUND. The authors used multiplex PCR to determine the *agr* group membership of 18 European glycopeptide heterointermediate and intermediate-resistant *Staphylococcus aureus* strains. Of the 15 *agr* group I strains, 13 were resistant and two were susceptible to methicillin. The remaining three strains, like the US and Japanese control strains, belonged to *agr* group II.

INTERPRETATION. VISA and hVISA can have either the group I or group II polymorphism at the accessory gene regulator locus.

Comment

This study looked at six VISAs from France, Belgium, Japan and the US and 16 hVISAs from France and Japan. In keeping with previous studies, hVISA/VISA isolated in the US or Japan had the group II *agr* polymorphism |7|. However, 15 out of 18 strains isolated in Europe had *agr* group I. This suggests that the development of reduced susceptibility to vancomycin is unrelated to *agr* group.

Vancomycin susceptibility within methicillin-resistant *Staphylococcus aureus* lineages

Howe RA, Monk A, Wootton M, Walsh TR, Enright MC. *Emerg Infect Dis* 2004; **10**: 855–7

BACKGROUND. MRSA with reduced vancomycin susceptibility VISA has been reported from many countries. Whether resistance is evolving regularly in different genetic backgrounds or in a single clone with a genetic predisposition, as early results suggest, is unclear. The researchers studied 101 MRSA with reduced vancomycin susceptibility from nine countries by multilocus sequence typing (MLST), characterization of SCCmec (staphylococcal chromosomal cassette mec) and *agr*. They found nine genotypes by MLST, with isolates within all five major hospital MRSA lineages. Most isolates (88/101) belonged to two of the earliest MRSA clones that have global prevalence. The results show that reduced susceptibility to vancomycin has emerged in many successful epidemic lineages with no clear clonal disposition. Increasing antimicrobial resistance in genetically distinct pandemic clones may lead to MRSA infections that will become increasingly difficult to treat.

INTERPRETATION. Reduced susceptibility to vancomycin has emerged in all five pandemic MRSA lineages.

Comment

The strains tested in this study were from the US, Japan, Europe and China. The results suggest that the development of the low-level resistance seen in VISA/hVISA can emerge in diverse strains of *S. aureus*. The representation of such characteristics as *agr* group presumably depends on the *agr* group of the MRSA strains circulating locally.

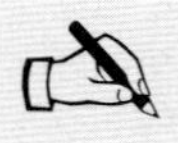

Nucleotide substitutions in *Staphylococcus aureus* strains, Mu50, Mu3, and N315

Ohta T, Hirakawa H, Morikawa K, *et al. DNA Res* 2004; **11**: 51–6

BACKGROUND. A specific phenotype of *Staphylococcus aureus* strains Mu50 and Mu3 is characterized by a thickened cell wall and moderate resistance to vancomycin. The N315 strain is a prototype of MRSA, but it is methicillin-susceptible despite carrying the *mecA* resistance gene. Here, the researchers revised differences in the sequences of Mu50 and N315, referencing that of Mu3, which were assumed to be of one lineage. The 362 open reading frames (ORFs) diverse between Mu50 and N315 were picked up, and the corresponding ones in three strains were resequenced. This defined 213 ORFs diverse between Mu50 and N315 and nine between Mu50 and Mu3. The fixed diversities of 174 ORFs (except for 39 silent ORFs from 213), including nucleotide substitution, frame shift and truncation, were grouped into three major functional categories, which were transport (14.9% in the 174 diverse ORFs), metabolism of carbohydrates (5.7%) and RNA synthesis (9.6%). The other gene categories had small diversities. These gene categories seemed to be functionally decisive for the Mu50-specific characters, the thickened cell wall and moderate vancomycin resistance. All of the diverse genes and the high-quality sequence of Mu50 can be viewed at the website http://133.5.48.239/VRSA/.

INTERPRETATION. There are many genetic differences seen between the whole-genome sequences of strain N315 (a fully vancomycin-susceptible MRSA) compared with Mu50 (the archetypal VISA). These are predominantly in genes encoding products involved in transport, carbohydrate metabolism or RNA synthesis.

Comment

This study is an attempt to compare the whole genome of a fully vancomycin-sensitive *S. aureus*, an hVISA and a VISA with the implication that genomic differences may be related to the mechanism of vancomycin resistance. A potential problem, however, is that the strains that are compared are not particularly related: N315 was isolated in 1982, Mu50 in 1997 and Mu3 in 1996. Thus, the genomic difference found may be unrelated to vancomycin resistance. Also, this type of genetic comparison does not give any information about the levels of expression of different genes. It is possible that the VISA/hVISA phenotype is the result of altered expression of genes under regulatory control rather than mutations.

Microarray transcription analysis of clinical *Staphylococcus aureus* isolates resistant to vancomycin

Mongodin E, Finan J, Climo MW, Rosato A, Gill S, Archer GL. *J Bacteriol* 2003; **185**: 4638–43

BACKGROUND. The transcriptomes of VISA clinical isolates HIP5827 and Mu50 (MIC 8 µg/ml) were compared with those of highly vancomycin-resistant *S. aureus* (VRSA; MIC 32 µg/ml) passage derivatives by microarray. There were 35 genes with increased transcription and 16 genes with decreased transcription in common between the two VRSA compared with those of their VISA parents. Of the 35 genes with increased transcription, 15 involved purine biosynthesis or transport, and the regulator (purR) of the major purine biosynthetic operon (purE-purD) was mutant. The authors hypothesize that increased energy (adenosine triphosphate [ATP]) is required to generate the thicker cell walls that characterize resistant mutants.

INTERPRETATION. Progressive increases in resistance to vancomycin that occur by mutation and selection are accompanied by increases in cell wall thickness and in the transcription of genes involved in purine biosynthesis and cell wall autolysis to meet the energetic and constructive demands of new cell wall biosynthesis.

Comment

This study investigated changes in gene expression associated with increased resistance to vancomycin. Only one isogenic set of strains was investigated and therefore it is unclear whether the results can be extrapolated to other VISAs. An increase in the transcription of genes involved in cell wall hydrolysis is described, although autolysis has been reported to be decreased in most VISA strains studied |6,11,14|. Thus, the isolates examined may not be representative of all VISAs. The fact that an increase in transcription of genes involved in purine synthesis was seen does not necessarily imply that this is involved in the primary mechanism of vancomycin resistance. It may be that this is merely a result of the underlying mechanism that is generating a thickened cell wall.

The clinical importance of hVISA

The three strains of VRSA reported were all associated with a poor response to vancomycin, as would be expected given their level of resistance. More than 20 VISAs have now been reported from around the world, and although there has not been a controlled study they also appear to be less responsive to vancomycin therapy. However, there has been considerable controversy as to whether hVISA is clinically relevant and therefore whether it should be sought by diagnostic laboratories. There have been many case reports of hVISA infections which have not responded to vancomycin therapy |3|, but there seems to be a significant publication bias, as in

most cases strains are discovered to be hVISA only after patients have failed vancomycin therapy. The lack of standardized methods for screening and confirmation of
hVISA in the laboratory has made performance of a controlled study of outcomes
difficult. A study by the Centers for Disease Control and Prevention in the US compared outcomes of 15 patients with infections caused by MRSA with vancomycin
MICs of 4 mg/l (SA-RVS [*S. aureus*-Reduced Susceptibility to Vancomycin]) with
those of patients with fully vancomycin-susceptible MRSA |15|. Patients with
SA-RVS were less likely to respond to vancomycin and had similar clinical presentations to patients with VISA. Although the SA-RVS strains were on the borderline of
susceptibility to vancomycin it was not reported whether they were hVISA.

During the last year, further reports have sought to define the clinical importance
of hVISA but seem to give conflicting evidence.

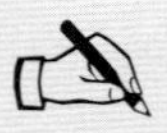

Clinical features associated with bacteremia due to heterogeneous vancomycin-intermediate *Staphylococcus aureus*

Charles PG, Ward PB, Johnson PD, Howden BP, Grayson ML. *Clin Infect Dis*
2004; **38**: 448–51

BACKGROUND. The authors assessed all episodes of MRSA bacteraemia at their
hospital during a 12-month period (*n* = 53) and compared those due to hVISA (*n* = 5,
9.4%) with those due to VS-MRSA (*n* = 48). Patients with hVISA bacteraemia were
more likely to have infections with a high bacterial load (*P* = 0.001), failure of
vancomycin treatment (persistent fever and bacteraemia for >7 days after the start
of therapy; *P* <0.001), and initially low serum vancomycin levels (*P* = 0.006). These
clinical markers of hVISA bacteraemia may help focus diagnostic efforts and
treatment.

INTERPRETATION. Bacteraemic infection with hVISA is associated with vancomycin
treatment failure.

Comment

This is one of the few reports to study systematically the clinical relevance of hetero-
resistance to vancomycin in *S. aureus*. The implication from the data summarized in
Table 7.3 is that there is a clear association between hVISA and the failure of vancomycin therapy. The authors report that hVISA is associated with high bacterial load
infections, which they define as the presence of prosthetic device infection, an
undrained abscess due to MRSA, or endocarditis confirmed by echocardiogram. It is
also noted that the patients with hVISA had initially subtherapeutic vancomycin
serum concentrations, although these were subsequently corrected. The main criticism of this study is that only the last isolate from each patient was investigated. Thus,
while the implication is that hVISA leads to the failure of vancomycin therapy, it
may be that the hVISA phenotype develops as a result of a persistent infection and is

possibly favoured by the presence of a high bacterial load infection or exposure to subtherapeutic concentrations of vancomycin. Vaudaux *et al.* used a tissue cage rat model of chronic MRSA infection and found that, after 3 weeks of infection and in the absence of antimicrobial exposure, fully vancomycin-susceptible MRSA developed into hVISA |**16**|. This suggests that the expression of a phenotype linked with persistent infection is associated with the hVISA phenotype. A study investigating clinical outcomes in patients with hVISA from initial blood culture isolates is needed to establish whether there is a causal relationship between the hVISA phenotype and clinical failure of vancomycin.

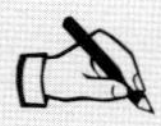

Vancomycin treatment failure associated with heterogeneous vancomycin-intermediate *Staphylococcus aureus* in a patient with endocarditis and in the rabbit model of endocarditis

Moore MR, Perdreau-Remington F, Chambers HF. *Antimicrob Agents Chemother* 2003; **47**: 1262–6

BACKGROUND. Heterogeneous resistance to vancomycin is thought to precede the emergence of intermediate susceptibility to vancomycin in *S. aureus*, but the clinical significance of heterogeneous resistance is unknown. Paired *S. aureus* isolates from a patient with endocarditis who relapsed after vancomycin treatment were tested for heterogeneous resistance to vancomycin. The pretreatment and the relapse clinical isolates (strains SF1 and SF2 respectively) were genotyped by PFGE. Susceptibility to vancomycin was assessed by the broth dilution method, population analysis and time-kill studies, and in the rabbit model of endocarditis. Strains SF1 and SF2 had similar genotypes, and the vancomycin MICs for the strains were ≤2 mg/l. SF2

Table 7.3 Clinical features of 53 cases of bacteraemia due to hVISA and VS-MRSA

		hVISA infection	VS-MRSA infection	*P*
Clinical vancomycin treatment failure	Proportion (%) of episodes	5/5 (100)	1/48 (2.1)	<0.001
Time until afebrile	Median days (range)	24 (13–77)	2 (0–19)	<0.001
Duration of bacteraemia	Median days (range)	26 (9–87)	3.5 (1–7)	0.002
Duration of inpatient stay	Median days (range)	83 (34–187)	20 (1–284)	0.006
High bacterial load infection	Proportion (%) of episodes	5/5 (100)	10/48 (21)	0.001
Low serum trough vancomycin concentration during first week	Proportion (%) of episodes	5/5 (100)	11/36 (31)	0.006
Survival at 1 month	Proportion (%) of episodes	4/5 (80)	31/48 (65)	0.7

Source: adapted from Charles *et al.* (2004).

exhibited heterogeneous resistance to vancomycin. Vancomycin eradicated SF1 in the rabbit model of endocarditis, whereas SF2 persisted at pretreatment levels.

INTERPRETATION. Vancomycin treatment failure in this patient with endocarditis was attributable to the emergence of heterogeneous resistance to vancomycin.

Comment

The clinical case in this report was of a 47-year-old male injection drug user who had positive blood cultures with MRSA (strain SF1) and a vegetation on the tricuspid valve. His course was complicated by septic pulmonary emboli and vertebral osteomyelitis and he was treated with vancomycin at therapeutic levels. Soon after completing a 6-week course of vancomycin, he re-presented with septic arthritis of the elbow, from which MRSA (strain SF2) was cultured. A further 6-week course of vancomycin with the addition of rifampicin led to clinical and microbiological cure. There have been many case reports that have correlated hVISA with a poor outcome |4,17–21|. However, this is the first report to test the isolates in an animal model. As can be seen from Table 7.4, vancomycin was effective in reducing vegetation titres for the original isolate (SF1) but had no effect on vegetation titres for the strain (SF2) obtained when the patient relapsed. The authors speculate about why SF1 was so readily eradicated from the rabbit vegetation but must have persisted in the patient in order for selection to occur. It is presumed that this was due to the higher organism load in the patient, which gives a greater chance that a heterogeneous subpopulation will survive.

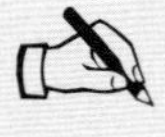

Prevalence, molecular epidemiology, and clinical significance of heterogeneous glycopeptide-intermediate *Staphylococcus aureus* in liver transplant recipients

Bert F, Clarissou J, Durand F, *et al. J Clin Microbiol* 2003; **41**: 5147–52

Table 7.4 Vegetation titres before treatment and after 4 days of vancomycin therapy in aortic valves of rabbits infected with SF1 or SF2

Strain	Titre ($\log_{10}$ cfu/g)	
	Before treatment	**Vancomycin**
SF1	7.35 ± 1.15 (3)	0.21 ± 0.43 (7)
SF2	7.01 ± 1.2 (3)	6.9 ± 0.9 (5)

The values are mean ± standard deviation, with the number of rabbits tested given in parentheses.
cfu, colony-forming units.
Source: adapted from Moore *et al.* (2003).

BACKGROUND. The authors investigated the prevalence, molecular epidemiology and clinical significance of heterogeneous glycopeptide-intermediate *Staphylococcus aureus* (hGISA) isolates in 48 liver transplant recipients infected or colonized with MRSA over a 5-year period. Strains were screened for hGISA on Müller–Hinton agar containing 5 mg/l of teicoplanin. Heterogeneous glycopeptide resistance was confirmed by the E-test method with a dense inoculum and a simplified method of population analysis. hGISA strains were found in 13 (27%) of the 48 patients studied. Eleven of the 13 strains shared a common multiresistant phenotype with homogeneous methicillin resistance and gentamicin resistance, and they were closely related according to the results of PFGE. Only two of the 13 patients infected or colonized with hGISA strains had previously received glycopeptide therapy. Most patients were successfully treated with vancomycin, but one patient who failed to respond to vancomycin subsequently died. These results suggest that the high prevalence of hGISA among our patients was due to the clonal spread of a multiresistant strain.

INTERPRETATION. This study reports a high prevalence of hGISA in liver transplant patients, related to the dissemination of a multi-drug-resistant strain. Although glycopeptide resistance was potentially involved in the death of one patient who failed to respond to vancomycin, most patients infected or colonized with hGISA were successfully treated with vancomycin.

Comment

This study suggests that heterogeneous resistance to glycopeptides does not affect the outcome of glycopeptide therapy. The patients are all immunocompromised following liver transplant and the infections in patients with hVISA are comparable with those in patients with fully susceptible MRSA. Although the methods of detection and confirmation of hVISA seem robust, the rate of hVISA is relatively high in this study at 27% of MRSA and PFGE typing suggests a clonal outbreak. Thus it is possible that the findings in respect of the outcome of vancomycin therapy may be a characteristic of the outbreak strain and may not be generalizable.

Conclusion

Undoubtedly, the most important recent development in this area has been the emergence in S. *aureus* of high-level vancomycin resistance conferred by transfer of the *vanA* gene from VRE. The level of resistance in the three strains so far described is variable and it is particularly concerning that standard susceptibility test methods have not always been able to identify resistance. Clearly, this raises the possibility that resistant strains have emerged elsewhere but, as yet, remain unidentified. Epidemiological studies of the first two cases found no evidence of spread either to contacts or the environment; this is perhaps due to loss of fitness associated with the development of resistance. However, the emergence of further resistant strains is inevitable and now is the time to re-enforce controls on the use of vancomycin and teicoplanin and to develop robust screening strategies in diagnostic laboratories to ensure early identification of resistance.

As regards VISA/hVISA, epidemiological studies suggest that this low-level resistance has developed in many different strains from around the world. The mechanism of resistance was initially studied in a relatively limited number of strains, but as more strains are investigated conflicting results are emerging. It appears clear that vancomycin resistance in VISA/hVISA is associated with a thickened cell wall, but the underlying mechanism remains unclear and may be different in different strains.

Although the last year has seen the first systematic studies using rigorous methods to confirm the hVISA phenotype, results have been conflicting. It remains to be proved that testing of initial clinical isolates for the hVISA phenotype would have any predictive value in terms of the outcome of vancomycin therapy. As ever, further studies are required.

References

1. Uttley AHC, Collins CH, Naidoo J, George RC. Vancomycin-resistant enterococci. *Lancet* 1988; i: 57–8.

2. Hiramatsu K. The emergence of *Staphylococcus aureus* with reduced susceptibility to vancomycin in Japan. *Am J Med* 1998; **104**: 7S–10S.

3. Walsh TR, Howe RA. The prevalence and mechanisms of vancomycin resistance in Staphylococcus aureus. *Annu Rev Microbiol* 2002; **56**: 657–75.

4. Hiramatsu K, Aritaka N, Hanaki H, Kawasaki S, Hosoda Y, Hori S, Fukuchi Y, Kobayashi I. Dissemination in Japanese hospitals of strains of *Staphylococcus aureus* heterogeneously resistant to vancomycin. *Lancet* 1997; **350**: 1670–3.

5. Reipert A, Ehlert K, Kast T, Bierbaum G. Morphological and genetic differences in two isogenic *Staphylococcus aureus* strains with decreased susceptibilities to vancomycin. *Antimicrob Agents Chemother* 2003; **47**: 568–76.

6. Boyle-Vavra S, Carey RB, Daum RS. Development of vancomycin and lysostaphin resistance in a methicillin-resistant *Staphylococcus aureus* isolate. *J Antimicrob Chemother* 2001; **48**: 617–25.

7. Sakoulas G, Eliopoulos GM, Moellering RC Jr, Wennersten C, Venkataraman L, Novick RP, Gold HS. Accessory gene regulator (agr) locus in geographically diverse *Staphylococcus aureus* isolates with reduced susceptibility to vancomycin. *Antimicrob Agents Chemother* 2002; **46**: 1492–502.

8. Hiramatsu K, Hanaki H, Ino T, Yabuta K, Oguri T, Tenover FC. Methicillin-resistant *Staphylococcus aureus* clinical strain with reduced vancomycin susceptibility. *J Antimicrob Chemother* 1997; **40**: 135–6.

9. Finan JE, Archer GL, Pucci MJ, Climo MW. Role of penicillin-binding protein 4 in expression of vancomycin resistance among clinical isolates of oxacillin-resistant *Staphylococcus aureus*. *Antimicrob Agents Chemother* 2001; **45**: 3070–5.

10. Peschel A, Vuong C, Otto M, Gotz F. The D-alanine residues of *Staphylococcus aureus* teichoic acids alter the susceptibility to vancomycin and the activity of autolytic enzymes. *Antimicrob Agents Chemother* 2000; **44**: 2845–7.

11. Sakoulas G, Eliopoulos GM, Moellering RC Jr, Novick RP, Venkataraman L, Wennersten C, DeGirolami PC, Schwaber MJ, Gold HS. *Staphylococcus aureus* accessory gene regulator (agr) group II: is there a relationship to the development of intermediate-level glycopeptide resistance? *J Infect Dis* 2003; **187**: 929–38.

12. Jarraud S, Lyon GJ, Figueiredo AM, Gerard L, Vandenesch F, Etienne J, Muir TW, Novick RP. Exfoliatin-producing strains define a fourth agr specificity group in *Staphylococcus aureus*. *J Bacteriol* 2000; **182**: 6517–22.

13. Moore PC, Lindsay JA. Genetic variation among hospital isolates of methicillin-sensitive *Staphylococcus aureus*: evidence for horizontal transfer of virulence genes. *J Clin Microbiol* 2001; **39**: 2760–7.

14. Sieradzki K, Tomasz A. Inhibition of cell wall turnover and autolysis by vancomycin in a highly vancomycin-resistant mutant of *Staphylococcus aureus*. *J Bacteriol* 1997; **179**: 2557–66.

15. Fridkin SK, Hageman J, McDougal LK, Mohammed J, Jarvis WR, Perl TM, Tenover FC. Epidemiological and microbiological characterization of infections caused by *Staphylococcus aureus* with reduced susceptibility to vancomycin, United States, 1997–2001. *Clin Infect Dis* 2003; **36**: 429–39.

16. Vaudaux P, Francois P, Berger-Bachi B, Lew DP. *In vivo* emergence of subpopulations expressing teicoplanin or vancomycin resistance phenotypes in a glycopeptide-susceptible, methicillin-resistant strain of *Staphylococcus aureus*. *J Antimicrob Chemother* 2001; **47**: 163–70.

17. Howe RA, Bowker KE, Walsh TR, Feest TG, MacGowan AP. Vancomycin-resistant *Staphylococcus aureus*. *Lancet* 1998; **351**: 602.

18. Marchese A, Balistreri G, Tonoli E, Debbia EA, Schito GC. Heterogeneous vancomycin resistance in methicillin-resistant *Staphylococcus aureus* strains isolated in a large Italian hospital. *J Clin Microbiol* 2000; **38**: 866–9.

19. Trakulsomboon S, Danchaivijitr S, Rongrungruang Y, Dhiraputra C, Susaemgrat W, Ito T, Hiramatsu K. First report of methicillin-resistant *Staphylococcus aureus* with reduced susceptibility to vancomycin in Thailand. *J Clin Microbiol* 2001; **39**: 591–5.

20. Ward PB, Johnson PD, Grabsch EA, Mayall BC, Grayson ML. Treatment failure due to methicillin-resistant *Staphylococcus aureus* (MRSA) with reduced susceptibility to vancomycin. *Med J Aust* 2001; **175**: 480–3.

21. Wong SS, Ho PL, Woo PC, Yuen KY. Bacteremia caused by staphylococci with inducible vancomycin heteroresistance. *Clin Infect Dis* 1999; **29**: 760–7.

8

Burkholderia cepacia complex

MILES DENTON

Introduction

Until the early 1980s *Burkholderia cepacia* was a little-known phytopathogen, first identified in 1950 as the cause of onion rot [1] (Fig. 8.1). Its inherent resistance to many antimicrobial agents and ability to grow in a variety of environments, including distilled water and disinfectants, have allowed it to flourish in the nosocomial setting [2]. It can cause a variety of infections, particularly bacteraemia and pneumonia, in immunocompromised patients and patients in the intensive care unit. However, it

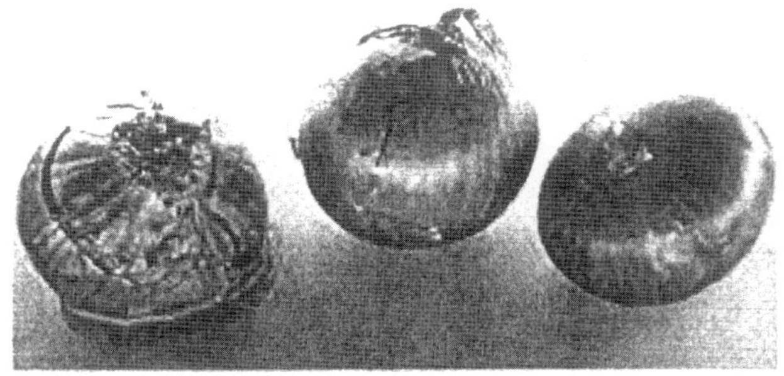
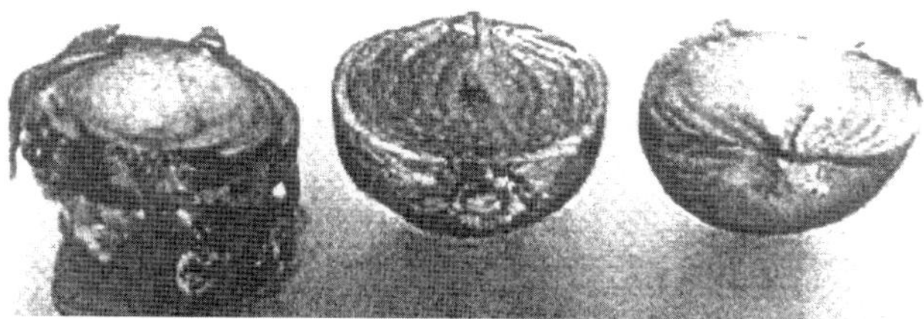

Fig. 8.1 *B. cepacia* causes an onion rot known as slippery skin (1). The onions shown were inoculated with three strains of *B. cepacia*. Rot occurred in onion 1 (left), which was inoculated with a strain originally isolated from onions. Rot did not occur with environmental isolates tested or with strains from CF lung. Reproduced from Holmes *et al.* [11].

came to prominence when associated with a rapidly progressive, fulminant pneumonitis ('cepacia syndrome') in patients with cystic fibrosis (CF), which resulted in
death in around 20% of those patients unfortunate enough to become infected with
the bacterium |3|. Its prevalence in UK CF clinics is variable; some of them report no
more than 7% |4–6|, but prevalence is much higher in CF clinics affected by outbreaks
|7,8|. Global prevalence is also variable. In Italy the prevalence varies between 4 and
30% |9| and in Canada it varies between 5 and 25% |10|.

Taxonomy

The taxonomy of *B. cepacia* has been revised significantly in recent years and there
are now at least nine closely related species (sometimes referred to as 'genomovars')
in what is now called the *Burkholderia cepacia* complex (|12,13| and Vermis *et al.*,
2004 below) (Table 8.1). The most prevalent strains in CF are *Burkholderia cenocepacia* and *B. multivorans*. Although *B. cenocepacia* is most associated with cepacia syndrome and unit-wide outbreaks, there have been anecdotal reports of transmission
and mortality associated with other members of the *B. cepacia* complex.

Proposal to accommodate *Burkholderia cepacia* genomovar VI as *Burkholderia dolosa* sp. nov

Vermis K, Coenye T, LiPuma JJ, Mahenthiralingam E, Nelis HJ, Vandamme P.
Int J Syst Evol Microbiol 2004; **54**: 689–91

BACKGROUND. Eighteen isolates of *B. cepacia* complex genomovar VI were
obtained from samples from CF patients worldwide and the environment. Following a
series of phenotypic and genotypic studies which allowed the differentiation of
B. cepacia complex genomovar VI from other members of the *B. cepacia* complex,

Table 8.1 The genomovar and species names of members of
the *Burkholderia cepacia* complex

Genomovar	Species name
I	*Burkholderia cepacia*
II	*Burkholderia multivorans*
III	*Burkholderia cenocepacia*
IV	*Burkholderia stabilis*
V	*Burkholderia vietnamiensis*
VI	*Burkholderia dolosa*
VII	*Burkholderia ambifaria*
VIII	*Burkholderia athina*
IX	*Burkholderia pyrrocinia*

the authors have proposed the name *Burkholderia dolosa* (*dolosa*: deceitful, unwilling, referring to the absence of growth on a *B. cepacia*-selective medium). The description of the organism is as follows: Gram-negative, small (1.5–2.5 μm long), motile, rod-shaped cells; unable to assimilate tryptamine, azelaic acid and salicin; isolates fail to grow on the *B. cepacia*-selective medium PCAT (*Pseudomonas cepacia* azelaic acid medium); the G+C content of the DNA is 66.9–67.7 mol%. Compared with other *B. cepacia* complex bacteria, strains generate unique 16S rDNA (ribosomal deoxyribonucleic acid) restriction fragment length polymorphism (RFLP) and *recA* RFLP patterns and can be identified using a specific 16S rDNA-based polymerase chain reaction (PCR) assay.

INTERPRETATION. *B. cepacia* complex is difficult to identify using phenotypic methods alone. Common kits utilizing biochemical reactions are unreliable and studies have highlighted the problems of misidentifying these organisms |**14**|. This can lead to inappropriate management and infection control interventions in CF units. At present it is therefore recommended that all suspect isolates of *B. cepacia* complex are confirmed using molecular methods.

Comment

This study now formalizes the names of all nine of the currently described species within the *B. cepacia* complex. It is not clear how clinically significant *B. dolosa* will be in comparison with other members of the complex. It has already been responsible for one outbreak in a North American CF unit |**15**|. Further studies are awaited.

Burkholderia cepacia complex genomovars: utilization of carbon sources, susceptibility to antimicrobial agents and growth on selective media

Vermis K, Vandamme PA, Nelis HJ. *J Appl Microbiol* 2003; **95**: 1191–9

BACKGROUND. This study investigated the relationship between genomovar status and carbon source utilization, antibiotic susceptibility and growth ability on selective media of 142 clinical and environmental *B. cepacia* complex isolates belonging to all nine genomovars. Carbon source utilization and growth on selective media was assessed using agar plate multipoint inoculation. MICs (minimum inhibitory concentrations) were determined using agar dilution. There was significant variability in the utilization of carbon sources both between and within the different genomovars. *B. dolosa* (genomovar VI) grew on a very limited number of carbon sources. In general, environmental isolates tended to be nutritionally more versatile than clinical or CF isolates. Not surprisingly, the isolates exhibited high levels of resistance to a wide range of antimicrobial agents. Susceptibilities differed for the individual genomovars, *B. dolosa* showing the highest antimicrobial resistance. In general, whilst there were individual differences, the susceptibility of environmental isolates was not significantly different from that of clinical or CF isolates. *B. cepacia*-selective agar (BCSA) |16| and Mast *B. cepacia* medium supported the growth of *B. cepacia* complex isolates more efficiently than LAB M *B. cepacia* medium and Oxoid *B. cepacia* medium.

INTERPRETATION. There are no reliable phenotypic methods for differentiating between members of the *B. cepacia* complex. Microbiology laboratories will need to continue their reliance on molecular methods. For most routine laboratories, this will require referral of isolates to reference laboratories.

Comment

The differentiation of *B. cepacia* complex from other non-fermentative bacteria using phenotypic methods alone is difficult. Commonly used kits, such as API 20NE, are unreliable. This study confirmed that identifying the different members of the *B. cepacia* complex from each other with phenotypic methods is also extremely difficult. Apart from the poor growth capabilities of *B. dolosa*, no reliable phenotypic characteristics could be found in order to reliably distinguish between the genomovars. The finding that BCSA and Mast *B. cepacia* medium were more efficient than either LAB M or Oxoid selective *B. cepacia* media for isolating *B. cepacia* complex suggests that microbiology laboratories should review their current choice of medium, particularly if they are providing a clinical service to a CF unit.

Identification of *Pseudomonas aeruginosa*, *Burkholderia cepacia* complex, and *Stenotrophomonas maltophilia* in respiratory samples from cystic fibrosis patients using multiplex PCR

da Silva Filho LV, Tateno AF, Vellosos L de F, *et al*. *Pediatr Pulmonol* 2004; **37**: 537–47

BACKGROUND. A multiplex PCR method was developed to identify *B. cepacia* complex (along with *Pseudomonas aeruginosa* and *Stenotrophomonas maltophilia*) directly in sputum and oropharyngeal samples from patients with CF. Two hundred and fifty-seven samples from 106 patients were simultaneously cultured on selective media and subjected to multiplex PCR using primer pairs targeting specific genomic sequences for each species. *B. cepacia* complex was cultured from 11/257 (4.3%) samples. The identity of the isolates was *B. cenocepacia* (six), *B. multivorans* (two), *B. vietnamiensis* (two) and one indeterminate. The multiplex PCR for *B. cepacia* complex was positive on 10/257 (3.9%) samples. Five samples were both culture- and PCR-positive (three *B. cenocepacia* and two *B. multivorans*), six were culture-positive but PCR-negative (three *B. cenocepacia*, two *B. vietnamiensis* and one indeterminate) and five were culture-negative but PCR-positive. Using culture on selective media as the gold standard, this multiplex PCR method for *B. cepacia* complex had a sensitivity of 45.5%, a specificity of 97.6%, a positive predictive value of 50% and a negative predictive value of 97.5%.

INTERPRETATION. This multiplex PCR method had good specificity and negative predictive value but had poor sensitivity. This suggests that it is likely to be some time before culture can be replaced by molecular methods for the detection of *B. cepacia* complex in clinical samples.

Comment

Although the method demonstrated a reasonable negative predictive value, it lacked sensitivity. There were five samples that were PCR-positive but culture-negative. These samples were subjected to sequencing of 16S rDNA amplicons but it was not clear from the paper what the resulting identifications were. There were no follow-up data to ascertain whether these patients subsequently became culture-positive either. There was also no mention of cost or turnaround times of the respective methods. PCR methods for the direct detection of *B. cepacia* complex in clinical samples require significant further development before they can be considered a real alternative to existing culture methods using selective media.

Epidemiology

The epidemiology of *B. cepacia* complex has been an area of intense study. It has not been particularly easy to find strains that are associated with clinical disease in the environment |**17–19**|. However, early studies were hampered by the lack of accurate taxonomy.

One study looked at the prevalence of *B. cepacia* complex in the homes and other social areas frequented by CF and non-CF patients |**18**|. *B. cepacia* was recovered from five of 27 homes examined (18%) and from 20 of 509 (4%) samples taken outside of homes. Another survey of 55 environmental sites yielded only twelve *B. cepacia* isolates. None of these displayed phenotypic properties of multiresistant epidemic strains isolated from CF patients, the environmental isolates being more sensitive to antimicrobial agents |**17**|. However, more recent studies have isolated genomovar III strains from a variety of environmental niches |**20**|, including one strain from a soil sample associated with clinical disease in patients |**21**|.

B. cepacia has been isolated from three of 35 home-use nebulizers |**22**|. One of two strains found on one patient's nebulizer had a genotype identical to the one colonizing his sputum. The other two patients had not grown *B. cepacia* from sputum cultures. *B. cepacia* is also disseminated into the air and onto bedding during physiotherapy and can be detected up to 45 min later |**23**|. The roles of these routes in transmission are uncertain.

The difficulty in finding environmental reservoirs has led to the belief that clusters of cases in CF units must be due to patient-to-patient transmission. The presence of single clones which have infected large numbers of patients has been shown in all of the studies, including one which spread throughout CF clinics in Canada and the UK |**24–26**|. This clone, known as the ET-12 intercontinental clone |**19**|, is associated with the presence of cell-surface pili with unique 'cable' morphology |**27**|. Another genetic marker, referred to as *Burkholderia cepacia* Epidemic Strain Marker (BCESM), has also been associated with transmissible strains |**28**|. ET-12 has been identified as a strain of *B. cenocepacia* and has been closely associated with 'cepacia syndrome'. However, not all virulent, transmissible strains of *B. cepacia* complex are identified as *B. cenocepacia*, nor are all of these strains positive for cable pilus or BCESM |**27**|.

However, many patients also possess unique strains, suggesting widespread inter-strain variation in transmission capability. This may also explain the findings of a small number of studies that could not demonstrate transmission between patients who were not segregated |29|.

Epidemiology of *Burkholderia cepacia* complex colonisation in cystic fibrosis patients

De Boeck K, Malfroot A, Van Schil L, *et al.*; Belgian *Burkholderia cepacia* Study Group. *Eur Respir J* 2004; **23**: 851–6

BACKGROUND. Belgian CF clinics routinely screen sputum samples from all their patients for the presence of *B. cepacia* complex every 3 months. This study compared isolates obtained in 1993 with those obtained in 1999 to determine changes to the genomovar status and evaluate clinical outcomes of colonized and non-colonized patients. Isolates were examined using *recA* RFLP analysis and pulsed-field gel electrophoresis (PFGE). In 1993, 12 of 465 Belgian CF patients were colonized with *B. cepacia* complex (six *B. cenocepacia*, three *B. multivorans* and three *B. stabilis*). Four were colonized with the same *B. cenocepacia* strain and two with the same *B. stabilis*. After 5 years, three patients with *B. cenocepacia* and one with *B. multivorans* had died. Three patients from the 1993 cohort were only transiently colonized with *B. cepacia* complex (two *B. cenocepacia* and one *B. stabilis*). In 1999, twelve of 650 Belgian CF patients were colonized with *B. cepacia* complex (nine *B. multivorans*, two *B. cenocepacia* and one *B. stabilis*). Three patients were colonized with the same *B. multivorans* strain. After 4 years, three patients with *B. multivorans* and one with *B. cenocepacia* had died. Patients colonized with *B. cepacia* complex had significantly worse lung function (FVC [forced vital capacity] and FEV$_1$ [forced expiratory volume in one second]) than controls.

INTERPRETATION. *B. cenocepacia* has been replaced by *B. multivorans* as the predominant *B. cepacia* complex species isolated from Belgian CF patients.

Comment

This study highlights the changing pattern of *B. cepacia* complex now seen in many (but not all) CF centres. For years the predominant genomovar seen in CF centres was *B. cenocepacia*, particularly in those affected by outbreaks with transmissible strains such as ET-12. These strains were also the ones most closely associated with 'cepacia syndrome'. The introduction of effective infection control measures and the unfortunate death of many *B. cenocepacia*-positive patients may have contributed to a reduction in the numbers of this genomovar. However, this study highlights that other species within the *B. cepacia* complex, particularly *B. multivorans*, can also be associated with significant morbidity and mortality. The number of patients colonized with this genomovar is increasing and some also share the same genotype. Whether this represents patient-to-patient transmission or exposure to common environmental sources remains uncertain. Further studies are required.

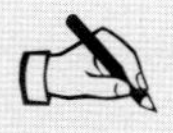

Molecular analysis of *Burkholderia cepacia* complex strains from a Portuguese cystic fibrosis center: a 7-year study

Cunha MV, Leitao JH, Mahenthiralingam E, *et al*. *J Clin Microbiol* 2003; **41**: 4113–20

BACKGROUND. A systematic molecular analysis was made of 113 *B. cepacia* complex isolates obtained from 23 patients with CF attending the Santa Maria Hospital in Lisbon, Portugal, over a 7-year period. Twelve of the 23 patients were infected with *B. cenocepacia*, eight with *B. cepacia* (genomovar I), four with *B. stabilis* and two with *B. multivorans*. All four genomovars were associated with poor clinical outcome, including the cepacia syndrome, and could give rise to both chronic and transient infections. The epidemic strain marker BCESM was found only in *B. cenocepacia* but the cable pilus gene *cblA* was found in both *B. cepacia* and *B cenocepacia*. There was no clear association between the presence of these markers and transmissibility.

INTERPRETATION. This study confirms that members of the *B. cepacia* complex other than *B. cenocepacia* and *B. multivorans* are also associated with poor clinical outcome and transmission in patients with CF.

Comment

In this study *B. cepacia* and *B. stabilis* were associated with poor clinical outcome. Previous studies had mainly implicated *B. cenocepacia* and *B. multivorans*. Further studies are required in order to understand what patient and other factors determine clinical outcome. It was clear from this study that BCESM and cable pili are unreliable indicators of prognosis and transmission. This study also highlighted the geographical variation observed between countries with respect to the predominant genomovars. Whether this relates to environmental factors, such as climate, requires further study.

Epidemiology of *Burkholderia cepacia* complex species recovered from cystic fibrosis patients: issues related to patient segregation

McDowell A, Mahenthiralingam E, Dunbar KE, Moore JE, Crowe M, Elborn JS. *J Med Microbiol* 2004; **53**: 663–8

BACKGROUND. In this study *B. cepacia* complex isolates from 131 patients with CF, obtained between 1997 and 2001, were identified using molecular methods, genotyped using RAPD (random amplification of polymorphic DNA) and PFGE, and screened for the presence of the putative transmissibility markers *cblA* and BCESM.

The patients were from four centres in Ireland (50 isolates), nine centres in Great Britain (46 isolates) and one centre in mainland Europe (35 isolates). Of the isolates, 103/131 (79%) were identified as *B. cenocepacia* and 23/131 (18%) as *B. multivorans*. The five remaining isolates were *B. vietnamiensis* (three), *B. cepacia* (one) and *B. stabilis* (one). The *recA* analysis of the *B. cenocepacia* isolates revealed that 91% were of lineage III-A. Genotyping revealed that 58/103 *B. cenocepacia* isolates were the ET-12 strain, 57 (98%) of which were shown to be positive for both *cblA* and BCESM. Although all 35 isolates obtained from the CF centre in mainland Europe were identified as *B. cenocepacia* and 33/35 were identical on genotyping, this strain was genetically distinct from ET-12. This strain contained BCESM but not *cblA*. Genotyping also revealed two clusters of *B. multivorans*, one involving four patients and the other involving two patients. Both were negative for transmissibility markers, as were all the other *B. cenocepacia* isolates with unique genotypes. The sensitivity and specificity of putative strain markers is shown in Table 8.2.

INTERPRETATION. In Great Britain and Ireland the most prevalent members of the *B. cepacia* complex among CF patients are *B. cenocepacia* and *B. multivorans*. The ET-12 strain of *B. cenocepacia* appears to be limited to Great Britain and Ireland. The ET-12 strain was not found in the unnamed mainland European CF centre.

Comment

Taken along with the studies of De Boeck *et al.* in Belgium and Cunha *et al.* in Portugal, a picture is emerging of geographical differences in the epidemiology of *B. cepacia* complex across Europe. Although *B. cenocepacia* is still the most prevalent genomovar in many European CF centres, epidemic lineages appear to be different. In the US, unlike Europe, most epidemic lineages of *B. cenocepacia* belong to the *recA* lineage III-B [27]. The reasons for these geographical differences warrant further study. This study also concurred with the findings of Cunha *et al.* that BCESM and *cblA* are unreliable markers of the virulence and transmissibility for *B. cepacia* complex strains. It is therefore recommended that segregation within CF units is based on the presence or absence of *B. cepacia* complex infection, not on the basis that a patient has *B. cenocepacia* positive for transmissibility markers.

Table 8.2 Sensitivity and specificity of putative strain markers for transmissible strains of *B. cenocepacia* and all *B. cepacia* complex isolates combined

	Transmissible *B. cenocepacia*	All transmissible *B. cepacia* complex
BCESM sensitivity	100%	94%
BCESM specificity	33%	76%
cblA sensitivity	63%	59%
cblA specificity	100%	100%

Clinical

B. cepacia complex is associated with significant morbidity and mortality in immunocompromised patients and patients with CF |2|. Whether this relates more to immune factors in the host or to virulence factors in the organism is poorly understood. Prior infection with *B. cepacia* complex has been used as a contra-indication to lung transplantation because of the poor clinical outcome of many of the patients.

Prevalence and clonality of *Burkholderia cepacia* complex genomovars in UK patients with cystic fibrosis referred for lung transplantation

De Soyza A, Morris K, McDowell A, *et al. Thorax* 2004; **59**: 526–8

BACKGROUND. An extensive study was conducted to determine the prevalence and clonality of *B. cepacia* complex genomovars isolated from patients referred for lung transplant assessment at the Freeman Hospital, Newcastle, between 1989 and 2002 and, where appropriate, to ascertain if strain type was related to transplant outcome. Thirty-two referred patients were found to have presumptive *B. cepacia* complex on phenotypic analysis. However, on further molecular analysis, three were identified as other non-fermenters. Of the 29 patients confirmed to have *B. cepacia* complex, 16 were infected with *B. cenocepacia* (14 type III-A and two type III-B), eleven with *B. multivorans* and two with *B. vietnamiensis*. Thirteen of the *B. cenocepacia* isolates were the highly transmissible ET-12 strain. All the other patients were infected with unique strains. All reported deaths following transplantation (five) were associated with the ET-12 strain. Patients transplanted with other genomovars all had good clinical outcomes despite the fact that four patients had persistence of the same *B. multivorans* or *B. vietnamiensis* strain in respiratory samples up to one year after transplantation.

INTERPRETATION. This study confirms previous reports highlighting poorer transplantation outcomes for patients infected with *B. cenocepacia*, particularly the ET-12 strain. It also indicates the importance of accurate identification of *B. cepacia* complex in patients undergoing transplantation, because this can have a major bearing on prognosis.

Comment

Some transplant centres consider *B. cepacia* complex infection as an absolute contra-indication for surgery. Despite these findings, the transplant unit at the Freeman Hospital continues to transplant patients with CF who are infected with *B. ceno-cepacia*. However, they have modified their management of such patients by omitting T-cell ablation at induction, reducing trough target cyclosporin levels, washing the pleural cavities with the surface disinfectant taurolidine, and commencing a 48-h multi-antibiotic regimen (chosen on the basis of recent sensitivities). Two patients infected with *B. cenocepacia* ET-12 have now been successfully transplanted using this approach and are alive after 1 year.

Virulence associated with outbreak-related strains of *Burkholderia cepacia* complex among a cohort of patients with bacteremia

Woods CW, Bressler AM, LiPuma JJ, *et al*. *Clin Infect Dis* 2004; **38**: 1243–50

BACKGROUND. Host and pathogen features associated with mortality were evaluated for 53 patients with *B. cepacia* complex bacteraemia. All cases occurred between May 1996 and May 2002 at the Duke University Medical Center, North Carolina, US. Isolates were identified to species level by 16S rDNA and *recA*-based species-specific PCR and *recA* RFLP. Genotyping was performed using PFGE. Of the 53 patients identified, only nine (17%) had CF and 25 (47%) died within 14 days of the bacteraemia. Patients with CF were significantly less likely to die within 14 days of bacteraemia, as were those who were recipients of lung transplants. Conversely, all five bone marrow transplant recipients with *B. cepacia* complex bacteraemia died. Patients with a primary bacteraemia of unknown source did significantly worse than those with an identifiable source, such as pneumonia. Removal of central lines or changing them within 7 days of the bacteraemia was associated with reduced mortality. However, this association did not reach statistical significance when those who died within 24 h of bacteraemia were excluded.

INTERPRETATION. Although previous treatment with an antibiotic to which the isolate was susceptible was not associated with improved outcome, initiation of therapy with trimethoprim–sulphamethoxazole after isolation of *B. cepacia* complex from blood was associated with reduced mortality. Molecular speciation demonstrated that *B. cenocepacia* accounted for 39/53 (74%) of the cases of bacteraemia. The other 14 cases were caused by *B. multivorans* (six), *B. cepacia* (five), *B. vietnamiensis* (two) and *B. stabilis* (one). *B. cenocepacia* also accounted for 21/25 (84%) of deaths and was associated with an increased risk of 14-day mortality relative to other genomovars. Genotyping revealed that two strains of *B. cenocepacia* accounted for 27/53 (51%) bacteraemias and 18/25 (72%) of deaths. A point source for either outbreak strain could not be identified. When combined in multivariate analysis, bacteraemia caused by the two outbreak strains was strongly associated with 14-day mortality.

Comment

This study is the largest single investigation of *B. cepacia* complex bacteraemia and the first to document high rates of attributable mortality in patients without CF. Most previous studies of *B. cepacia* complex bacteraemia have been much smaller and have reported much lower case–fatality rates. This may reflect the patient population, most of whom had significant underlying comorbid factors; for example, bone marrow and solid-organ transplants. Patients without CF were at increased risk of death from *B. cepacia* complex. This may be explained by their older age and the fact that most would not have previously colonized with the bacterium and had an opportunity to form antibodies. The close association between *B. cenocepacia*, particularly outbreak strains, and 14-day mortality concurs with the evidence from infections in patients with CF that this is the most virulent and transmissible genomovar of the complex. In 44/53 cases the *B. cepacia* complex isolate was susceptible to trimethoprim–sulphamethoxazole and commencement of this agent was associated with reduced mortality. This suggests that trimethoprim–sulphamethoxazole should be considered to be the first-line choice for *B. cepacia* complex bacteraemia. In addition, changing or removing central lines should also be considered in these cases.

Treatment

B. cepacia strains isolated from CF patients are generally multiresistant, most strains being resistant to aminoglycosides, quinolones, cefotaxime, imipenem, chloramphenicol, tetracycline and trimethoprim–sulphamethoxazole |26|. The use of aminoglycosides has been associated with an increased risk of *B. cepacia* colonization |30|. It is also inherently resistant to colistin, but the use of this drug in nebulizers does not appear to increase the risk of colonization |4|. However, more than three-quarters of strains are sensitive to ceftazidime, meropenem, piperacillin and piperacillin–tazobactam |26|. Strains of *B. cepacia* from chronically colonized patients can have variable antibiotic susceptibility over time and this is associated with changes in outer membrane proteins |31|. The possession of rough lipopolysaccharide |32| and β-lactamases with penicillinase |33| and carbapenemase activity |34,35| may also contribute to resistance. More recent studies have demonstrated the presence of class 1 integrons carrying aminoglycoside acetyltransferase-encoding genes |36|. Many clinical strains isolated from patients with CF are resistant to all available classes of antimicrobials. However, recent studies have failed to show a clear association between resistance and genomovar status within the *B. cepacia* complex |37|. Whilst the clinical impact of this resistance remains uncertain, clinicians still have difficulty in selecting the most appropriate therapy in these cases |38|. Synergy testing has been suggested as a means of optimizing therapy, but this has yet to be shown to improve clinical outcome |39|.

In vitro activity and synergy of bismuth thiols and tobramycin against *Burkholderia cepacia* complex

Veloria WG, Domenico P, LiPuma JJ, Davis JM, Gurzenda E, Kazzaz JA.
J Antimicrob Chemother 2003; **52**: 915–19

BACKGROUND. Bismuth–thiols (BTs) are agents with antibiofilm activity against Gram-positive and -negative bacteria. The thiol component functions as a lipophilic carrier that promotes bismuth uptake into bacteria, enhancing the effects of

bismuth up to 1000-fold and resulting in cell death. They also inhibit exoenzymes and biofilm formation. The study determined the susceptibility of 25 strains each of *B. multivorans* and *B. cenocepacia* to six BTs and examined their synergistic effects in combination with tobramycin. Tested strains showed a wide range of susceptibilities to the six BTs. A MIC$_{90}$ of 15.6 μM was obtained for two BTs, although these levels would be toxic in the clinical setting. One BT (bismuth ethanedithiol) was studied in combination with tobramycin. At concentrations of 2 μM this BT reduced the MIC and MBC (minimum bacteriocidal concentration) of tobramycin against all strains, achieving synergy in many instances. Most strains became susceptible to tobramycin at clinically achievable concentrations in the presence of non-toxic bismuth ethanedithiol levels.

INTERPRETATION. Against *B. cepacia* complex isolates, BTs appear to have only moderate activity. Given that BTs are cytotoxic at concentrations greater than 10 μM, they are probably too toxic to be considered as direct therapeutic agents. However, when used at the subtherapeutic level of 2 μM they may have a role in facilitating synergy with other agents against *B. cepacia* complex.

Comment

Pulmonary infections in CF are treated primarily with antibiotic therapy. Treatment can reduce bacterial density and virulence factor production, leading to decreased inflammation and clinical improvement. Unfortunately, *B. cepacia* complex is often multiresistant and refractory to antibiotics. There is therefore an urgent need for novel agents and combinations with clinical activity against this bacterium. BTs are one of a number of novel compounds that exhibit activity against multiresistant pathogens. It would also be interesting to know if the findings of this study (BTs in combination with aminoglycosides) could be replicated with other antibiotic classes, such as the β-lactams. The antibiofilm activity of BTs also needs further study. Biofilms are an important feature of chronic infection with *Pseudomonas aeruginosa* in patients with CF as well as a wide range of infections relating to prosthetic devices in other patient groups.

Conclusion

The taxonomy of *Burkholderia cepacia* complex continues to evolve and the proposal to name genomovar VI as *Burkholderia dolosa* is the latest development in this rapidly changing field. However, the absence of reliable, phenotypic methods of identification means that most laboratories will still need to refer isolates suspected to be *B. cepacia* to reference laboratories for confirmation of identity using molecular methods.

Burkholderia cenocepacia and *Burkholderia multivorans* continue to be the most commonly isolated species of *B. cepacia* in CF units. However, geographical differences are emerging in the relative prevalence of each species. There is also evidence that members of the *B. cepacia* other than *B. cenocepacia* or *B. multivorans* are associated with poor clinical outcome and transmission in patients with CF. Previously identified virulence markers such as BCESM and *cblA* have also been shown to be unreliable markers of virulence and transmissibility for *B. cepacia* strains. Thus, species and virulence factor identification can no longer be used as reliable prognostic or infection control markers. It is therefore recommended that segregation within CF units be based on the presence or absence of *B. cepacia* infection, not on the basis that a patient has transmissibility marker-positive *B. cenocepacia*. Whilst there is evidence that *B. cenocepacia* (particularly the ET-12 strain) may be associated with worse clinical outcome after lung transplantation, one transplant centre has demonstrated successful clinical outcome if a modified immunosuppression regimen is used. Treatment of *B. cepacia* remains problematic given the high levels of antibiotic resistance seen with the organism. Novel agents, such as bismuth thiols, may be of use in combination with other agents but further studies are needed. Clinical studies suggest that treatment with cotrimoxazole is associated with lower mortality in patients with *B. cepacia* bacteraemia. Removal of intravenous catheters may also improve outcome in this setting.

References

1. Burkholder WH. Sour skin, a bacterial rot of onion bulbs. *Phytopathology* 1950; **40**: 115–17.

2. Spencer RC. The emergence of epidemic, multiple-antibiotic-resistant *Stenotrophomonas (Xanthomonas) maltophilia* and *Burkholderia (Pseudomonas) cepacia. J Hosp Infect* 1995; 30(Suppl): 453–64.

3. Isles A, Maclusky I, Corey M, Gold R, Prober C, Fleming P, Levison H. *Pseudomonas cepacia* infection in cystic fibrosis: an emerging problem. *J Pediatr* 1984; **104**: 206–10.

4. Simmonds EJ, Conway SP, Ghoneim ATM, Ross H, Littlewood JM. *Pseudomonas cepacia*: a new pathogen in patients with cystic fibrosis referred to a large centre in the United Kingdom. *Arch Dis Child* 1990; **65**: 874–7.

5. Gladman G, Connor PJ, Williams RF, David TJ. Controlled study of *Pseudomonas cepacia* and *Pseudomonas maltophilia* in cystic fibrosis. *Arch Dis Child* 1992; **67**: 192–5.

6. Taylor RFH, Dalla Costa L, Kaufmann ME, Pitt TL, Hodson ME. *Pseudomonas cepacia* pulmonary infection in adults with cystic fibrosis: is nosocomial acquisition occurring? *J Hosp Infect* 1992; **21**: 199–204.

7. Whiteford ML, Wilkinson JD, McColl JH, Conlon FM, Michie JR, Evans TJ, Paton JY. Outcome of *Burkholderia (Pseudomonas) cepacia* colonisation in children with cystic fibrosis following a hospital outbreak. *Thorax* 1995; **50**: 1194–8.

8. Ledson MJ, Gallagher MJ, Jackson M, Hart CA, Walshaw MJ. Outcome of *Burkholderia cepacia* colonization in an adult cystic fibrosis centre. *Thorax* 2002; **57**: 142–5.

9. Agodi A, Mahenthiralingam E, Barchitta M, Giannino V, Sciacca A, Stefani S. *Burkholderia cepacia* complex infection in Italian patients with cystic fibrosis: prevalence, epidemiology, and genomovar status. *J Clin Microbiol* 2001; **39**: 2891–6.

10. Speert DP, Henry D, Vandamme P, Corey M, Mahenthiralingam E. Epidemiology of *Burkholderia cepacia* complex in patients with cystic fibrosis, Canada. *Emerg Infect Dis* 2002; **8**: 181–7.

11. Holmes A, Govan J, Goldstein R. Agricultural use of *Burkholderia* (*Pseudomonas*) *cepacia*: a threat to human health? *Emerg Infect Dis* 1998; **4**(2): 221–7.

12. Coenye T, Vandamme P, Govan JRW, LiPuma JJ. Taxonomy and identification of the *Burkholderia cepacia* complex. *J Clin Microbiol* 2001; **39**: 3427–36.

13. Mahenthiralingam E, Baldwin A, Vandamme P. *Burkholderia cepacia* complex infection in patients with cystic fibrosis. *J Med Microbiol* 2002; **51**: 533–8.

14. Brisse S, Stefani S, Verhoef J, Van Belkum A, Vandamme P, Goessens W. Comparative evaluation of the BD Phoenix and VITEK 2 automated instruments for identification of isolates of the *Burkholderia cepacia* complex. *J Clin Microbiol* 2002; **40**: 1743–8.

15. Biddick R, Spilker T, Martin A, LiPuma JJ. Evidence of transmission of *Burkholderia cepacia*, *Burkholderia multivorans* and *Burkholderia dolosa* among persons with cystic fibrosis. *FEMS Microbiol Lett* 2003; **228**: 57–62.

16. Henry D, Campbell M, LiPuma J, Speert D. Identification of B. cepacia isolates from patients with cystic fibrosis and use of a simple new selective medium. *J Clin Microbiol* 1997; **35**: 614–19.

17. Butler SL, Doherty CJ, Hughes JE, Nelson JW, Govan JRW. Burkholderia cepacia and cystic fibrosis: do natural environments present a potential hazard? *J Clin Microbiol* 1995; **33**: 1001–4.

18. Mortensen JE, Fisher MC, LiPuma JJ. Recovery of Pseudomonas cepacia and other Pseudomonas species from the environment. *Infect Cont Hosp Epidemiol* 1995; **56**: 152–62.

19. Govan JRW, Hughes JE, Vandamme P. Burkholderia cepacia: medical, taxonomic, and ecological issues. *J Med Microbiol* 1996; **45**: 395–407.

20. Bevivino A, Dalmastri C, Tabacchioni S, Chiarini L, Belli ML, Piana S, Materazzo A, Vandamme P, Manno G. Burkholderia cepacia complex bacteria from clinical and environmental sources in Italy: genomovar status and distribution of traits related to virulence and transmissibility. *J Clin Microbiol* 2002; **40**: 846–51.

21. LiPuma JJ, Spilker T, Coenye T, Gonzalez CF. An epidemic Burkholderia cepacia complex strain identified in soil. *Lancet* 2002; **359**: 2002–3.

22. Hutchinson GR, Parker S, Pryor JA, Duncan-Skingle F, Hoffman PN, Hodson ME, Kaufmann ME, Pitt TL. Home-use nebulisers: a potential primary source of Burkholderia cepacia and other colistin-resistant, gram-negative bacteria in patients with cystic fibrosis. *J Clin Microbiol* 1996; **34**: 584–7.

23. Ensor E, Humphreys H, Peckham D, Webster C, Knox AJ. Is *Burkholderia cepacia* disseminated from cystic fibrosis patients during physiotherapy? *J Hosp Infect* 1996; **32**: 9–15.

24. Govan JR, Brown PH, Maddison J, Doherty CJ, Nelson JW, Dodd M, Greening AP, Webb AK. Evidence for transmission of *Pseudomonas cepacia* by social contact in cystic fibrosis. *Lancet* 1993; **342**: 15–19.

25. Mahenthiralingam E, Campbell ME, Henry DA, Speert DP. Epidemiology of *Burkholderia cepacia* infection in patients with cystic fibrosis: analysis by randomly amplified polymorphic DNA fingerprinting. *J Clin Microbiol* 1996; **34**: 2914–20.

26. Pitt TL, Kaufmann ME, Patel PS, Benge LC, Gaskin S, Livermore DM. Type characterization and antibiotic susceptibility of *Burkholderia (Pseudomonas) cepacia* isolates from patients with cystic fibrosis in the United Kingdom and the Republic of Ireland. *J Med Microbiol* 1996; **44**: 203–10.

27. LiPuma JJ, Spilker T, Gill LH, Campbell PW 3rd, Liu L, Mahenthiralingam E. Disproportionate distribution of *Burkholderia cepacia* complex species and transmissibility markers in cystic fibrosis. *Am J Resp Crit Care Med* 2001; **164**: 92–6.

28. Mahenthiralingam E, Simpson DA, Speert DP. Identification and characterization of a novel DNA marker associated with epidemic *Burkholderia cepacia* strains recovered from patients with cystic fibrosis. *J Clin Microbiol* 1997; **35**: 808–16.

29. Hardy KA, McGowan KL, Fisher MC, Schidlow DV. *Pseudomonas cepacia* in the hospital setting: lack of transmission between cystic fibrosis patients. *J Pediatr* 1986; **109**: 51–4.

30. Govan JR, Nelson JW. Microbiology of lung infection in cystic fibrosis. *Br Med Bull* 1992; **48**: 912–30.

31. Larsen GY, Stull TL, Burns JL. Marked phenotypic variability in *Pseudomonas cepacia* isolated from a patient with cystic fibrosis. *J Clin Microbiol* 1993; **31**: 788–92.

32. Simpson IN, Finlay J, Winstanley DJ, Dewhurst N, Nelson JW, Butler SL, Govan JR. Multi-resistant isolates possessing characteristics of both *Burkholderia (Pseudomonas) cepacia* and *Burkholderia gladioli* from patients with cystic fibrosis. *J Antimicrob Chemother* 1994; **34**: 353–61.

33. Trepanier S, Prince A, Huletsky A. Characterization of the penA and penR genes of *Burkholderia cepacia* 249 which encode the chromosomal class A penicillinase and its LysR-type transcriptional regulator. *Antimicrob Agents Chemother* 1997; **41**: 2399–405.

34. Simpson IN, Hunter R, Govan JR, Nelson JW. Do all *Pseudomonas cepacia* produce carbapenemases? *J Antimicrob Chemother* 1993; **32**: 339–41.

35. Baxter IA, Lambert PA. Isolation and partial purification of a carbapenem-hydrolyzing metallo-beta-lactamase from *Pseudomonas cepacia*. *FEMS Microbiol Lett* 1994; **122**: 251–6.

36. Crowley D, Daly M, Lucey B, Shine P, Collins JJ, Cryan B, Moore JE, Murphy P, Buckley G, Fanning S. Molecular epidemiology of cystic fibrosis-linked *Burkholderia cepacia* complex isolates from three national referral centres in Ireland. *J Appl Microbiol* 2002; **92**: 992–1004.

37. Nzula S, Vandamme P, Govan JR. Influence of taxonomic status on the in vitro antimicrobial susceptibility of the *Burkholderia cepacia* complex. *J Antimicrob Chemother* 2002; **50**: 265–9.

38. Conway SP, Brownlee KG, Denton M, Peckham DG. Antibiotic treatment of multidrug-resistant organisms in cystic fibrosis. *Am J Respir Med* 2003; **2**: 321–32.

39. Chernish RN, Aaron SD. Approach to resistant gram negative bacterial pulmonary infections in patients with cystic fibrosis. *Curr Opin Pulm Med* 2003; **9**: 509–15.

Part III

Emerging infections

9

Typhoid fever

CHRISTIANE DOLECEK

Introduction

Typhoid fever is a systemic infection with the facultative intracellular Gram-negative bacterium *Salmonella enterica* subspecies *enterica* serovar Typhi (*S. typhi*), which is restricted to the human host. In developing countries typhoid fever is common, and as a result of the emergence and alarming spread of microbial resistance it is increasingly difficult to treat. Current estimates from the World Health Organization (WHO) suggest that the worldwide incidence of typhoid fever is approximately 21 million cases annually, with more than 210 000 deaths.

The diagnosis of *S. typhi* infection is made following a careful history and clinical examination and can be confirmed by blood culture (with a sensitivity of approximately 50%) or bone marrow aspirate culture (sensitivity is approximately 80%). Bone marrow culture can allow the isolation of *S. typhi* even after the start of antibiotic treatment. Serological tests are available and can be helpful, but need to be interpreted carefully.

Antimicrobial resistance among *S. typhi* and the non-Typhi *Salmonella* to traditional first-line antibiotics, such as ampicillin, chloramphenicol and trimethoprim–sulphonamide combinations has emerged in the last few decades. These multidrug-resistant (MDR) strains have been responsible for numerous outbreaks in countries in the Indian subcontinent, south-east Asia and Africa. In all MDR strains so far examined, the multiple drug resistance has been encoded by plasmids of the H1 incompatibility group. Consequently, the fluoroquinolone class of drugs (which derive from nalidixic acid, the prototype quinolone, which has been available since the 1960s) have become the treatment of choice for typhoid fever. The fluoroquinolones show excellent tissue penetration, accumulation in monocytes and macrophages and high drug levels in the gall bladder. However, there have been recent reports from Vietnam, India and Tajikistan of the emergence of *S. typhi* isolates that respond less well to the fluoroquinolones. These isolates are resistant to nalidixic acid (which itself is never used for the treatment of typhoid fever, but the *in vitro* sensitivity to this old antibiotic is a useful laboratory screening tool to predict a poorer clinical response to the fluoroquinolones), and exhibit higher minimum inhibitory concentrations (MICs) for the fluoroquinolones than nalidixic acid-sensitive strains, but are still within the current breakpoints for fluoroquinolone susceptibility in disc sensitivity testing according to the current National Committee for Clinical Laboratory Standards (NCCLS) guidelines. This reduced susceptibility to the fluoroquinolones results in a poor clinical response to treatment, characterized by longer fever clearance times and a higher rate of relapse. Quinolone resistance is frequently caused by single point mutations in the quinolone resistance-determining region of the *GyraseA* gene of *S. typhi*. The emergence of MDR *S. typhi* isolates with reduced susceptibility to fluoroquinolones is a major setback. Our treatment options are limited and we face the real danger of untreatable typhoid fever.

S. typhi infections seen in Europe and the US are usually acquired abroad (mostly from the Indian subcontinent, south-east Asia and South America) and reflect the global problem of drug resistance.

I have reviewed 14 papers from a period of 18 months between November 2002 and April 2004. I believe these papers represent the most important publications during this period. The topics are diverse and cover clinical studies, microbial resistance, epidemiology, experiences with the current registered vaccines and new approaches to vaccination.

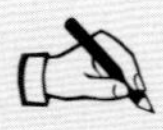

Background document: the diagnosis, treatment and prevention of typhoid fever. Communicable Disease Surveillance and Response, Vaccines and Biologicals

World Health Organization, 2003 (WHO/V&B/03.07)
http://www.who.int/vaccines-documents/

BACKGROUND. This is the current position paper of the WHO on typhoid fever, with detailed chapters on the epidemiology, diagnosis, clinical management, treatment and prevention of typhoid fever.

INTERPRETATION. The definitive diagnosis of typhoid fever depends on the isolation of *S. typhi* from blood, bone marrow or a specific anatomical lesion. Because a low level of bacteraemia (between 1 and 10 bacteria per ml of blood) is characteristic of typhoid fever, a large volume of blood is one of the most important factors in the successful isolation of *S. typhi*. The authors suggest a volume of 10–15 ml for schoolchildren and adults, and 2–4 ml for toddlers and preschool children. Antimicrobial susceptibility testing is crucial for the guidance of clinical management. It is recommended that antimicrobial susceptibility testing is performed against a fluoroquinolone, nalidixic acid (strains that are nalidixic acid-resistant show reduced susceptibility to fluoroquinolones, even when still within the current breakpoints for fluoroquinolone susceptibility), a third-generation cephalosporin, any other drug currently used for treatment and the previous first-line antibiotics to which the strains could be resistant (chloramphenicol, ampicillin, trimethoprim–sulphamethoxazole, streptomycin and tetracycline). The WHO guidelines recommend the fluoroquinolones (Table 9.1) as the first choice in the treatment of fully sensitive and MDR *S. typhi* in adults, and that they may also be used in children. Full fluoroquinolone resistance is still rare; azithromycin, a third-generation cephalosporin or a 10- to 14-day course of high-dose fluoroquinolones is effective in these cases.

Table 9.1 Treatment of uncomplicated typhoid fever

Susceptibility	Optimal therapy			Alternative effective drugs		
	Antibiotic	**Daily dose mg/kg**	**Days**	**Antibiotic**	**Daily dose mg/kg**	**Days**
Fully sensitive	Fluoroquinolone e.g. ofloxacin or ciprofloxacin	15	5–7*	Chloramphenicol Amoxicillin TMP-SMX	50–75 75–100 8–40	14–21 14 14
Multidrug resistance	Fluoroquinolone or cefixime	15 15–20	5–7 7–14	Azithromycin Cefixime	8–10 15–20	7 7–14
Quinolone resistance†	Azithromycin or ceftriaxone	8–10 75	7 10–14	Cefixime	20	7–14

* Three-day courses are also effective, particularly so in epidemic containment.
† The optimum treatment for quinolone-resistant typhoid fever has not been determined. Azithromycin or a third-generation cephalosporin or a 10- to 14-day course of high-dose fluoroquinolones are effective. Combinations of these are now being evaluated.
Source: WHO (2003).

Comment

The four chapters of this paper give a state-of-the-art overview of the current issues concerning typhoid fever, including diagnosis, treatment, epidemiology and prevention. The document is targeted at public health professionals, clinicians and laboratory specialists, but it will also find an interested readership amongst medical students. Important points discussed are:

1. the importance of taking a good volume of blood (or bone marrow) for culture to help increase the sensitivity of detection of *S. typhi*;

2. the importance of undertaking *in vitro* antimicrobial sensitivity testing to guide therapy;

3. the recommendation that the fluoroquinolones are the drugs of choice for the treatment of typhoid fever; and

4. the recommendation to public health authorities to exploit the two currently available improved typhoid vaccinations, parenteral Vi polysaccharide and oral Ty21a, in large nursery- or school-based immunization programmes to reduce the burden of disease.

There are, however, still a number of clinical issues that remain unresolved in typhoid fever, such as the antibiotics of choice in severe/complicated typhoid fever, and whether the addition of dexamethasone reduces mortality in typhoid fever patients with severe disease.

Typhoid fever

Parry CM, Hien TT, Dougan G, White NJ, Farrar JJ. *N Engl J Med* 2002; **347**: 1770–82 [review]

BACKGROUND. In 2001, the complete 4.8 million base pairs of the genomic sequence of an MDR strain of *S. typhi* (CT 18) were determined. The strain was isolated from a young girl in the Mekong Delta region of Vietnam. CT 18 harbours two plasmids, the larger of which is pHCM1, an *inc*H1 conjugative plasmid about 218 kilobases (kb) in length, which encodes resistance to chloramphenicol, ampicillin, trimethoprim, sulphonamides and streptomycin. The smaller plasmid, pHCM2, is 106 kb in length and phenotypically cryptic |1|.

INTERPRETATION. This review gives a comprehensive summary of the pathogenesis, routes of transmission, clinical picture, complications and treatment of typhoid fever. Clinical complications of typhoid fever are most likely to occur in patients who have been ill for more than 2 weeks. Gastrointestinal bleeding is the most common, occurring in up to 10% of patients; it results from a necrotic Peyer's patch eroding the wall of an enteric blood vessel. In most cases the bleeding is slight and does not require blood transfusion, but in about 2% of cases the bleeding is clinically significant and can be rapidly fatal if a large vessel is involved. Intestinal perforation is the most serious complication, occurring in about 1–3% of hospitalized patients. Perforation is manifested as acute abdomen or as worsening of abdominal pain, a rising pulse and falling blood pressure. The incidence of typhoid encephalopathy varies among countries, and patients can present as apathetic, agitated or delirious. A reduced level of consciousness, often accompanied by shock, is associated with high mortality. The fluoroquinolones are the drugs of choice for the treatment of typhoid fever and the authors recommend their use at the highest possible dose for a minimum of 10–14 days to treat *S. typhi* that shows reduced susceptibility to the fluoroquinolones.

Comment

This paper gives an excellent overview of the current issues concerning typhoid fever and is highly recommended for further reading. The big problem in typhoid fever—the emerging antibiotic resistance—is covered in depth by this paper. The authors also discuss controversial issues like the use of dexamethasone to reduce mortality in severe typhoid, and they address the lack of evidence-based data to establish which is the best treatment in severe typhoid fever. Measurements to control typhoid fever need to be implemented to control the spread of drug resistance and reduce the burden of disease. Mass vaccination in schoolchildren or smaller children (with the upcoming Vi-conjugate vaccine) as part of the WHO's Expanded Program of Immunization would be effective strategies to control typhoid fever.

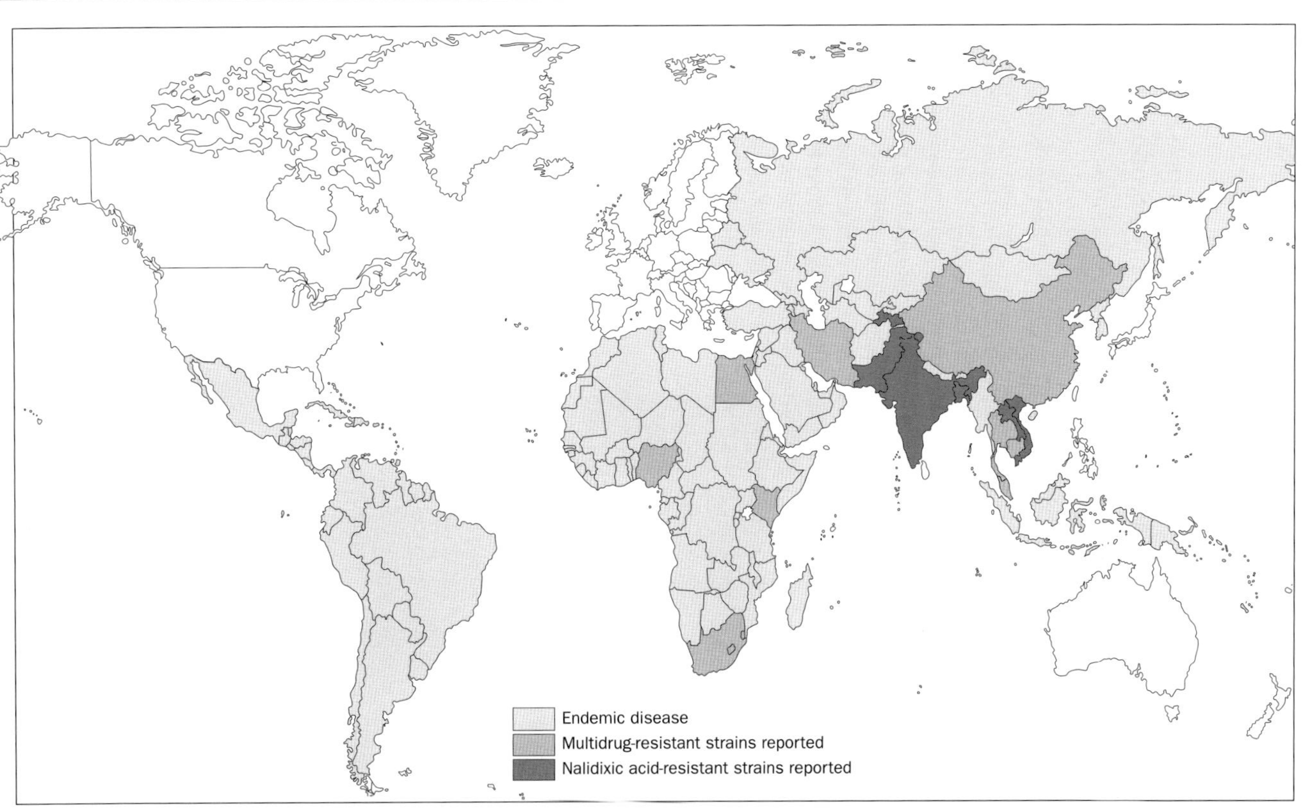

Fig. 9.1 Global distribution of resistance to *Salmonella enterica* serotype Typhi, 1990 to 2002. Source: Parry *et al.* (2002).

Clinical studies and antimicrobial resistance

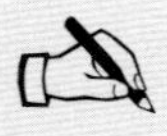

Persistence of Salmonellae in blood and bone marrow: randomized controlled trial comparing ciprofloxacin and chloramphenicol treatments against enteric fever

Gasem MH, Keuter M, Dolmans WM, Van Der Ven-Jongekrijg J, Djokomoeljanto R, Van Der Meer JW. *Antimicrob Agents Chemother* 2003; **47**: 1727–31

BACKGROUND. This paper reports a randomized controlled trial from Semarang, Indonesia, involving 55 adult patients with clinically suspected enteric fever to compare chloramphenicol treatment (500 mg four times a day orally) for 14 days and ciprofloxacin treatment (500 mg twice a day orally) for 7 days. Blood and bone marrow cultures and cytokine profiles during therapy were done to compare the clinical and bacteriological efficacies of these drugs. Fifty of the 55 patients had *Salmonella typhi*, and five patients had *Salmonella paratyphi* A isolated from their blood and/or bone marrow. All strains isolated were susceptible to both antibiotics. Twenty-seven patients received chloramphenicol and 28 received ciprofloxacin. Patients were considered clinically cured if they were afebrile within 7 days of antibiotic therapy.

INTERPRETATION. No significant differences in clinical cure and time to defervescence were found between the two groups. Two treatment failures were found in the chloramphenicol group and one failure in the ciprofloxacin group. The mean (SD) time to defervescence was 5.7 ± 2.2 days (range 3–12 days) in the chloramphenicol group and 5.1 ± 1.4 days (range 2–8 days) in the ciprofloxacin group. No relapse was found in either group, but long-term follow-up (beyond day 14) was not systematically pursued. Comparing the bacteriological response to therapy, there was no statistical difference between the elimination of *Salmonella* in blood between chloramphenicol and ciprofloxacin, but ciprofloxacin was more effective in the elimination of S. *typhi* and S. *paratyphi* A from bone marrow than chloramphenicol ($P < 0.05$). The persistence of *Salmonella* in the bone marrow culture was 100% for the chloramphenicol group and 67% for the ciprofloxacin group after 5 days of antibiotic therapy. Sequential blood samples were taken and stimulated with lipopolysaccharide (LPS) to look at *ex vivo* production of cytokines (TNF-α, IL-1β and IL-1 receptor antagonist). There were no significant differences in the restoration of LPS-stimulated production of TNF-α and IL-1β between the two groups, however LPS-induced IL-1β production on day 8 was significantly higher in the ciprofloxacin group.

Comment

The fluoroquinolones are currently recommended for the treatment of typhoid fever because they are less toxic and more effective than chloramphenicol. In this study all isolates were found to be sensitive to chloramphenicol and to the fluoroquinolones. Four S. *typhi* isolates were co-trimoxazole-resistant and one was ampicillin-resistant.

One of the *S. paratyphi* A isolates was resistant to amoxycillin and one to co-trimoxazole. This is the only published trial directly comparing chloramphenicol with the fluoroquinolones for the treatment of typhoid fever. It was a small study and the authors relied on surrogate markers to define treatment success, i.e. the capacity to eliminate *S. typhi* from bone marrow and the restoration of cytokine production, which is suppressed during the acute phase of typhoid infection and restored during convalescence. As a result, the answer to the question of whether the fluoroquinolone antibiotics, e.g. ciprofloxacin, are more effective than chloramphenicol for the treatment of typhoid fever remains unsolved. The small number of patients and the lack of follow-up did not allow a clear statement. The sample sizes were too small to show either superiority or equivalence. The argument is that, as a result of their rapid bactericidal effect and high intracellular concentrations in human phagocytic cells and bone marrow tissues, the fluoroquinolones are more effective. This remains an important question that a larger study with rigorous follow-up to identify carriers should be designed to answer.

Re-evaluating fluoroquinolone breakpoints for *Salmonella enterica* serotype Typhi and for non-Typhi salmonellae

Crump JA, Barrett TJ, Nelson JT, Angulo FJ. *Clin Infect Dis* 2003; **37**: 75–81

BACKGROUND. Antimicrobial resistance of *S. typhi* and non-Typhi *Salmonella* to traditional first-line antibiotics, such as ampicillin, chloramphenicol and trimethoprim–sulphonamide combinations, has emerged worldwide in the past few decades. Consequently, the quinolone antimicrobial agents, particularly the fluoroquinolones, have become the drugs of choice. Since the 1990s an increasing number of nalidixic acid-resistant *S. typhi* and non-Typhi *Salmonella*, isolated from humans or food animals, have been reported in the literature.

INTERPRETATION. In 1996 to 1997, 20 (6.8%) out of 293 *S. typhi* isolates reported to the Center for Disease Control and Prevention were nalidixic acid-resistant, by 2000, 41 (23.2%) out of 177 were nalidixic acid-resistant. Eighty per cent of *S. typhi* infections are acquired abroad, reflecting the global increase in nalidixic acid resistance. A similar increase in the prevalence of nalidixic acid resistance has been noted among non-Typhi *Salmonella* isolates. These infections are usually acquired domestically and their reservoir is food animals. Such *Salmonella* isolates typically have decreased susceptibility to fluoroquinolones, although MICs are usually within the susceptible range of the NCCLS criteria. The current breakpoints for Enterobacteriaceae (including *Salmonella*) for ciprofloxacin are ≥4 mg/l (resistant) and ≤1 mg/l (susceptible). The breakpoints for nalidixic acid are ≥32 mg/l (resistant) and ≤16 mg/l (susceptible). This reduction in susceptibility results in a poor clinical response to treatment. In 1997, a typhoid trial conducted in Vietnam showed that the median time to fever clearance was 156 h for patients infected with nalidixic acid-resistant *S. typhi* and 84 h for those infected with nalidixic acid-susceptible *S. typhi* ($P \leq 0.001$). Furthermore 33% of the nalidixic acid-resistant *S. typhi* infections required retreatment, whereas only 0.8% of the infections caused by nalidixic acid-susceptible *S. typhi* required retreatment. In an outbreak of infection with MDR *S.*

typhimurium DT104 caused by contaminated pork in Denmark during 1998, ciprofloxacin therapy lacked clinical effect for five (19%) of 27 patients. Two patients died with intestinal perforations and three patients had persistent diarrhoea, despite receiving ciprofloxacin therapy at recommended doses. The outbreak strain was resistant to nalidixic acid, but had MICs for ciprofloxacin of 0.06–0.12 mg/l. The authors recommend that laboratories test extra-intestinal *Salmonella* isolates for nalidixic acid resistance, and that short-course fluoroquinolone therapy should be avoided in the case of nalidixic acid-resistant *Salmonella* infections.

Comment

Nalidixic acid-resistant *S. typhi* and non-Typhi *Salmonella* infections exhibit a decreased clinical response to fluoroquinolones. This manifests in significantly longer fever clearance times, longer hospital admissions and a higher rate of relapse. The authors suggest that testing for resistance to nalidixic acid should be used as a screening tool and, if resistance is demonstrated, short-course (2–3 days) fluoro-quinolone therapy should be avoided. A better understanding of the pharmaco-dynamics of nalidixic acid-resistant bacteria and further clinical studies are needed to establish whether higher doses of fluoroquinolones taken for 7–10 days would reduce clinical and bacteriological failure rates. These clinical and bacteriological data strongly suggest that the current NCCLS fluoroquinolone breakpoints for resistance need to be re-evaluated for *Salmonella*.

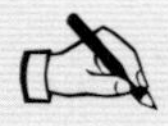

Is it time to change fluoroquinolone breakpoints for *Salmonella* spp.?

Aarestrup FM, Wiuff C, Molbak K, Threlfall EJ. *Antimicrob Agents Chemother* 2003; **47**: 827–9

BACKGROUND. Infections with *Salmonella* spp. are one of the most common causes of human gastroenteritis worldwide. Non-Typhi *Salmonella* infections are primarily caused by the consumption of contaminated food of animal origin. The use of fluoroquinolone antibiotics in animals since the early 1990s led to an increased incidence of human infections with nalidixic acid-resistant *Salmonella* strains, which exhibited decreased susceptibility to fluoroquinolones. The authors of this paper cite case reports and trials from different countries, including Denmark, France, India, Spain, the UK and Vietnam, that support evidence that the treatment efficacy of fluoroquinolones is reduced in humans infected with strains of *Salmonella* that show decreased susceptibility to fluoroquinolones.

INTERPRETATION. The current NCCLS breakpoints for resistance for Enterobacteriaceae (including *Salmonella*) for ciprofloxacin are ≥4 mg/l (resistant) and ≤1 mg/l (susceptible). The breakpoint for resistance for its veterinary equivalent, enrofloxacin, is ≥2 mg/l. The paper summarizes two case reports from *S. typhi* infections in Denmark and the UK that failed to respond to ciprofloxacin treatment; MICs for these strains were 0.19 and 0.5 mg/l (for ciprofloxacin). A trial from India showed that 32 out of 140 children infected with *S. typhi* did not respond adequately to treatment with ciprofloxacin; MICs for these strains were between 0.0625 and 0.5 mg/l. In a trial from Vietnam undertaken in 1996, 18 out of 150 culture-confirmed patients were infected with nalidixic acid-resistant *S. typhi*, which showed higher clinical failure rates, when treated with ofloxacin. The MICs for these strains for ofloxacin were between 0.125 and 1 mg/l. The study also cites the experience in Denmark in 1998, where, in an outbreak of infection with MDR *S. typhimurium* DT104 caused by contaminated pork, ciprofloxacin therapy failed in five (19%) out of 27 patients (see also the previous paper). The authors suggest that the breakpoint for resistance for *Salmonella* should be changed to ≥0.125 mg/l for fluoroquinolones. Ideally, *Salmonella* strains would be screened first for nalidixic acid resistance and then the MICs for the relevant fluoroquinolone would be determined for all nalidixic acid-resistant isolates.

Comment

This is the second paper included in this chapter that argues for the need to change the current NCCLS breakpoints for resistance to the fluoroquinolones. Clinical and bacteriological data suggest that the current NCCLS fluoroquinolone breakpoints for resistance are misleading and need to be re-evaluated for *Salmonella*. The current breakpoints for fluoroquinolones are too generous and may obscure the true prevalence of resistance amongst *Salmonella* strains. The breakpoint suggested by the authors, of ≥0.125 mg/l for resistance to the fluoroquinolones, also reflects our clinical experience. The implications of reclassifying a substantial proportion of *Salmonella* isolates as fluoroquinolone-non-susceptible are far-reaching. It might be that parts of the world would lose the fluoroquinolone class of antibiotics for the treatment of *S. typhi* and non-Typhi *Salmonella* altogether. Alternatives for treatment might be too expensive or lack the excellent tissue penetration and quick bacteriological clearance that the fluoroquinolones show for the nalidixic acid-susceptible isolates. Generally, the two major mechanisms fuelling drug resistance are the uncontrolled and indiscriminate use of antibiotics in many countries and the use of antibiotics in food animals. Tighter regulations in both areas would help to sustain an otherwise excellent class of antibiotics for use in humans.

Short-course azithromycin for the treatment of uncomplicated typhoid fever in children and adolescents

Frenck RW Jr, Mansour A, Nakhla I, *et al*. *Clin Infect Dis* 2004; **38**: 951–7

BACKGROUND. This study from Egypt recruited 149 children and adolescents (3–17 years of age) with clinical typhoid fever who were treated with either oral azithromycin (20 mg/kg per day; maximum dose, 1000 mg/day) or intravenous ceftriaxone (75 mg/day; maximum dose, 2.5 g/day) daily for 5 days. Blood and stool specimens were obtained for culture before the initiation of therapy and were repeated on days 4 and 8 of treatment. *S. typhi* was isolated from 68 patients, 32 of whom were receiving azithromycin.

INTERPRETATION. Both antibiotic therapies were highly effective. Mean ($\pm$ SD) time to defervescence was 4.5 $\pm$ 1.9 days for patients who received azithromycin and 3.6 $\pm$ 1.6 days for patients who received ceftriaxone (P = non-significant). Clinical cure (defined as the resolution of all typhoid-related symptoms within 7 days of initiating therapy) was achieved in 30 (94%) of 32 patients in the azithromycin group and in 35 (97%) of 36 patients in the ceftriaxone group (P = non-significant). Clinical failures in both groups were due to mild gastrointestinal symptoms or persistent fever that resolved without any additional treatment. Microbiological cure (defined as a sterile blood culture on day 8, 3 days after discontinuation of antibiotic therapy) was achieved in every patient treated with azithromycin and in 35 (97%) of patients treated with ceftriaxone (P = 0.5). Antibiotic susceptibility testing was performed on all the *S. typhi* isolates. No isolate was resistant to either ceftriaxone or ciprofloxacin, one isolate was resistant to co-trimoxazole, two were resistant to chloramphenicol and three were resistant to ampicillin. Only one isolate was MDR, with resistance to chloramphenicol, ampicillin and co-trimoxazole. Seven isolates had an MIC of $\geq$8 mg/l for azithromycin, classifying them as resistant. Four of these 'resistant' isolates were from patients randomized to the azithromycin group, and all of these patients achieved clinical and microbiological cure. Mean time to clearance of bacteraemia was longer in the azithromycin group than in the ceftriaxone group. None of the patients treated with ceftriaxone had *S. typhi* recovered from blood cultures on day 4 of therapy, whereas twelve patients (37.5%) treated with azithromycin had *S. typhi* recovered from their blood on day 4. All these twelve isolates were susceptible to azithromycin. No patient who received azithromycin had a relapse, compared with six patients who received ceftriaxone. A 5-day course of azithromycin was found to be an effective treatment for uncomplicated typhoid fever in children and adolescents.

Comment

This is an important study (although not the first one) that looks at alternatives to the fluoroquinolones to treat typhoid fever. Azithromycin, a macrolide antibiotic, shows excellent tissue penetration and secretion into the biliary tree, and achieves concentrations in macrophages and neutrophils that are more than 100-fold higher than concentrations in serum. These properties make it an excellent choice for the treatment of a principally intracellular infection such as typhoid fever. The disadvantage is that azithromycin is considerably more expensive than the fluoroquinolones. Previous studies in Egypt and Vietnam showed that oral azithromycin was highly effective against uncomplicated typhoid fever in adults and children |2|. One problem is that the appropriate breakpoint recommendations for azithromycin are still not clear, as in this study, so patients may show satisfactorily clinical and microbiological responses even if isolates are intermediate or resistant according to current guidelines. Six (19%) out of 32 patients who received intravenous ceftriaxone therapy had a confirmed relapse; this is consistent with other reports in the literature. Because of the need for parenteral administration and the high relapse rate, ceftriaxone is not an ideal option for the routine treatment of typhoid fever.

Adjunctive treatment with antipyretics

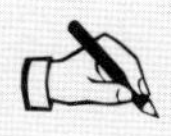

Double-blind comparison of ibuprofen and paracetamol for adjunctive treatment of uncomplicated typhoid fever

Vinh H, Parry CM, Hanh VT, *et al. Pediatr Infect Dis J* 2004; **23**: 226–30

BACKGROUND. The prolonged, high fever is characteristic of infection with S. typhi, especially in children. The benefits of non-steroidal drugs in this role have not been quantified. There have been concerns about the safety of antipyretics in typhoid. In 1956 Dowdle reported five adults with typhoid fever who developed sweating, collapse and bradycardia after a sudden decrease in temperature with the use of aspirin. None of these patients needed intravenous fluids and the symptoms resolved within hours. This report has discouraged the use of antipyretics in typhoid fever. In this double-blind randomized study, 80 Vietnamese children with uncomplicated typhoid fever were randomized to receive identical syrup preparations of ibuprofen (10 mg/kg) or paracetamol (12 mg/kg) every 6 h until 36 h after defervescence. Children with a nalidixic acid-susceptible isolate of S. typhi were treated with ofloxacin (15 mg/kg/day) for 3 days and those with a nalidixic acid-resistant isolate were treated for 7 days.

INTERPRETATION. S. typhi was isolated from 36 of 40 children randomized to ibuprofen (eleven isolates were nalidixic acid-resistant) and 37 of 40 randomized to paracetamol (13 isolates were nalidixic acid-resistant). The median and range of fever clearance time (Table 9.2) was shorter in the ibuprofen group than the paracetamol group (68, 4–260 vs 104, 12–404; $P = 0.055$) as was the area under the temperature time curve above 37°C (74, 0–237 vs 127, 0–573; $P = 0.013$). The differences occurred predominantly in the children infected with a nalidixic acid-resistant S. typhi (Table 9.3), whose infections responded more slowly to antibiotic treatment. There were no major side effects associated with the use of either drug. Excessive sweating after defervescence occurred in two children in the ibuprofen group and one child in the paracetamol group, but this was not accompanied by a fall in blood pressure or bradycardia. One child who received ibuprofen had slight melaena for 2 days, but with no significant change in haematocrit. There were no convulsions. No differences between the two treatment arms in the concentrations of circulating IL-6 and TNF-α during the course of treatment were found. The antipyretic effect of ibuprofen is superior to that of paracetamol in children with typhoid fever, particularly those with prolonged fever. Both antipyretics appeared to be safe.

Comment

This is a well-designed and important study that contributes to the management of children (and adults) with typhoid fever. To our knowledge this is the first study giving evidence of which antipyretic is best to use to reduce the prolonged fever in children. In a previous, unpublished study by the same authors, the median fever clearance time in children infected with a nalidixic acid-resistant strain of S. *typhi* was an unpleasant 207 h; therefore a placebo arm was not included in this study.

Table 9.2 Response to treatment with ofloxacin in combination with either ibuprofen or paracetamol

Outcome variable	Ibuprofen (*n* = 40)	Paracetamol (*n* = 40)	*P*
Clinical failure (%)	1 (3)	4 (10)	0.359
Microbiological failure (%)	0 (0)	0 (0)	1.00
Relapse (%)	2 (5)	1 (3)	0.513
Faecal culture-positive (%)	0/23 (0)	2/25 (8)	0.490
Fever clearance time (h)*	68 (4–260)†	104 (12–404)	0.055
Area under the temperature time curve (°C above 37°C h)*	74 (0–237)	127 (0–573)	0.013
Duration of hospital admission after start of treatment (days)*	8 (4–14)	8 (4–20)	0.281
Children with possible side effects	13	7	0.197
Diarrhoea	8	4	0.348
Abdominal pain	4	2	0.675
Sweating	3	1	0.615
Coryza	1	1	1.00
Melaena	1	0	1.00
Epistaxis	0	1	1.00

* Continuous variables expressed as medians with range.
† Numbers in parentheses, range.
Source: Vinh *et al.* (2004).

Table 9.3 Response to treatment with ofloxacin in combination with either ibuprofen or paracetamol. The fever response is differentiated by the nalidixic acid susceptibility of the infecting isolate

Outcome variable	Ibuprofen	Paracetamol	*P*
Children with nalidixic acid-susceptible typhoid fever	*n* = 25	*n* = 24	
Fever clearance time (h)*	68 (8–148)†	68 (28–232)	0.383
Area under the temperature time curve (°C above 37°C h)*	69 (3–230)	96 (19–362)	0.073
Duration of hospital admission after start of treatment (days)*	7 (4–12)	7 (5–12)	0.846
Children with nalidixic acid-resistant typhoid fever	*n* = 11	*n* = 13	
Fever clearance time (h)	116 (4–260)	164 (88–404)	0.207
Area under the temperature time curve (°C above 37°C h)	128 (0–237)	169 (83–573)	0.026
Duration of hospital admission after start of treatment (days)*	9 (5–14)	9 (8–20)	0.331

* Continuous variables expressed as medians with range.
† Numbers in parentheses, range.
Source: Vinh *et al.* (2004).

Epidemiology

Association between *Helicobacter pylori* infection and increased risk of typhoid fever

Bhan MK, Bahl R, Sazawal S, *et al. J Infect Dis* 2002; **186**: 1857–60

BACKGROUND. *Helicobacter pylori* infection has been reported to increase the risk of cholera. The aim of this nested case–control study was to find out whether *H. pylori* infection would increase susceptibility to *S. typhi* infection as a result of the induced hypochlorhydria. Eighty-three case subjects of culture-proven typhoid fever were identified in a 1-year surveillance of subjects aged 0–40 years in an urban slum community in south Delhi. Two age- and sex-matched neighbourhood control subjects were concurrently selected for each case subject. Data on family and personal characteristics, socio-economic indicators and the previous 3 weeks' consumption of food and drinks were collected from case subjects and matched control subjects by trained field workers. Serum anti-*H. pylori* immunoglobulin (Ig) G antibodies were measured in case and neighbourhood control subjects with a commercially available enzyme-linked immunosorbent assay (ELISA). To determine other risk factors, two additional community control subjects per case were selected to avoid overmatching for risk factors such as water and sanitation; these subjects were interviewed in the same way, but blood samples for serological testing of *H. pylori* were not obtained.

INTERPRETATION. Serum anti-*H. pylori* IgG antibodies were detected in 64% of case subjects (53 of 83) and 50% of neighbourhood control subjects. After adjusting for confounders (such as age, family size, source of water, open garbage within the house, food outside the home in the past 3 weeks) in a conditional logistic regression model, there remained a significant association between the presence of serum anti-*H. pylori* IgG antibodies and typhoid fever (adjusted odds ratio [OR] 2.03; 95% confidence interval 1.02–4.01). Illiteracy, being part of a nuclear family, non-use of soap, and consumption of ice-cream were also associated with a significantly greater risk of typhoid fever. This study provides the first empirical evidence that *H. pylori* infection is associated with an increased risk of typhoid fever.

Comment

This is an interesting study. To our knowledge it is the first to look at the risk of typhoid fever in individuals with previous or active infection with *H. pylori*, set up as a nested study within a cohort study for the surveillance of typhoid fever. The association found was only moderate, with an OR of 2 (two-fold risk). One weakness of the study is that the authors do not give data on the sensitivity and specificity of their serological test for *H. pylori* when compared with the gold standard (culture). Infection with *H. pylori* in the case subjects and control subjects might have been more common than shown in this study. *H. pylori* infections occur widely among children in developing countries. Studies have demonstrated that *H. pylori* infection is associated with an increased risk of cholera, diarrhoea and typhoid fever in childhood and an increased risk of gastroduodenal disease in adult life. Further big studies are probably needed to help in deciding whether its prevention should be a priority.

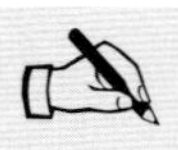

Estimating the incidence of typhoid fever and other febrile illnesses in developing countries

Crump JA, Youssef FG, Luby SP, *et al*. *Emerg Infect Dis* 2003; **9**: 539–44

BACKGROUND. The aim of this study was to set up a sensitive and specific surveillance system that measures the incidence and causes of febrile illness in Bilbeis District, Egypt. First, a household survey was conducted to determine patterns of health-seeking among persons with fever for more than 3 days. A contemporary census of all district health services and health providers from the Bilbeis District Health Office was obtained, recording one district fever hospital, eleven fever specialists and 68 primary care providers (general practitioners, internal medicine physicians and rural health unit doctors). The surveillance was conducted from July to October 2001 at the fever hospital, among the eleven fever specialists and among a random selection of ten (15%) of 68 other representative health providers. All persons above 6 months of age visiting a surveillance health provider during the 4-month study period and with current fever of more than 3 days' duration were invited to participate. After obtaining informed consent from the febrile patients, a brief questionnaire capturing demographic and clinical information was administered, and blood was collected for culture and serological testing. Health-care providers were trained in obtaining blood cultures, sterile technique and needle safety. Materials for venipuncture and blood culture were provided by the study. Training of laboratory technicians, new equipment and provision of all materials necessary to process blood cultures and identify bacteria strengthened the laboratory capacity of the microbiology unit at the central fever hospital in Bilbeis.

INTERPRETATION. In total, 449 patients were enrolled at the sentinel surveillance sites. *S. typhi* was isolated by blood culture from 19 (4.2%) patients. The median age of patients with typhoid fever was 22 years (range 5–60 years); five patients (26.3%) were female. *Brucella* spp. was isolated by blood culture from 15 (3.3%) patients, and brucellosis was confirmed by positive tube agglutination assay (titre ≥1:160) for another 16 (3.6%). The median age of patients with brucellosis was 31 years (range 11–60 years); twelve (38.7%) were female. *Escherichia coli* and *Haemophilus influenzae* serotype b were each isolated by blood culture from one patient. No non-Typhi *Salmonella* were isolated. In total, 302 (71%) of 432 patients were already using an antimicrobial agent at the time they sought treatment by a health provider, reflecting the global epidemic of community antibiotic abuse. After adjusting for the provider sampling scheme (only 15% of primary care providers in the district were included in the study, so their results were multiplied by 6.8), test sensitivity (a multiplier of 2.0 was applied to account for the estimated 50% test sensitivity of a single blood culture for the diagnosis of typhoid fever) and seasonality, the authors estimated that the incidence of typhoid fever was 13/100 000 persons per year, and the incidence of brucellosis was 18/100 000 persons per year in the district.

Table 9.4 Incidence estimates for typhoid fever and brucellosis, Bilbeis district, Egypt, 2001

Disease	No. of cases captured by surveillance site type Crude (adjusted*)				Test sensitivity multiplier	Seasonality multiplier	Total cases	Incidence (/100 000)
	Fever hospital	Fever specialist	Primary provider	Total				
Typhoid fever	6.0 (6.0)	13.0 (13.0)	0.0	19.0 (19.0)	2.0	2.2	83.6	12.6
Brucellosis	15.0 (15.0)	12.0 (12.0)	4.0 (27.2)	31.0 (54.2)	1.0	2.2	119.2	18.0

* Adjusted for health provider sampling scheme. No multiplier is applied for cases identified at the fever hospital and among fever specialists. A multiplier of 6.8 is applied for cases identified among primary providers.
Source: Crump et al. (2003).

Comment

The most reliable existing estimates of the typhoid fever incidence in Egypt were established during typhoid vaccine studies conducted more than two decades earlier. These studies documented an annual typhoid fever incidence of 209/100 000 persons in 1972–1973 and of 48/100 000 persons in 1978–1981 among school-aged children in Alexandria, Egypt. The study reported by Crump *et al.* (2003) among all age groups in a single district showed annual typhoid incidence rates that were lower, at 13/100 000 persons. This finding is consistent with a study design not targeted at a high-incidence population, improved management of diarrhoeal disease and the growing proportions of persons living in both rural and urban areas with access to safe water. The incidence and relative importance of the aetiological agents of febrile illness remain unknown in many parts of the world. The authors present a relatively simple and timely restricted surveillance tool for febrile illness that could be adapted for use in other countries and could be extended to include surveillance for other febrile illnesses, such as malaria. This data would be important for public health personnel in developing countries in order to guide priorities for the use of scarce health resources and to refine a policy on the empirical management of febrile illness. Such sentinel surveillance could be conducted every 5 years in a region to update the management of disease incidence and to guide syndrome-based patient management.

The global burden of typhoid fever

Crump JA, Luby, SP, Mintz ED. *Bull World Health Organ* 2004; **82**: 346–53
http://www.who.int/bulletin/volumes/82/5/en/346.pdf

BACKGROUND. The aim of this study was to use new data to make a revised estimate of the global burden of typhoid fever to guide public health decisions for disease control and prevention. A computer search of the multilingual scientific literature between 1996 and 2001 was carried out to find data on the incidence of typhoid fever. Studies were selected for inclusion if they were population-based (i.e. they captured cases at all levels of the healthcare system or by regular household visits) and confirmed the diagnosis of *S. typhi* by blood culture. Studies that were conducted during typhoid fever epidemics were not considered. A total of 22 studies were eligible.

INTERPRETATION. The world's population was divided into seventeen 5-year strata from 0–4 years to >80 years, and 21 regions. Where there were no eligible studies, data were extrapolated from neighbouring countries and regions. Age–incidence curves were used to adjust incidence rates measured among narrow age cohorts, such as schoolchildren, to the general population. Regions with a high incidence of typhoid fever (>100/100 000 cases/year) include south-central Asia and south-east Asia. Regions of medium incidence (10–100/100 000 cases/year) include the rest of Asia, Africa, Latin America and the Caribbean, and Oceania, except for Australia and New Zealand. Europe, North America, and the rest of the developed world have low incidences of typhoid fever

(<10/100 000 cases/year). The total number of typhoid fever cases in 2000 was calculated by age stratum for each region and the sum of total cases (Table 9.5) was calculated as the crude global typhoid fever burden (10 835 487). To adjust for the 50% sensitivity of blood culture for diagnosing typhoid fever, an adjustment factor of 2 was applied, producing a

Table 9.5 Crude typhoid fever incidence rates by region, 2000

Area/region	Typhoid cases	Population	Crude incidence*	Incidence classification
Africa				
Eastern Africa†	98 560	255 500 000	39	Medium
Middle Africa†	36 857	95 385 000	39	Medium
Northern Africa	58 210	175 037 000	33	Medium
Southern Africa	123 473	52 887 000	233	High
Western Africa†	91 737	241 102 000	38	Medium
Area total	**408 837**	**819 911 000**	**50**	**Medium**
Asia				
Eastern Asia	182 927	1 483 111 000	12	Medium
South-central Asia	9 299 064	1 495 977 000	622	High
South-eastern Asia	575 407	521 983 000	110	High
Western Asia†	61 481	187 463 000	33	Medium
Area total	**10 118 879**	**3 688 534 000**	**274**	**High**
Europe				
Eastern Europe	15 940	306 654 000	5	Low
Northern Europe	143	93 736 000	<1	Low
Southern Europe	2785	144 861 000	2	Low
Western Europe	276	184 077 000	<1	Low
Area total	**19 144**	**729 328 000**	**3**	**Low**
Latin America/Caribbean				
Caribbean†	19 889	37 757 000	53	Medium
Central America†	79 164	135 497 000	58	Medium
South America	174 465	341 434 000	51	Medium
Area total	**273 518**	**514 688 000**	**53**	**Medium**
Northern America				
Northern America	453	308 636 000	<1	Low
Area total	**453**	**308 636 000**	**<1**	**Low**
Oceania				
Australia/New Zealand	62	22 598 000	<1	Low
Melanesia†	3897	6 489 000	60	Medium
Micronesia†	326	539 000	60	Medium
Polynesia	371	626 000	59	Medium
Area total	**4656**	**30 252 000**	**15**	**Medium**
Global				
Crude total	10 825 487	6 091 349 000	178	High
Adjusted total	21 650 974	6 091 349 000	355	

* Per 100 000 persons per year.
† Regional incidence estimate derived by extrapolation.
Source: Crump *et al.* (2004).

global typhoid fever case burden estimate of 21 650 974. A conservative case–fatality rate of 1% was chosen on the basis of estimates from hospital-based typhoid fever studies, mortality data from countries with a reliable national typhoid fever surveillance system, and expert opinion. The burden of paratyphoid fever was derived by a proportional method. The study estimated that typhoid fever caused 21 650 974 illnesses and 216 510 deaths during 2000 and that paratyphoid fever caused 5 412 744 illnesses.

Comment

This paper makes a valuable contribution to updating the current incidence estimates. The previous estimate of the global burden of typhoid fever, of 16 million illnesses and 600 000 deaths annually, was presented at the Meeting of the Pan American Health Organization in 1984 and was published in 1986. This 1984 estimate was subject to several limitations. The methods were not outlined in detail so the study could not be reproduced (the estimate excluded China); incidence, risk and the denominator population have changed considerably in the meantime. As outlined in the paper, data from the African continent on the incidence of typhoid fever or other febrile illnesses remain scarce and further studies would be needed to improve the estimate (most studies reported from Africa use the Widal test and not blood culture, so they were not included in this analysis). One weakness of the study is that the mortality of typhoid fever had to be guessed – as 1% – but this is just a reflection of the lack of data.

Trends of multiple-drug resistance among *Salmonella* serotype Typhi isolates during a 14-year period in Egypt

Wasfy MO, Frenck R, Ismail TF, Mansour H, Malone JL, Mahoney FJ. *Clin Infect Dis* 2002; **35**: 1265–8

BACKGROUND. This study was carried out in a 1500-bed infectious disease hospital in Cairo, Egypt, that serves an estimated population of 16 million people. During a 14-year period, from 1987 to 2000, a total of 853 *S. typhi* isolates were identified in blood culture and underwent antibiotic susceptibility testing using the disc diffusion Kirby-Bauer method to determine multiple drug resistance (in this paper this is defined as resistance to more than two antibiotics: ampicillin, chloramphenicol and trimethoprim–sulphamethoxazole or tetracycline).

INTERPRETATION. Resistance to individual antibiotics varied dramatically during the reported period. For example, the prevalence of ampicillin-resistant isolates was 100% in 1993 but decreased to only 5% by 2000. The prevalence of MDR *S. typhi* isolates increased from 19% in 1987 to 100% in 1993, but subsequently decreased again to only 5% by 2000 (Table 9.6). The authors conclude that the observed resurgence of chloramphenicol susceptibility ($P = 0.002$) may suggest the re-use of this drug for the treatment of typhoid fever in Egypt.

Table 9.6 Percentage of MDR *Salmonella* serotype Typhi isolates recovered from patients with typhoid fever at a hospital in Cairo, Egypt, during a 14-year period, according to the results of susceptibility testing

Percentage of MDR *S.* Typhi isolates (total no. of *S.* Typhi isolates)

Year	Amp	Chl	TMP-SMX	Em	Tet	MDR
1987	19 (75)	20 (60)	NA	80 (70)	NA	19 (60)
1988	24 (58)	25 (28)	24 (28)	75 (2)	11 (28)	24 (28)
1989	45 (51)	30 (10)	45 (38)	69 (51)	41 (41)	45 (51)
1990	65 (48)	59 (48)	29 (48)	92 (48)	NA	60 (48)
1991	65 (114)	61 (93)	55 (111)	90 (93)	56 (111)	61 (127)
1992	66 (114)	28 (114)	53 (114)	100 (110)	49 (114)	53 (114)
1993	100 (27)	100 (27)	100 (27)	NA	NA	100 (27)
1994	45 (20)	45 (20)	45 (20)	NA	NA	45 (9)
1995	62 (50)	62 (50)	62 (50)	NA	NA	62 (31)
1996	4 (29)	4 (29)	4 (29)	NA	NA	14 (4)
1997	20 (85)	15 (85)	22 (83)	NA	19 (42)	15 (83)
1998	15 (41)	15 (41)	17 (41)	NA	NA	15 (41)
1999	9 (100)	9 (100)	9 (100)	NA	NA	9 (100)
2000	5 (41)	5 (41)	5 (41)	NA	NA	5 (41)
Total	43.4 (853)	33 (746)	37.4 (730)	88 (400)	43.5 (336)	37.7 (764)

Multiple drug resistance (MDR) was defined as resistance to more than two antibiotics, including ampicillin and chloramphenicol. Amp, ampicillin; Chl, chloramphenicol; TMP-SMX, trimethoprim–sulphamethoxazole; Em, erythromycin; Tet, tetracycline; NA, not available.
Source: Wasfy *et al.* (2002).

Comment

This paper demonstrates the importance of antibiotic susceptibility monitoring for the treatment of infectious diseases in general. Antibiotic resistance patterns among *S. typhi* isolates in Egypt changed significantly over relatively short periods, reflecting changes in treatment policies and therefore the withdrawal of drug pressure. It is postulated that, in the absence of antibiotic pressure, *S. typhi* strains lose their resistance plasmid. Other parts of the world, for instance India and Bangladesh, reported similar increases in the prevalence of chloramphenicol-susceptible *S. typhi* isolates. The disadvantage of administering chloramphenicol for the treatment of typhoid fever is the long course of treatment (2–3 weeks), the large number of tablets (an adult would often have to take >250 capsules) and the small but real risk of agranulocytosis (1:10 000).

Vaccines

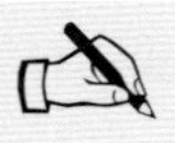

Experience with registered mucosal vaccines

Dietrich G, Griot-Wenk M, Metcalfe IC, Lang AB, Viret JF. *Vaccine* 2003; **21**: 678–83

BACKGROUND. This paper reviews the immune responses and protective efficacy elicited by the two registered live oral vaccines, *S. typhi* Ty21a and *Vibrio cholerae* CVD 103-HgR-, which are employed as vaccines against typhoid fever and cholera, respectively. Ty21a, developed in the 1970s by chemical mutagenesis of the pathogenic *S. typhi* strain Ty2, is available in two commercial forms, as enteric coated capsules and as a liquid formulation; both formulations are given in three doses within 1 week (in the US and Canada four enteric coated capsules are given). *S. typhi* is a facultative intracellular bacterium characterized by mucosal invasion and systemic spreading. Both antibody (mucosal IgA and serum IgG) and cell-mediated immune (CMI) responses are involved in protection against typhoid fever. Ty21a induces local immune responses through colonization and multiplication of the vaccine bacteria in the host, and induces CMI responses through its invasive properties.

INTERPRETATION. Three doses of Ty21a induce seroconversion (defined as greater than a two-fold rise over baseline) in about 70% of vaccinated subjects, as measured by serum IgG antibodies and gut-derived IgA antibodies against the bacterial LPS. Vaccination with Ty21a elicits strong CD4$^+$ T-helper type 1 response and strong CD8$^+$ cytotoxic T cells that are able to lyse *S. typhi*-infected autologous target cells. These CMI responses were found to last at least 2 years after immunization. The protective efficacy and safety of Ty21a has been shown in a field trial in Chile. Three doses of the enteric coated capsules led to a protective efficacy of 67% during the first 3 years after vaccination and 62% protective efficacy over a period of 7 years |3|.The liquid formulation showed even better protective efficacy, three doses resulting in 77% protection over 3 years and 78% protection over 7 years.

Comment

The ideal vaccine against enteric pathogens would elicit a strong, long-lasting immune response at the site of infection as well as at the systemic level. The currently registered live attenuated bacterial vaccine strain Ty21a seems to fulfil all these criteria, is safe and shows protective efficacy of about 70%. If this vaccine were applied in regions or countries where typhoid is endemic, this would greatly reduce transmission and help to stop the spread of antimicrobial drug resistance. Ty21a is licensed only for children over 6 years of age (although in the meantime data have been presented on its safety and immunogenicity in children between 3 and 5 years). One weakness of this review article is that it does not consider the problems that a live vaccine such as Ty21a could pose to the immune-compromised host.

A further improvement in this field would be the development of a single-dose oral vaccine against typhoid fever. This is discussed in the next paper.

Vaccination and efficacy: experience with a one-dose oral live vaccine

Concomitant induction of CD4+ and CD8+ T-cell responses in volunteers immunized with *Salmonella enterica* serovar typhi strain CVD 908-htrA

Salerno-Goncalves R, Wyant TL, Pasetti MF, *et al*. *J Immunol* 2003; **170**: 2734–41

BACKGROUND. This study evaluates whether immunization with *S. typhi* strain CVD 908-htrA (a Δ aroC Δ aroD Δ htrA mutant), a leading live oral typhoid vaccine candidate, elicits specific CD4$^+$ and CD8$^+$ immune responses. Previous studies have shown that this auxotrophic mutant of *S. typhi* is clinically safe and highly immunogenic in Phase I and Phase II human clinical trials in a single dose |4|. In a previous trial, 80 adult volunteers received either high-dose (4.5 × 10^8 colony-forming units [c.f.u.]) or low-dose (0.5 × 10^8 c.f.u.) CVD 908-htrA or placebo. After 28 days a crossover took place. Peripheral blood mononuclear cells (PBMC) from 30 volunteers were used to look at the cell-mediated immune response.

INTERPRETATION. Potent cytotoxic T-cell (CTL) responses and interferon-γ (IFN-γ) secretion by CD8$^+$ T cells were detected after immunization with CVD 908-htrA in high and low doses. *S. typhi*-specific CTL were observed in six of eight vaccinated subjects (four high dose and two low dose) after immunization. Mean (±SD) increases in the frequency of IFN-γ spot-forming cells (SFC) in the presence of *S. typhi*-infected targets were 221 ± 41 and 233 ± 87 SFC/10^6 PBMC in the high- and low-dose groups, respectively. Strong CD4$^+$ T-cell responses were also observed. Increases in IFN-γ production in response to soluble *S. typhi* flagella occurred in 82 and 38$^\%$ of the volunteers who received the high and low doses, respectively. These data demonstrate the concomitant induction of both CD4- and CD8-mediated CMI and support the continuing evaluation of CVD 908-htrA as a typhoid vaccine candidate.

Comment

Both antibody and cell-mediated immune responses are involved in the protection against typhoid fever. This paper demonstrates the induction of cellular immunity against *S. typhi* CVD 908-htrA strain, a promising candidate for a one-dose oral vaccine. The development of such a vaccine would greatly facilitate administration and distribution in developing countries. Temperature-stable vaccines that can be administered needle-free |5| would have big advantages for the global community.

Vaccination and efficacy: Vi conjugate vaccine trial in children under 5 years of age

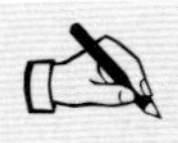

Persistent efficacy of Vi conjugate vaccine against typhoid fever in young children

Mai NL, Phan VB, Vo AH, *et al. N Engl J Med* 2003; **349**: 1390–1 [letter]

BACKGROUND. In 2001, the authors published a large double-blind randomized trial evaluating the safety, immunogenicity and efficacy of a new conjugate vaccine consisting of the capsular polysaccharide of *S. typhi*, Vi, bound to the non-toxic recombinant *Pseudomonas aeruginosa* exotoxin A (Vi-rEPA) in children between 2 and 5 years of age |6|. The trial was carried out in the Dong Thap province in the Mekong Delta region in Vietnam, where the incidence of typhoid fever was 413 per 100 000 for children younger than 15, and 358 per 100 000 for children between 2 and 4 years old. Two injections of either Vi-rEPA or saline were given to 11 091 children at a 6-week interval; 771 children received only one injection. Active surveillance took place over a period of 27 months. Typhoid fever was diagnosed by blood culture from children who had had fever for more than 3 days. In total there were four cases of typhoid fever among the 11 091 children who received two injections and 47 cases in children in the placebo group (91.5% vaccine efficacy). There was one case of typhoid fever among the 771 children who received only one injection of vaccine and eight cases in the placebo group (87.7% vaccine efficacy). In total, there were five cases of typhoid fever in the vaccine group and 56 in the placebo group (91.1% efficacy; 95% confidence interval 78.6–96.5%). Levels of serum IgG Vi antibodies in the vaccinated children had increased by a factor of 10 or more 4 weeks after the second vaccination. The Vi-rEPA vaccine was safe and immunogenic and had greater than 90% efficacy.

INTERPRETATION. In this letter, published in 2003, the authors report the results from a further 19-month period of passive surveillance after unblinding the data. Over the entire 46-month period, the vaccine showed an efficacy of 89%. There were no deaths or complications. After 46 months a crossover vaccination in the placebo group took place. A total of 5232 children in the placebo group received Vi-rEPA in January 2002. Only one injection was offered, because the levels of IgG anti-Vi antibodies induced by one injection in children 5–8 years old were similar to those induced by two injections in those 2–5 years old. There was a tendency towards age-related persistence of IgG anti-Vi antibodies, with higher levels found in the older children. At 46 months, the geometric mean level of IgG anti-Vi antibodies had decreased to 3.66 ELISA units among children in the vaccine group. It was therefore estimated that the protective levels of IgG anti-Vi antibodies would be approximately 3.5 ELISA units.

Comment

This large and superbly conducted trial involving more than 12 000 children in 16 communes in an endemic region in Vietnam targeted the age group of 2- to

5-year-old children. Previous epidemiological studies in Vietnam and other parts of south-east Asia have shown that the incidence of typhoid fever is highest in children under 5 years old. The currently registered typhoid vaccines do not protect young children. Ty21a, the oral *S. typhi* vaccine, is not licensed for use in children under 6 years and, because of its T-cell-independent properties, the currently used parenteral Vi-based vaccine is immunogenic only in children over 2 years of age. In this study, the capsular polysaccharide of *S. typhi*, Vi, was bound to a non-toxic recombinant protein, and the resulting conjugate enhanced the immunogenicity of Vi and gave it T-cell-dependent properties. The protective efficacy of Vi-rEPA was 89% over 4 years, the highest reported efficacy for any typhoid vaccine. The authors are planning to study the safety and immunogenicity of Vi-rEPA in infants or 9 months or younger. Ideally this vaccine could become part of the WHO's Expanded Program of Immunization in typhoid endemic countries. The disadvantages of the conjugate vaccines are their high cost, which makes them unaffordable in many developing countries, and their parenteral administration, which poses logistic problems. From this point of view, an oral live (attenuated) vaccine would be preferable because it would be cheaper and easier to administer, it induces immunity at the site of infection, and it expresses a broad cocktail of antigens.

Conclusion

Typhoid fever is a disease of poverty and remains endemic in many parts of the world. Antimicrobial resistance is a major problem in treating typhoid fever, the indiscriminate and uncontrolled use of antibiotics in many countries helping to fuel drug resistance. The options for treatment are increasingly limited. There is a very real danger that we will return to the pre-antibiotic era (when approximately 30% of patients with typhoid fever died) if resistance continues to evolve and spread.

The overall burden of disease is greatest in developing countries, where poor infrastructure and problems with the water supply and sanitation prevent its eradication. In these countries, typhoid fever contributes significantly to the overall morbidity and mortality. As is true for many diseases that mostly affect the poorest people, interventions that could have a big impact on the prevention of typhoid fever are well established and available, but sadly they are difficult or impossible to implement. It is difficult to overcome poverty: peace, stable government, investment in infrastructure and public health are urgently needed but hard to achieve. In this era of increasing drug resistance and in the absence of dramatic changes in infrastructure in the poorest countries, vaccination may be the only effective intervention.

The current available vaccines, the oral Ty21a and the parenteral Vi conjugate, offer a protective efficacy of about 70–90%, which is a reasonable degree of protection. Mass vaccinations in endemic areas and the subsequent development of immunity in the population could greatly reduce transmission and have a significant impact on the incidence of this disease.

References

1. Parkhill J, Dougan G, James KD, Thomson NR, Pickard D, Wain J, Churcher C, Mungall KL, Bentley SD, Holden MT, Sebaihia M, Baker S, Basham D, Brooks K, Chillingworth T, Connerton P, Cronin A, Davis P, Davies RM, Dowd L, White N, Farrar J, Feltwell T, Hamlin N, Haque A, Hien TT, Holroyd S, Jagels K, Krogh A, Larsen TS, Leather S, Moule S, O'Gaora P, Parry C, Quail M, Rutherford K, Simmonds M, Skelton J, Stevens K, Whitehead S, Barrell BG. Complete genome sequence of a multiple drug resistant *Salmonella enterica* serovar Typhi CT18. *Nature* 2001; **413**: 848–52.

2. Chinh NT, Parry CM, Ly NT, Ha HD, Thong MX, Diep TS, Wain J, White NJ, Farrar JJ. A randomized controlled comparison of azithromycin and ofloxacin for treatment of multidrug-resistant or nalidixic acid-resistant enteric fever. *Antimicrob Agents Chemother* 2000; **44**: 1855–9.

3. Levine MM, Ferreccio C, Cryz S, Ortiz E. Comparison of enteric-coated capsules and liquid formulation of Ty21a typhoid vaccine in randomised controlled field trial. *Lancet* 1990; **336**: 891–4.

4. Tacket CO, Sztein MB, Wasserman SS, Losonsky G, Kotloff KL, Wyant TL, Nataro JP, Edelman R, Perry J, Bedford P, Brown D, Chatfield S, Dougan G, Levine MM. Phase 2 clinical trial of attenuated Salmonella enterica serovar Typhi oral live vector vaccine CVD 908-htrA in U.S. volunteers. *Infect Immunol* 2000; **68**: 1196–201.

5. Levine MM. Can needle-free administration of vaccines become the norm in global immunization? *Nat Med* 2003; **9**: 99–103.

6. Lin FY, Ho VA, Khiem HB, Trach DD, Bay PV, Thanh TC, Kossaczka Z, Bryla DA, Shiloach J, Robbins JB, Schneerson R, Szu SC. The efficacy of a Salmonella typhi Vi conjugate vaccine in two-to-five-year-old children. *N Engl J Med* 2001; **344**: 1263–9.

10

Tuberculosis

ROBERT DAVIDSON

Introduction

About one-third (2 billions) of the world's population has latent tuberculosis (TB), caused by *Mycobacterium tuberculosis* infection. From this pool, about 9 million cases of active TB emerge annually, resulting in approximately 2–3 million deaths. The number of cases of active TB is expected to rise, fuelled mainly by the HIV pandemic and an increase in the urban population.

Drug-resistant TB

The increase in TB is paralleled by the increase in multidrug-resistant TB (MDRTB); that is, patients whose infection is caused by *M. tuberculosis* resistant to both isoniazid and rifampicin. Isoniazid and rifampicin are the two most powerful anti-TB drugs, with excellent early bactericidal activity (able to kill *M. tuberculosis* in a rapidly dividing state, rendering the patient non-infectious) and excellent sterilizing activity (ability to kill 'persisters'—*M. tuberculosis* in a slowly metabolizing state). *M. tuberculosis* bacilli were thought to undergo random chromosomal mutations that rendered them resistant to drugs.

Acquired drug resistance for *M. tuberculosis* is almost always caused by inadequate treatment. This can include failure of the patient to take the prescribed drugs, failure of the physician to prescribe appropriately, and failure of the healthcare system to ensure that drugs are available. There has been much interest in optimizing the performance of TB control programmes, and specifically the advantages of directly observed therapy, short-course (DOTS) over self-administered therapy (see Davies and [1]). Where MDRTB is prevalent, WHO recommends DOTS-plus (Table 10.1). The second-line anti-TB drugs used in DOTS-plus are kanamycin, amikacin or capreomycin; prothionamide or ethionamide; ciprofloxacin or ofloxacin; para-amino salicylic acid; and cycloserine [2]. The choice of drugs needs to be made once sensitivity testing has been done on cultured *M. tuberculosis*, or empirically if culture and sensitivity data are not available. However, fewer than 25% of patients globally with smear-positive TB are being treated by DOTS, and there is concern that a DOTS-plus programme, if competing with a DOTS programme, may increase rather than decrease the numbers who die of TB (see Sterling *et al.*). A programme to treat MDRTB in a poor area of Lima, Peru, has been successful (see Mitnick *et al.*), though at a cost of about US$15000 per patient and with heavy support from colleagues at the Program in Infectious Disease and Social Change, Department of Social Medicine, Harvard Medical School, Boston, MA, USA.

New drugs for TB

The pipeline for TB drugs is empty. The current best hope is that antimicrobials developed for the lucrative market of resistant bacterial infections in the West will also have activity against *M. tuberculosis*. An example too expensive to enter trials (at about US$80 per 600 mg tablet) is linezolid. More affordable, and very promising, is a new quinolone, moxifloxacin (see Gosling *et al.*), which seems to have early bactericidal activity as good as that of rifampicin.

Diagnosis of TB infections and tracking outbreaks

In the West, the mainstay of prevention of TB is the identification and treatment of those latently infected with *M. tuberculosis*. This is problematic, because tuberculin skin testing (the method in use for the last 100 years) lacks sensitivity (in both active and latent TB) and specificity (environmental mycobacteria and BCG can produce false-positive tuberculin skin tests). The development of an *ex vivo* enzyme-linked immunospot (ELISPOT) assay that detects immune responses to an antigen specific to *M. tuberculosis*, ESAT-6, is a significant advance.

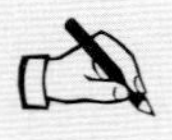

The role of DOTS in tuberculosis treatment and control
Davies PD. *Am J Respir Med* 2003; **2**: 203–9

BACKGROUND. DOTS consists of five distinct elements: political commitment; microscopy services; drug supplies; surveillance and monitoring systems, and the use of highly efficacious regimens; and direct observation of treatment. What is of concern is that in some trials cure rates less than 70% were achieved even in the direct observation arm. With no new drugs or adjuvant treatment available to bring the length of treatment down to substantially less than 6 months, DOTS offers the best means we have at our disposal for TB control.

INTERPRETATION. DOTS is not an end in itself but a means of ensuring that patients with TB complete therapy and of preventing drug resistance from developing in the community. A main criticism of DOTS is that although observational studies show the benefits of DOTS, some properly conducted randomized, controlled trials of DOTS have shown no benefit, and cure rates as low as 65%. It is impossible to design a study of DOTS against the previous self-administered, poorly resourced programs. As soon as a study is implemented, the attention to patients in the control (non-DOTS) arm inevitably improves from the previous non-trial service situation.

Comment

When rates of TB were declining in the 1970s and 1980s, physicians saw no need to change the habits of a lifetime, and self-administration of TB drugs was practised in most places. The upsurge of TB from 1986, especially in New York, required a radical change and there were no new drugs. The focus became that of ensuring that patients adhered to treatment. The difference in the way the term 'DOTS was defined by WHO and interpreted by many observers has led to some misunderstanding. WHO generally uses the term to mean the five components of DOTS (Table 10.1). But the word 'DOTS' is an acronym for directly observed therapy, short course. Many

Table 10.1 DOTS and DOTS-plus

DOTS is a package of five points:

- Commitment of governments to a national tuberculosis programme
- Detection of cases through case-finding by sputum smear microscopy examination of patients with suspected tuberculosis in general health services
- Standardized short-course chemotherapy with the first-line drugs isoniazid, rifampicin, pyrazinamide, and ethambutol (or streptomycin) for, at least, all smear-positive cases of tuberculosis under proper conditions of case management
- Regular, uninterrupted supply of all essential anti-tuberculosis drugs
- A monitoring system for programme supervision and evaluation

In addition:
- Mycobacterial cultures and drug susceptibility testing are not required
- Treatment is started on the basis of symptoms or a positive smear
- Second-line drugs are not used
- Three categories of treatment regimens exist; all are directly observed
- In the developing world, mycobacterial cultures and susceptibility testing are generally not performed, so drug resistance is not detected even if it is present

In DOTS-plus:
- Second-line anti-tuberculosis drugs (more toxic and expensive and less effective than first-line drugs) are used. The regimen includes two or more drugs to which the isolate is susceptible, including one drug given parenterally for 6 months or more. Total duration of treatment is 18–24 months; treatment is observed directly

The treatment regimen is either:
- Individualized according to drug susceptibility test results of the *M. tuberculosis* isolate identified on culture; or
- Given as a standardized regimen to patients who fail supervised retreatment (for example, when culture and drug susceptibility testing are not performed)
- Mycobacterial cultures and drug susceptibility testing may be performed

Source: Sterling *et al.* (2003).

workers therefore interpret DOTS purely as direct supervision of therapy. DOTS uses rifampicin, isoniazid, pyrazinamide and ethambutol, either daily or two or three times weekly, for 26 weeks. Theoretically this results in a 95% cure rate and a relapse rate of less than 5% – mainly within 6 months – of organisms that retain their original susceptibility. In Africa, DOTS drug costs are about US$11 and the total cost is about US$41 per patient. DOTS is also suitable for HIV$^+$ patients, who seem to have only a modestly increased risk of relapse. Successful DOT programmes often have more than five components—the provision of incentives and enablers for patients; tracing of defaulters; legal sanctions; patient-centred approaches; decentralization of services; staff motivation; supervision; and extra funding. Extra financial input seems central to successful DOTS programmes. Some authors hold that, despite the burdens placed on the healthcare system and patient, the benefit from improved TB cure rates means that DOT programmes result in net savings to the community |1|. Others point out that, without large financial inputs, DOTS programmes are no more efficient that the old system of treating TB. However, when an existing programme has default and relapse rates of less than 5% there is unlikely to be further benefit from DOTS.

Impact of DOTS compared with DOTS-plus on multidrug resistant tuberculosis and tuberculosis deaths: decision analysis

Sterling TR, Lehmann HP, Frieden TR. *Br Med J* 2003; **326**: 574

BACKGROUND. Seventy-seven per cent of TB patients currently do not yet receive DOTS. The authors addressed the outcome of implementing a DOTS-plus strategy for patients with MDRTB which competed with DOTS for resources. A decision analysis with Monte Carlo simulation of a Markov decision tree was used, the patient population having smear-positive pulmonary TB (Fig. 10.1). Analyses modelled different levels of programme effectiveness of DOTS and DOTS-plus, and high (10%) and intermediate (3%) proportions of primary MDRTB. The model predicted that in an area with 3% primary MDRTB, with a DOTS programme 276 people would die from TB over a 10-year period (24 MDRTB and 252 sensitive *M. tuberculosis*). Optimal implementation of DOTS-plus would result in 1.5% fewer deaths. If implementation of DOTS-plus were to result in a decrease of just 5% in the effectiveness of DOTS, 16% more people would die with TB than under DOTS alone. In an area with 10% primary MDRTB, 10% fewer deaths would occur under optimal DOTS-plus than under optimal DOTS, but 16% more deaths would occur if implementation of DOTS-plus were to result in a 5% decrease in the effectiveness of DOTS.

INTERPRETATION. Under optimal implementation, fewer TB deaths would occur under DOTS-plus than under DOTS. However, if implementation of DOTS-plus were associated with even minimal decreases in the effectiveness of treatment, substantially more patients would die than under DOTS.

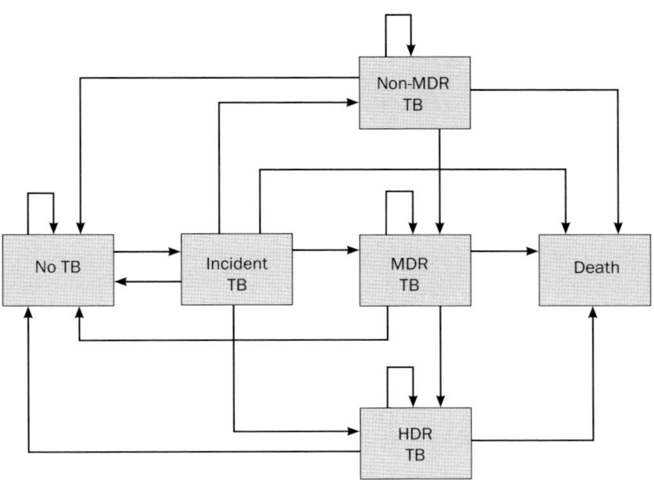

Non-MDR TB = *M tuberculosis* susceptible to first line antituberculosis
agents or isolates not resistant to isoniazid and rifampicin

MDR TB = *M tuberculosis* resistant to isoniazid and rifampicin

HDR TB = *M tuberculosis* resistant to isoniazid, rifampicin, plus at
least one second line antituberculosis agent

Fig. 10.1 Transition states of the Markov analysis. Source: Sterling *et al.* (2003).

Comment

For DOTS, the marginal cost per patient was US$10. For DOTS-plus, the costs were
US$200 for culture and sensitivity testing plus US$2000 for second-line agents. It is a
striking finding that if DOTS-plus were to divert resources from DOTS such that
DOTS was just 5% less effective than under optimal conditions, 16% more TB
patients would die. If the effectiveness of the control programme were to be decreased
by 10%, 128 more patients would die. DOTS-plus would therefore be beneficial as a
programme only if it were truly 'plus'—that is, if it did not divert resources from
DOTS. Even in that case, the cost per death from TB averted would be US$68 860.

Programmes and principles in treatment of multidrug-resistant tuberculosis

Mukherjee JS, Rich ML, Socci AR, *et al. Lancet* 2004; **363**(9407): 474–81

BACKGROUND. MDRTB presents an increasing threat to the global control of TB.
Many crucial management issues in MDRTB treatment remain unanswered. The
existing scientific research on MDRTB treatment consists of 13 retrospective cohort

studies. Eleven studies were done in developed countries, one in Peru and one in Turkey. Nine cohorts were treated at tertiary referral hospitals and four in outpatient clinics. In all cohorts except one, treatment regimens were individually tailored to drug susceptibility testing results and previous treatment history. In the Peru cohort a standard drug regimen (ethambutol, pyrazinamide, kanamycin, ciprofloxacin and ethionamide) was used, irrespective of drug susceptibility testing. This resulted in a low cure rate (48%) at a cost per disability-adjusted life year saved of US$211 and an average total treatment cost per patient of US$2381.

INTERPRETATION. MDRTB can and should be addressed therapeutically in resource-poor settings; starting the treatment early is crucial; aggressive treatment regimens and high-end dosing are recommended, given the lower potency of second-line anti-TB drugs; and strategies to improve treatment adherence, such as directly observed therapy, should be used.

Comment

Opportunities to treat MDRTB in developing countries are now possible through the Global Fund to Fight AIDS, TB, and Malaria, and the Green Light Committee for Access to Second-line Anti-tuberculosis Drugs |1|. As treatment of MDRTB becomes necessary in resource-poor areas, evidence-based guidelines for the treatment of MDRTB is necessary to guide clinicians and programmes. Without the two most potent drugs, rifampicin and isoniazid, the treatment of MDRTB becomes difficult since second-line drugs are less potent and often not well tolerated. Patients with MDRTB frequently have advanced disease with chronic thick-walled cavities that are difficult for antibiotics to penetrate. There is a hierarchy of effectiveness of drugs, and the principles of treating MDRTB are shown in Table 10.2.

Table 10.2 Recommendations for the design of MDRTB treatment regimens

The individualized treatment is based on drug sensitivity testing or drugs thought to be sensitive. Drugs are added until five adequate drugs are found.
More than five can be used if a drug's sensitivity is unclear or if the regimen contains few bactericidal drugs.

1 Use any first-line oral agent to which the isolate is sensitive: isoniazid, rifampicin, ethambutol or pyrazinamide.
2 Use an injectable to which an isolate is sensitive—an aminoglycoside or capreomycin. Injectable agents should be used for >6 months after culture conversion since they are frequently one of only two bactericidal components of treatment regimen.
3 Use a quinolone. If the isolate is resistant to a lower-generation quinolone but sensitive to higher-generation quinolones, consider use of the latter. Quinolones have been used in randomized controlled trials.
4 Add as many bacteriostatic second-line agents as needed to make up the five-drug regimen. Among the second-line agents, ethionamide and cycloserine are generally used first because of their efficacy, side effect profile and price, shown through *in vivo* and *in vitro* evidence, and their historical use in tuberculosis. p-aminosalicylic acid is frequently used in patients with higher-grade resistance.
5 Other drugs. If the regimen does not contain five adequate medications, consider the use of additional agents, such as amoxicillin or clavulanate and clofazimine, depending on clinical status, disease burden, degree, pattern of resistance, and other factors.

Source: Mukherjee *et al.* (2004).

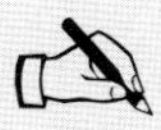

Community-based therapy for multidrug-resistant tuberculosis in Lima, Peru

Mitnick C, Bayona J, Palacios E, *et al*. *N Engl J Med* 2003; **348**: 119–28

BACKGROUND. Despite the prevalence of MDRTB in nearly all low-income countries surveyed, effective therapy has been deemed too expensive and considered not to be feasible outside referral centres. This study evaluated the results of community-based therapy for MDRTB in a poor section of Lima, Peru. The authors conducted a retrospective review of the charts of the first 75 patients enrolled in the programme between 1 August 1996 and 1 February 1999 and identified predictors of poor outcomes. The infecting strains of *M. tuberculosis* were resistant to a median of six drugs. Among the 66 patients who completed 4 or more months of therapy, 83% (55) were probably cured at the completion of treatment. Five of these 66 patients (8%) died while receiving therapy. Only one patient continued to have positive cultures after 6 months of treatment. All patients in whom treatment failed or who died had extensive bilateral pulmonary disease. In a multiple Cox proportional hazards regression model, the predictors of the time to treatment failure or death were a low haematocrit (hazard ratio [HR] 4.09; 95% confidence interval [CI], 1.35–12.36) and a low body mass index (HR 3.23; 95% CI 0.90–11.53). Inclusion of pyrazinamide and ethambutol in the regimen (when susceptibility was confirmed) was associated with a favourable outcome (HR for treatment failure or death 0.30; 95% CI 0.11–0.83).

INTERPRETATION. Community-based outpatient treatment of MDRTB can yield high cure rates even in resource-poor settings. Early initiation of appropriate therapy can preserve susceptibility to first-line drugs and improve treatment outcomes.

Comment

Among the 66 patients who completed 4 or more months of therapy, 83% were probably cured at the completion of treatment (that is, they had 12 months of negative sputum cultures). In Peru, MDRTB occurs in about 3% of cases among patients not previously treated for TB and about 15% of cases among those previously treated. Rates of cure of MDRTB with standardized short-course chemotherapy range from 5 to 60%, and repeated courses of standard therapy make matters worse by adding to the risk of resistance to pyrazinamide and ethambutol, and by increasing chronic scarring and thick-walled cavities, which drugs cannot penetrate. This study is different from those of MDRTB treatment in that it was community-based. However, this was not a 'normal' TB programme at all; it is apparent that a huge amount of input from the Harvard-based investigators took place; for example, drug susceptibility testing (which guided treatment) took place in Boston. The costs per patient were US$504 to US$32 383 (mean US$15 681 per patient). The authors state 'these costs were low—approximately 10% of those for hospitalized patients', which brings home the contrast between the rich and poor nations. Peru has a per capita annual income of US$4400; that of people in Malawi is US$180.

The bactericidal activity of moxifloxacin in patients with pulmonary tuberculosis

Gosling RD, Uiso LO, Sam NE, *et al*. *Am J Respir Crit Care Med* 2003; **168**: 1342–5; Epub 13 August 2003

BACKGROUND. Patients in whom acid-fast bacilli, smear-positive pulmonary TB was newly diagnosed were randomized to receive 400 mg moxifloxacin, 300 mg isoniazid or 600 mg rifampin daily for 5 days. Sixteen-hour overnight sputum collections were made for the 2 days before and for 5 days of monotherapy. Bactericidal activity was estimated by the time taken to kill 50% of viable bacilli (vt50) and the fall in sputum viable count during the first 2 days, designated as the early bactericidal activity (EBA). The mean vt50 of moxifloxacin was 0.88 days (95% CI 0.43–1.33 days) and the mean EBA was 0.53 (95% CI 0.28–0.79). For the isoniazid group, the mean vt50 was 0.46 days (95% CI 0.31–0.61 days) and the mean EBA was 0.77 (95% CI 0.54–1.00). For rifampin, the mean vt50 was 0.71 days (95% CI 0.48–0.95 days) and the mean EBA was 0.28 (95% CI 0.15–0.41).

INTERPRETATION. Using the EBA method, isoniazid was significantly more active than rifampin (*P* <0.01) but not moxifloxacin. Using the vt50 method, isoniazid was more active than both rifampin and moxifloxacin (*P* = 0.03). Moxifloxacin has activity similar to rifampin in human subjects with pulmonary TB, suggesting that it should undergo further assessment as part of a short-course regimen for the treatment of drug-susceptible TB.

Comment

The fluoroquinolones (ciprofloxacin, ofloxacin and moxifloxacin) are bactericidal drugs that inhibit DNA gyrase and are active against *M. tuberculosis*, including strains resistant to first-line drugs. Clinical studies have shown promise with quinolones in sensitive TB, and they are central to the treatment of MDRTB. Moxifloxacin has better *in vitro* activity than ciprofloxacin and ofloxacin and has good activity in a mouse model of TB. TB drugs need to be assessed more simply and quickly than by awaiting the cure and relapse rates in clinical trials in combination therapy. EBA is important early in the course of treatment by ensuring a rapid reduction in the infective load. This can be measured by using the drug as monotherapy for a few days and quantifying the reduction in bacillary load in sputum. In this Phase II EBA study in Tanzania, small groups of patients gave two sputum samples before therapy was started, and one sputum sample daily thereafter for 5 days during which they received moxifloxacin alone. Thereafter they received standard TB treatment. The EBA of moxifloxacin (a $\log_{10}$ fall of 0.53 in sputum bacillary load per day) was similar to that of rifampicin (0.28) and higher than that published for ciprofloxacin and ofloxacin (0.20–0.30). No other drug is as powerful as isoniazid (EBA 0.77). This study suffers from a small sample size, and it is a pity that drug susceptibility studies on the sputa were not carried out. Nonetheless, it seems that moxifloxacin is indeed the best quinolone for TB, and its once-daily dosing and affordable price make it attractive.

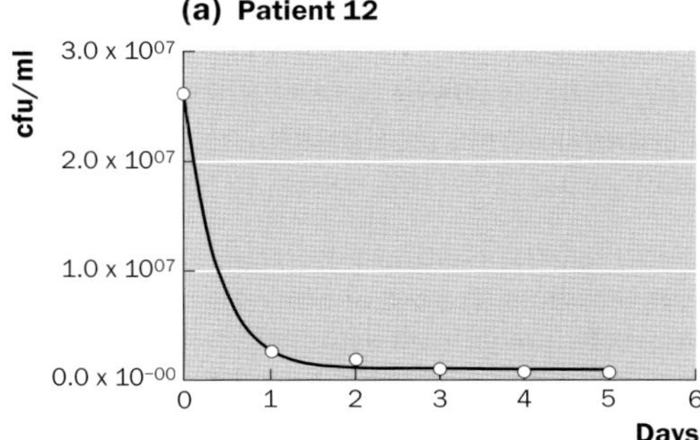

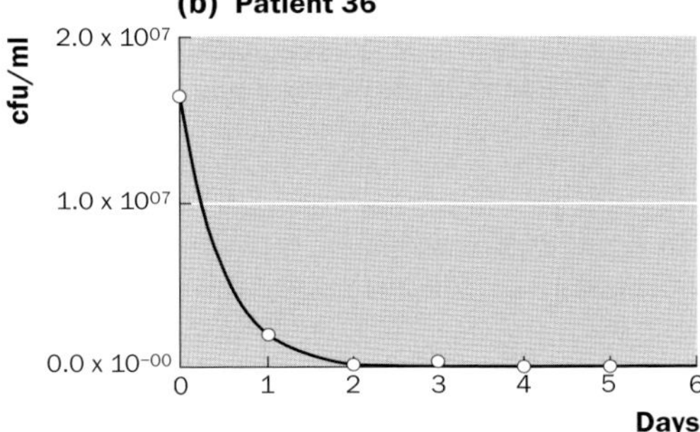

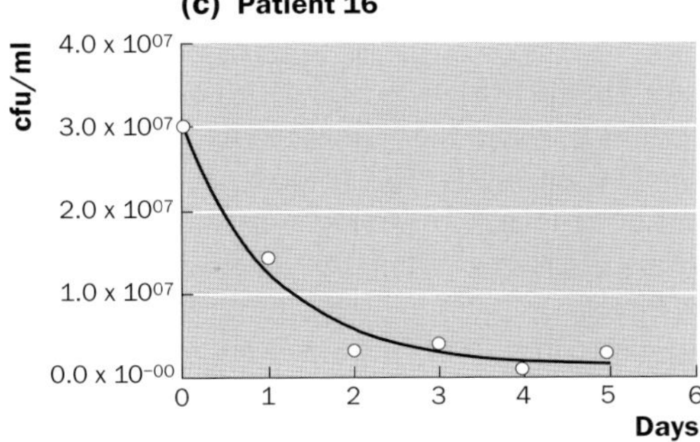

Fig. 10.2 (a) The fall in sputum viable count for a patient treated with isoniazid. (b) The fall in sputum viable count for a patient treated with moxifloxacin. (c) The fall in sputum viable count for a patient treated with rifampin. cfu, colony-forming units.
Source: Gosling *et al.* (2003).

Comparison of T-cell-based assay with tuberculin skin test for diagnosis of *Mycobacterium tuberculosis* infection in a school tuberculosis outbreak

Ewer K, Deeks J, Alvarez L, *et al. Lancet* 2003; **361**: 1168–73

BACKGROUND. The diagnosis of latent TB infection relies on the tuberculin skin test (TST), which has many drawbacks. However, to find out whether new tests are better than TST is difficult because of the lack of a gold standard test for latent infection. A sensitive ELISPOT assay was developed to detect T cells specific for *M. tuberculosis* antigens that are absent from *M. bovis* BCG and most environmental mycobacteria. The authors postulated that if the ELISPOT is a more accurate test of latent infection than TST, it should correlate better with the degree of exposure to *M. tuberculosis*. In the setting of a large TB outbreak in a UK school, resulting from one infectious index case, 535 students were tested for *M. tuberculosis* infection with TST and ELISPOT. Although agreement between the tests was high (89% concordance; κ = 0.72; P <0.0001), ELISPOT correlated significantly more closely with *M. tuberculosis* exposure than did TST on the basis of measures of proximity (P = 0.03) and duration of exposure (P = 0.007) to the index case. TST was significantly more likely to be positive in BCG-vaccinated than in non-vaccinated students (P = 0.002), whereas ELISPOT results were not associated with BCG vaccination (P = 0.44).

INTERPRETATION. ELISPOT offers a more accurate approach than TST for the identification of individuals who have latent TB infection and could improve TB control through more precise targeting of preventive treatment.

Comment

The ELISPOT test is the possible update of the TST. ELISPOT correlated significantly more closely with *M. tuberculosis* exposure than did TST on the basis of measures of proximity (P = 0.03) and duration of exposure (P = 0.007) to the index case (Fig. 10.3). The gold standard for the assessment of latent TB infection is the later development of TB disease, which will be known by following up ELISPOT-positive contacts in ongoing studies internationally. If ELISPOT were used to guide preventive treatment, in this school outbreak 31 children in the study would have been denied treatment and a further 27 would have received treatment; the key is whether those receiving treatment were those who needed it. The prevalence of latent TB infection is enormous—80% of a sample of normal adults in Mumbai and 69% in Lusaka have a positive ELISPOT. Thus, only in the West can preventive treatment be given to patients at risk; in high-burden countries, improving the treatment of active TB remains the priority. Patients with active TB produce less interferon-γ than TB contacts. This does not adversely affect ELISPOT results, since diagnostic sensitivity was 96% in adults with culture-confirmed active TB in the UK and 92% in HIV-1-positive adults with smear-positive pulmonary TB in Zambia. In the school

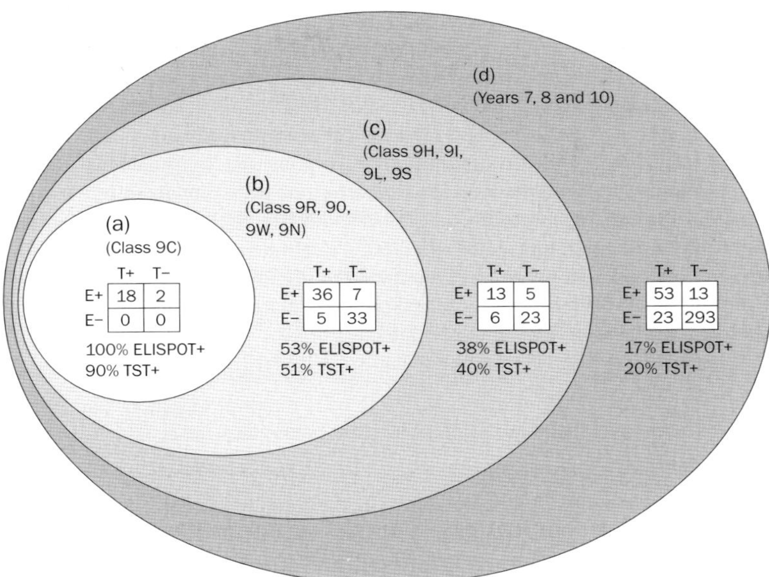

Fig. 10.3 TST and ELISPOT results for students stratified by decreasing proximity to index case based on school year and class. T+, TST positive; T−, TST negative; E+, ELISPOT positive; ELISPOT−, ELISPOT negative. (a) Students in the same class as the index case. (b) Students in classes in the same year who regularly shared lessons with the index case. (c) Students in the four remaining classes in the same year who shared only weekly school events but no lessons with the index case. (d) Students in different years who shared no school events with the index case. Source: Ewer *et al.* (2003).

outbreak described, 27 of 30 children with active TB were ELISPOT-positive. (The three ELISPOT-negative children did not have a bacteriological diagnosis, but were diagnosed presumptively on the basis of positive TSTs and suggestive chest radiography.) Better diagnosis of latent TB infection could help TB control in high-burden countries by improving diagnosis in children and in HIV-1-positive people, and by enhancing epidemiological surveys to assess the effect of TB control measures.

Transcriptional adaptation of *Mycobacterium tuberculosis* within macrophages: insights into the phagosomal environment

Schnappinger D, Ehrt S, Voskuil MI, *et al. J Exp Med* 2003; **198**: 693–704

BACKGROUND. Little is known about the biochemical environment in phagosomes harbouring an infectious agent. To assess the state of this organelle the authors studied the transcriptional responses of *M. tuberculosis* in macrophages from wild-type and nitric oxide (NO) synthase 2-deficient mice before and after immunological activation. The intraphagosomal transcriptome was compared with the transcriptome of *M. tuberculosis* in standard broth culture and during growth in diverse conditions designed to simulate features of the phagosomal environment. Genes expressed differentially as a consequence of intraphagosomal residence included an interferon-γ- and NO-induced response that intensifies an iron-scavenging programme, converts the microbe from aerobic to anaerobic respiration, and induces a dormancy regulon. Induction of genes involved in the activation and β-oxidation of fatty acids indicated that fatty acids furnish carbon and energy. Induction of σE-dependent, sodium dodecyl sulphate-regulated genes and genes involved in mycolic acid modification pointed to damage and repair of the cell envelope. Sentinel genes within the intraphagosomal transcriptome were induced similarly by *M. tuberculosis* in the lungs of mice.

INTERPRETATION. The microbial transcriptome thus served as a bioprobe of the *M. tuberculosis* phagosomal environment, showing it to be nitrosative, oxidative, functionally hypoxic, carbohydrate-poor, and capable of perturbing the pathogen's cell envelope.

Inhibition of respiration by nitric oxide induces a *Mycobacterium tuberculosis* dormancy program

Voskuil MI, Schnappinger D, Visconti KC, *et al. J Exp Med* 2003; **198**: 705–13

BACKGROUND. An estimated two billion persons are latently infected with *M. tuberculosis*. The host factors that initiate and maintain this latent state and the mechanisms by which *M. tuberculosis* survives within latent lesions are compelling but unanswered questions. One such host factor may be NO, a product of activated macrophages that exhibits antimycobacterial properties. Evidence for the possible significance of NO comes from murine models of TB showing progressive infection in animals unable to produce the inducible isoform of NO synthase and in animals treated with a NO synthase inhibitor. Here, the authors show that oxygen and low, non-toxic concentrations of NO competitively modulate the expression of a 48-gene regulon, which is expressed *in vivo* and prepares bacilli for survival during long periods of *in vitro* dormancy. NO was found to reversibly inhibit aerobic respiration and growth. A haem-containing enzyme, possibly the terminal oxidase in the respiratory pathway, probably senses and integrates NO and oxygen levels and signals the regulon.

INTERPRETATION. These data lead to a model postulating that, within granulomas, inhibition of respiration by NO production and oxygen limitation constrains *M. tuberculosis* replication rates in persons with latent TB.

Comment

The stage of clinical latency before infection, and of persistence after initial bactericidal activity of TB drugs, is of surpassing importance for the epidemiology and control of TB. The eradication of bacilli in latent and healing lesions by antimicrobials is notoriously slow, and this probably reflects the metabolic state of the bacillus. This multinational group of investigators has published two articles back-to-back which seek to unravel the biology of *M. tuberculosis* in its dormant or persistent state within long-lived phagosomes of host macrophages. It appears that, when *M. tuberculosis* senses low oxygen concentrations and the presence of sublethal amounts of NO, it holds its breath and goes to sleep. NO induces an *M. tuberculosis* genetic programme (a regulon of 48 genes) that adapts the organism for survival during extended periods of dormancy. The findings that NO competes with oxygen to inhibit respiration, slow growth and induce the dormancy regulon provide the basis for a model that describes the relationship between the tissue concentrations of NO and oxygen and the *in vivo* growth state of *M. tuberculosis* (Fig. 10.4). Granulomas, particularly if surrounded by an avascular fibrocalcific tissue, exemplify this circumstance. The bacilli respond to the decrease in respiration by initiating a transcriptional response that transforms the pathogen. This transformation stabilizes vital components of the bacterial cell and enables survival during extended periods of latency. In striking contrast to phagosomes containing most pyogens, which evolve and resolve over a few hours, the *M. tuberculosis*-containing phagosomes of macrophages are notable for their longevity and relative stability over several days *in vitro* and years *in vivo*. *M. tuberculosis* may achieve this effect by controlling phagosomal development, preventing its fusion with the lysosome, and reducing maximal acidification of the phagosomal contents. Whilst this may enable an understanding of the nature of phagosomes, a far more important result will be the identification of drug targets within *M. tuberculosis* that are not expressed on conventional culture media.

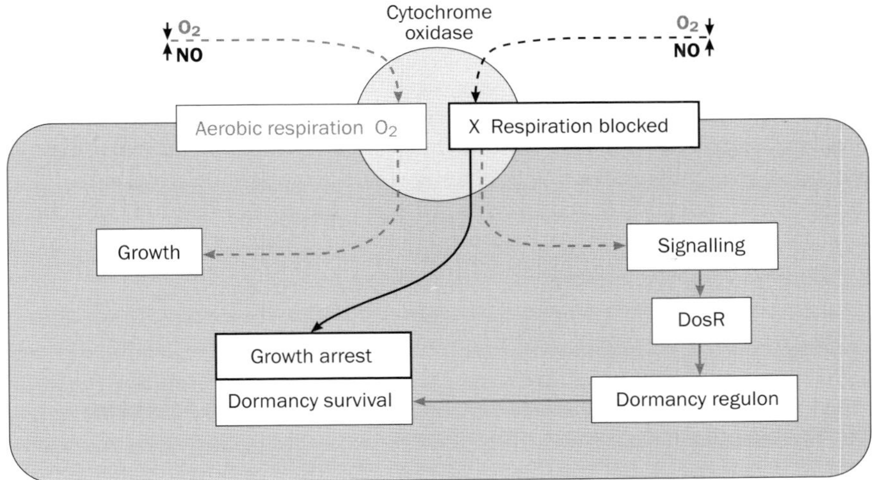

Fig. 10.4 Model of the control of respiration, growth and gene regulation by oxygen and NO. Cytochrome oxidase is posited as the sensor/integrator of oxygen/NO levels in this model. DosR, dormancy survival regulator. Source: Voskuil *et al.* (2003).

DnaE2 polymerase contributes to *in vivo* survival and the emergence of drug resistance in *Mycobacterium tuberculosis*

Boshoff HI, Reed MB, Barry CE 3rd, Mizrahi V. Cell 2003; **113**: 183–93

BACKGROUND. The presence of multiple copies of the major replicative DNA polymerase (DnaE) in some organisms, including important pathogens and symbionts, has remained an unresolved enigma. The authors postulated that one copy might participate in error-prone DNA repair synthesis. They found that UV irradiation of *M. tuberculosis* results in increased mutation frequency in the surviving fraction. They identified *dnaE2* as a gene that is upregulated *in vitro* by several DNA damaging agents, as well as during infection of mice. Loss of this protein reduces both the survival of the bacillus after UV irradiation and the virulence of the organism in mice.

INTERPRETATION. These data suggest that DnaE2, not a member of the known family of error-prone DNA polymerases, is the primary mediator of survival through inducible mutagenesis and can contribute directly to the emergence of drug resistance *in vivo*. These results may indicate a potential new target for therapeutic intervention.

Comment

An extremely low rate of mutation has been a noted feature of *M. tuberculosis* and contrasts with the inexplicably high frequency of emergence of drug resistance *in vivo*. Genetic mutation is one means of generating individual strains with enhanced fitness under conditions that threaten the continued survival of the bacterial population. A stress-inducible bacterial SOS response facilitates the generation of mutants during adverse conditions and is thought to occur through the induction of low-fidelity ('mutator') polymerases. This study clearly demonstrates that *M. tuberculosis* elevates mutational levels in response to DNA damage but does so by a mechanism that does not involve the induction of known error-prone polymerases. Error-prone DNA replication or the inaccurate repair of base-pair mismatches may contribute directly to the unexpectedly high rate of acquisition of drug resistance during infection.

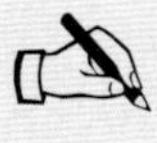

The complete genome sequence of *Mycobacterium bovis*

Garnier T, Eiglmeier K, Camus JC, *et al. Proc Natl Acad Sci USA* 2003; **100**: 7877–82; Epub 03 June 2003

BACKGROUND. *M. bovis* is the causative agent of TB in a range of animal species and man, with worldwide annual losses to agriculture of US$3 billion. The human burden of TB caused by the bovine tubercle bacillus is still largely unknown. *M. bovis* was also the progenitor for the *M. bovis* BCG vaccine strain, the most widely used human vaccine. Here the authors describe the 4 345 492-base pair genome sequence of *M. bovis* AF2122/97 and its comparison with the genomes of *M. tuberculosis* and *M. leprae*. Strikingly, the genome sequence of *M. bovis* is more than 99.95% identical to that of *M. tuberculosis*, but deletion of genetic information has led to a reduced genome size. Comparison with *M. leprae* reveals a number of common gene losses, suggesting the removal of functional redundancy. Cell wall components and secreted proteins show the greatest variation, indicating their potential role in host–bacillus interactions or immune evasion.

INTERPRETATION. There are no genes unique to *M. bovis*, implying that differential gene expression may be the key to the host tropisms of human and bovine bacilli. The genome sequence therefore offers major insight into the evolution, host preference and pathobiology of *M. bovis*.

Comment

Animal TB remains a huge problem, but to clinicians the value of having the *M. bovis* genome published is to compare it with strains pathogenic to humans: *M. tuberculosis* and *M. leprae*. Although the human and bovine tubercle bacilli can be differentiated by host range, virulence and physiological features, the genetic basis of these differences is unknown. *M. bovis* was also the progenitor of BCG, a strain that was attenuated by serial passage of *M. bovis* on potato slices soaked in ox bile and glycerol over 13 years. The precise mutations that led to attenuation of BCG are still unknown. It has long been thought that human TB had its origin as a zoonosis, with *M. bovis* jumping the species barrier and adapting to the human host to become *M. tuberculosis* at the time when cattle were domesticated 10 000–15 000 years ago. However, the genome sequence shows that *M. bovis* has lost genes since it evolved from a progenitor of the *M. tuberculosis* complex. Comparison of genomes among more and less pathogenic mycobacteria will have a major impact on the generation of vaccine candidates, diagnostic reagents and drugs against TB.

Conclusion

It is both ironic and fortunate that TB is transportable in its latent form in humans between continents, because it means that the endemic misery of disease in poor countries also effects the West, as an 'emerging disease'. This shared fate has enabled scientists in the West to obtain funds and devote energy to the solution of the problem of TB. Whilst purposeful drug development is still shamefully inadequate, moxifloxacin has luckily appeared as a powerful new agent. Our understanding of the biology of *M. tuberculosis* in its natural habitat (phagosomes within macrophages within granulomas) is galloping ahead and is likely to yield new drug targets soon. Improvement of TB treatment programmes has become a worthy topic of social and medical science, hopefully paving the way for the logical implementation of new vaccines and drug treatments when they become available. Also within sight is the arrival of surrogate markers for drug efficacy, so that years of follow-up in drug trials will not be needed to determine whether a new intervention is good at sterilizing persistent or latent *M. tuberculosis.* The ELISPOT assay for ESAT-6 may enable more accurate targeting of treatment of latent TB infection, and may also turn out to be a read-out for recovery from infection. Early bactericidal activity is a valuable low-tech method for identifying powerful new drugs, and counting of colonies in sputum might be replaced in time by a molecular surrogate of the viable bacterial load. The ingenuity of scientists seems poised to outwit *M. tuberculosis* over the next few decades.

References

1. Chan ED, Iseman MD. Current medical treatment for tuberculosis. *Br Med J* 2002; **325:** 1282–6.
2. World Health Organization website: http://www.who.int/gtb/policyrd/PDF/GLC_Application_Instructions.pdf

11

Haematopoietic stem cell transplantation

IAN KERRIDGE

Introduction

Infections are a major cause of morbidity and mortality following haematopoietic stem cell transplantation (HSCT). A number of factors are responsible for this, including myelosuppression resulting from transplant conditioning and from the underlying disease, mucosal damage caused by chemoradiotherapy, the presence of central venous catheters, the use of post-transplantation immunosuppression, and the immunosuppressive effect of graft-versus-host disease (GvHD) and its treatment [1–4]. In recent years, changes in transplantation practices, including the use of reduced intensity or non-myeloablative transplant conditioning and the increasing use of more intensive immunosuppressive regimens for the prevention and treatment of GvHD, such as alemtuzumab, daclizumab and infliximab, have also altered the pattern, incidence and severity of bacterial, fungal and viral infections in the post-transplantation setting.

Viral infections, in particular, have a high mortality rate in HSCT units and present particular problems, both because they cannot be easily prevented with anti-viral therapy and because spread cannot be prevented by HEPA (high-efficiency particulate air) filtration [5–7]. And while significant progress has been made in the prevention and management of many infections due to reactivation of pathogens, such as cytomegalovirus (CMV), little gain has been made in reducing the risk of infection contracted from hospital staff and the environment. The reasons for this are complex and include medical, occupational, financial and cultural factors. The end result is that while some infection control measures, such as hand washing, the wearing of masks and mandatory influenza vaccination of staff working in HSCT units, has become accepted practice throughout the developed world, other measures, including the monitoring of HSCT staff for viral shedding, the screening and exclusion of children from HSCT units and the relocation of staff who have symptoms of viral upper respiratory tract infection, have proven more contentious.

The papers chosen represent the major streams of recent research in viral infections in the post-transplantation setting. They include research into CMV, adenovirus, Epstein–Barr virus (EBV)-driven post-transplant lymphoproliferative disorder

(PTLD), molecular diagnostics, pre-emptive therapy, nosocomial infections, adoptive immunotherapy, novel antiviral agents and outpatient oral therapy for CMV.

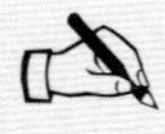

Outbreaks of infectious diseases in stem cell transplant units: a silent cause of death for patients and transplant programmes

McCann S, Byrne JL, Rovira M, *et al.*; Infectious Diseases Working Party of the EBMT. *Bone Marrow Transplant* 2004; **33**: 519–29

BACKGROUND. An outbreak of vancomycin-resistant enterococcal infection necessitated the closure of the National Blood and Bone Marrow Transplant Unit in Dublin. This prompted the European Group for Blood and Marrow Transplantation (EBMT) to investigate the occurrence of outbreaks of infection in stem cell transplant units over the 10 years from 1991 to 2001. The impacts of such outbreaks on patient morbidity and mortality and on the administration of the transplant programme were also considered.

INTERPRETATION. The initial questionnaire was returned by 41 of the 505 centres to which it was sent. Of the 41 centres that returned the questionnaire, 13 centres reported 23 outbreaks of infection involving 231 patients. There were ten bacterial, eight viral and five fungal outbreaks. These outbreaks apparently resulted in 56 deaths. All of those who died as a result of fungal and bacterial infections and the majority of those who died from viral infections were allograft recipients. The infection was reported to be hospital-acquired in all cases and cross-infection was a major factor in all the viral infections and half of the bacterial infections. All of the viral, four of the ten bacterial and three of the five fungal outbreaks occurred in rooms with HEPA filters. Twelve of the 13 transplant units reported partial or total closure as a result of infection. The authors considered that the low response to the initial questionnaire indicated the reluctance of physicians to report outbreaks of infection. The introduction of mandatory quality management systems (e.g. JACIE, the Joint Accreditation Committee ISCT-EBMT programme) should improve incident reporting. This change, together with systematic surveying of outbreaks in the future, should reduce the incidence of infectious outbreaks in stem cell transplant units.

Comment

While considerable attention has been paid to the infectious complications of HSCT, relatively little attention has been paid to the impact of outbreaks of infection in stem cell transplantation units and on transplant recipients.

This paper reports the results of an EBMT survey of transplant units regarding outbreaks of infections over a 10-year period from 1991 to 2001. While any conclusions drawn from this study are limited by the low response rate (12% of EBMT stem cell transplantation centres responded), the results do provide a snapshot of the range and impact of an extremely under-researched and under-reported problem.

Respondents to the survey reported a series of bacterial, viral and fungal outbreaks due to pseudomonas, serratia, vancomycin-resistant enterococcus, parainfluenza, respiratory syncytial virus (RSV), aspergillus, scedosporium and paecilomyces. Infections contributed to the deaths of 56 patients and twelve of 13 stem cell transplantation units reported partial or total closure as a consequence of the outbreak. These findings are significant because they illustrate the limitations of current infection control measures, such as HEPA filtration, and document how little has been achieved in reducing the risks of infection contracted from staff, the hospital environment and the community.

While the introduction of mandatory quality management systems, such as JACIE in Europe, will improve the reporting of hospital-acquired infections, much more substantial efforts will be needed to increase professional transparency where stem cell transplantation units exist in a climate characterized by fear of medical litigation, adherence to professional self-regulation and academic competition.

Induction of cytomegalovirus-specific CD4+ cytotoxic T lymphocytes from seropositive or negative healthy subjects or stem cell transplant recipients

Tazume K, Hagihara M, Gansuvd B, *et al. Exp Hematol* 2004; **32**: 95–103

BACKGROUND. Dendritic cells pulsed with crude CMV antigens were used to generate CMV-specific cytotoxic T lymphocytes (CTL) *in vitro*. Mononuclear cells from healthy CMV-seropositive or -seronegative volunteers and from stem cell transplant recipients were cultured with CD14+ monocyte-derived dendritic cells prepulsed with CMV antigen and then matured *in vitro* with lipopolysaccharide and tumour necrosis factor-α. The cells resulting after proliferation were checked for phenotype (CD4/CD8), and killing activity was measured by ^{51}Cr-release assay.

INTERPRETATION. The main proliferating cells from both seropositive and seronegative individuals, CD4+ T cells, killed antigen-pulsed autologous dendritic cells but not vehicle-pulsed autologous dendritic cells or CMV-pulsed allogeneic dendritic cells. Similar CTL induction was accomplished using mononuclear cells from stem cell transplant recipients. Significant killing of autologous CMV-infected fibroblasts required 16 h of incubation as opposed to the standard 4-h incubation. The killing was prevented either by a perforin inhibitor or by an anti-Fas ligand monoclonal antibody. CTL enhanced surface HLA-DR expression of CMV-infected fibroblasts, and their activity was neutralized by anti-HLA-DR monoclonal antibody. CMV-specific CD4+ CTL could be induced regardless of antiviral humoral immunity, even from immunosuppressed stem cell transplant recipients. After long-term (16 h) contact with CMV-infected target, these CTL showed perforin- and Fas/Fas ligand-mediated cytotoxicity.

Comment

While antiviral agents such as ganciclovir, foscarnet and cidofovir provide effective therapy for CMV infection, treatment is often complicated by significant toxicity, including pancytopenia and renal impairment, and may result in the emergence of drug-resistant strains. In recent years there has been considerable interest in adoptive cellular immunity as a means for preventing and treating CMV infection after transplantation. CMV-specific immunity is important for preventing CMV reactivation, including anti-CMV CD8$^+$ CTL and CMV-specific CD4$^+$ T cells, which contribute to the control of viral transmission by maintenance of the number and functional capacity of anti-CMV CD8$^+$ CTL, through direct cytotoxicity and through the secretion of antiviral cytokines such as interferon-γ (IFN-γ) and tumour necrosis factor-α |8,9|. The exact mechanism involved in CMV-specific CD4$^+$ CTL cytoxicity has not been fully characterized.

Infusions of CD8$^+$ CTL have previously been demonstrated to have clinical benefit in the prevention and treatment of post-transplant CMV infection |10|. Until recently, however, the generation of CMV-specific CTL was applicable only to selected donor– recipient pairs, was not possible in unrelated HSCT and was possible only in CMV-seropositive subjects. But as 30–40% of healthy adults aged 20–40 have not experienced a CMV infection and are CMV-seronegative, protocols for propagating anti-CMV CTL from both seropositive and seronegative people are needed.

This study represents a significant advance in adoptive immunotherapy as it demonstrates that CMV-specific CTL may be induced in both healthy CMV-seropositive and seronegative donors and in immunosuppressed HSCT recipients. Importantly, the CTL induced in these cases demonstrated effective CMV cytotoxicity. For those who believe that cellular immunotherapy represents the future of post-transplantation antimicrobial care, this research demonstrates that these benefits may be accessible to all patients, not only to selected patients with appropriate donors.

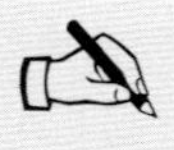

Molecular monitoring of adenovirus in peripheral blood after allogeneic bone marrow transplantation permits early diagnosis of disseminated disease

Lion T, Baumgartinger R, Watzinger F, *et al. Blood* 2003; **102**: 1114–20; Epub 2003 Apr 17

BACKGROUND. Transplant-related morbidity and mortality are high when adenovirus infection occurs in the course of allogeneic stem cell transplantation. Disseminated adenovirus disease is lethal in most instances. Any such infection, and the patients who are at high risk of disseminated disease, should therefore be detected as early as possible. In view of the large number of existing adenovirus types, the authors established real-time polymerase chain reaction (PCR) assays, permitting sensitive detection and quantification of all 51 currently known human adenovirus serotypes. More than 5000 samples were collected from 132 consecutive children undergoing stem cell transplantation. Samples from peripheral blood, stool, urine and throat were screened for adenovirus infection by PCR after transplantation.

INTERPRETATION. Thirty-six patients (27%) tested positive by PCR, revealing adenovirus types of the subgenera A, B, C, D and F. Detection of the virus at sites other than peripheral blood was not accompanied by clinical signs of viral disease except for enteritis in some patients whose stools were adenovirus-positive. Transplant-related mortality of these adenovirus-positive patients was not significantly different from that of adenovirus-negative patients. By contrast, 82% of the children with detectable adenovirus in peripheral blood died from infectious complications (P <0.001). Monitoring peripheral blood specimens using real-time PCR permitted early diagnosis of invasive adenovirus infection in all instances. In patients who developed disseminated adenovirus disease, the virus was detected in peripheral blood more than 3 weeks (median) before the onset of clinical symptoms. The detection of adenovirus in peripheral blood should allow early initiation of pre-emptive antiviral treatment.

Comment

Adenovirus can cause life-threatening infection in HSCT recipients, particularly children |**11**|. Infection can be asymptomatic, can cause localized disease, including enteritis, cystitis and upper respiratory tract infection, and can also cause severe, disseminated disease. The latter is almost always fatal, with a mortality rate greater than 60% |**12**|.

The diagnosis of adenovirus in immunocompromised HSCT recipients has traditionally been very difficult as serological tests are limited because of the hosts' impaired immunity, and the evaluation of positive cultures is a relatively insensitive and slow method |**13**|. PCR-based assays provide the possibility of rapid, specific and sensitive diagnosis of adenovirus infection.

This study used serial, real-time PCR to facilitate the preclinical diagnosis of invasive adenovirus infection in a population of paediatric HSCT recipients. The researchers used a panadenoviral PCR on the grounds that screening tests should be adequate for sensitive detection of all adenoviral serotypes, because all six species of adenovirus have been associated with deaths in the transplantation period, and because species differentiation is limited by major genetic differences between the different species |**14**|.

This study provides valuable information regarding the natural history, diagnosis and clinical presentation of adenovirus infection in the HSCT setting. Detection of adenovirus at sites other than the gut or peripheral blood was not associated with disease, except when adenovirus was detected at more than two sites, in which case it was strongly associated with invasive, life-threatening infection. Detection of adenovirus in the peripheral blood, even in the absence of tissue diagnosis, was highly predictive of subsequent disseminated infection and mortality. But, importantly, this study does not provide an indication of the association between adenovirus copy number and disease, as some patients developed clinical infection in the presence of quite low (<10^4 cells) peak levels. While this study adds to the growing evidence in support of adenoviral PCR monitoring in the post-transplantation setting, the actual level at which adenovirus infection is likely remains unclear, and the best distinction between latent and active infection is a ten-fold or greater increase in copy number on serial quantitative PCR. As more research is needed, at this stage the finding of a single positive PCR in peripheral blood does not provide definitive evidence of disease but certainly demands attention and consideration of antiviral therapy.

Donor CMV serologic status and outcome of CMV-seropositive recipients after unrelated donor stem cell transplantation: an EBMT megafile analysis

Ljungman P, Brand R, Einsele H, Frassoni F, Niederwieser D, Cordonnier C.
Blood 2003; **102**: 4255–60; Epub 2003 Aug 21

BACKGROUND. CMV has been a major cause of morbidity and mortality after allogeneic stem cell transplantation. The recipient's serological status is of paramount importance but the importance of the donor's serological status in CMV-seropositive recipients is controversial. The influence of the donor's CMV status was analysed in 7018 patients seropositive for CMV reported to the EBMT. Of these, 5910 patients had undergone HLA-identical sibling stem cell transplantation and 1108 patients had undergone unrelated donor stem cell transplantation. Survival, event-free survival, transplant-related mortality and the incidence of relapse were evaluated using univariate and multivariate proportional hazards models.

INTERPRETATION. Survival of patients receiving grafts from CMV-seropositive, HLA-identical sibling donors did not differ significantly from that of patients whose donors were seronegative (hazard ratio [HR] 1.04; $P = 0.37$; 95% confidence interval [CI] 0.95–1.14). However, when the donors were unrelated, the transplant recipients who received grafts from CMV-seropositive donors had an improved 5-year survival (35 versus 27%; HR 0.8; $P = 0.006$), improved event-free survival (30 versus 22%; HR 0.8; $P = 0.01$) and reduced transplant-related mortality (49 versus 62%; HR 0.7; $P <0.001$) compared with those whose donors were seronegative. The incidence of relapse was not affected by the CMV serological status of the donor. The effects of donor CMV status remained in multivariate analyses. The effect of donor status differed in different disease categories. In patients with chronic myelogenous leukaemia, T-cell depletion abrogated the beneficial effect of donor status. This suggests that the effect is mediated through transfer of donor immunity. These data suggest that, in unrelated stem cell transplantation, the donor's CMV status influences the outcome. For a CMV-seropositive patient, a seropositive donor may be preferable.

Comment

In recent years advances in antiviral therapy, diagnostics and pre-emptive therapy have reduced the mortality associated with CMV infection in HSCT recipients. However, CMV remains a significant complication of HSCT, particularly in patients receiving transplants from an HLA-mismatched or unrelated donor and in patients receiving immunosuppressive therapy for the prevention and treatment of GvHD. The major determinant of post-transplantation CMV reactivation remains the patient's CMV serostatus |**15**|. Where a patient is CMV-seronegative, the chances that they will develop *de novo* CMV infection is exceedingly small as long as they receive a stem cell inoculum from a CMV-seronegative donor and receive only CMV-negative, leukodepleted blood products. The influence of the donor's CMV serostatus on the outcome of transplantation in CMV-seropositive recipients is more controversial. This study throws doubt on the practice of preferential selection of CMV-seronegative donors for all transplant recipients.

Ljungman *et al.* report that CMV serostatus had no influence on overall survival and transplant-related mortality in patients receiving grafts from HLA-identical sibling donors but that patients receiving grafts from CMV-seropositive unrelated donors had improved survival, event-free survival and reduced transplantation-related mortality. This benefit was seen before day 100 and was independent of acute and chronic GvHD. The fact that this benefit was abrogated by T-cell depletion suggests that the probable mechanism is the transfer of mature CMV-specific effector cells or the transfer of T-cell precursors able to multiply and reconstitute T-cell immunity.

The clinical implications of these findings are unclear as recent studies of outcomes in unrelated donor transplants from the National Marrow Donor Program in the US found no effect of CMV donor serostatus |**16**|. Further studies will be required to clearly resolve questions about the preferable CMV serostatus of the donor in the unrelated donor setting. In the interim, however, this study provides support for those who believe that adoptive immunotherapy holds the key to managing the risk of infection in the post-transplantation period.

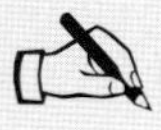

Cidofovir for adenovirus infections after allogeneic hematopoietic stem cell transplantation: a survey by the Infectious Diseases Working Party of the European Group for Blood and Marrow Transplantation

Ljungman P, Ribaud P, Eyrich M, *et al. Bone Marrow Transplant* 2003; **31**: 481–6

BACKGROUND. There is no established treatment for adenovirus, which is an important cause of morbidity and mortality after allogeneic HSCT. Cidofovir has *in vitro* efficacy against adenovirus. In a retrospective analysis, 45 patients (from ten centres) who were treated with cidofovir for adenovirus were studied. Of the group, 16 patients had definite adenovirus disease, 13 probable disease and 16 asymptomatic infections.

INTERPRETATION. Cidofovir therapy was successful in 31 patients (69%), ten with adenovirus disease, ten with probable disease and ten with asymptomatic infections. Treatment was unsuccessful in ten patients and four were not evaluable owing to early death from other causes. Overall survival was 76% at 28 days and 46% at 6 months after cidofovir therapy was started. Toxicity associated with cidofovir occurred in 18 patients (40%), renal toxicity in 14 patients and other types of toxicities in four patients. The authors concluded that cidofovir may be useful against adenovirus after allogeneic HSCT, but further studies are needed.

Comment

Adenovirus infections have become an increasingly important cause of mortality and morbidity following allogeneic HSCT. This is particularly the case in children, in T-cell depleted, unrelated donor or mismatched donor transplants, and in situations where the patient receives profound immunosuppression to prevent or treat acute GvHD |17,18|. The mortality associated with adenovirus infection varies widely, depending upon a number of patient and transplant-related variables, but has reported to be anywhere between 6 and 26% |19|.

Unfortunately, there is no unequivocally proven therapy for the prevention or treatment of adenovirus infection. While intravenous ribavirin is widely used for the treatment of invasive adenovirus infection, the efficacy of this agent remains in question. Given the mortality and morbidity associated with adenovirus infection in the transplant population, the toxicity of ribavirin to staff and patients and the absence of effective therapy, there is considerable interest in the assessment of alternative antiviral agents for the management of adenovirus infection.

Cidofovir is a nucleotide analogue with broad antiviral activity against viruses, including CMV, herpesvirus and adenovirus. This study demonstrates that cidofovir has potential as a safe and effective antiviral agent for the treatment of adenovirus infection. However, despite the promise suggested by the results of this study, questions remain. First, despite claims that cidofovir is relatively innocuous, a significant number of those who receive cidofovir develop nephrotoxicity and a number of these will show signs of renal impairment following discontinuation of cidofovir. Secondly, while cidofovir may provide effective treatment for adenovirus, the effectiveness of therapy is related to viral load, creating a strong argument for surveillance strategies, including PCR and the pre-emptive administration of cidofovir, to prevent the dissemination of adenovirus disease |20|.

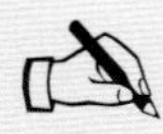

Low mortality rates related to respiratory virus infections after bone marrow transplantation

Machado CM, Boas LS, Mendes AV, *et al*. *Bone Marrow Transplant* 2003; **31**: 695–700

BACKGROUND. In bone marrow transplant patients, respiratory viruses are often the cause of severe respiratory disease. To determine the frequency of respiratory viruses, nasal washes were collected for a year from bone marrow transplant recipients with symptoms of upper respiratory tract infection. RSV, influenza A and B, adenovirus and parainfluenza viruses were determined by direct immunofluorescence assay. Ribavirin in aerosol form was given to patients with RSV pneumonia and to those with upper RSV infections who were considered at high risk of developing RSV pneumonia. Oseltamivir was given to those with influenza. In all, 392 episodes of upper respiratory tract infection in 179 patients were studied.

INTERPRETATION. Results of viral assays were positive in 68 patients (38%): RSV was detected in 18 patients (26%), influenza B in 17 (25%), influenza A in eleven (16%) and parainfluenza in seven (10%). Multiple respiratory virus infections or coinfection affected 14 patients (21%). RSV pneumonia developed in 56% of the patients with RSV upper respiratory tract infections. One of the 15 patients (7%) with RSV pneumonia died. Influenza pneumonia was diagnosed in three patients (7%). Peak infection times were autumn and winter for RSV infections and winter and spring for influenza. This study was not designed to evaluate antiviral interventions but patients treated with ribavarin or oseltamivir showed decreased rates of influenza and parainfluenza pneumonia and low mortality resulting from RSV pneumonia. Randomized trials are needed to assess the value of antiviral interventions such as aerosolized ribavirin and new neuraminidase inhibitors.

Comment

Community respiratory virus infections (RVI) due to RSV, influenza A and B, parainfluenza 1, 2 and 3, rhinovirus, adenovirus and coronavirus represent a major cause of morbidity and mortality in HSCT recipients, particularly during winter and autumn. The true extent of this problem is unclear, however, with prevalence rates of 1.8–36% reported in HSCT recipients. Most studies report data from developed countries in the northern hemisphere |**21**|.

This Brazilian study sought to quantify the prevalence, mortality and morbidity of RVI in HSCT recipients. The researchers found a low prevalence of RVI, with the peak RSV incidence in autumn and winter and the peak influenza A/B incidence in winter and spring. Importantly, they also found that 15% of patients had multiple episodes of RVI, that respiratory symptoms were frequently present throughout the year and that cases of influenza A/B also occurred during the summer months. Somewhat surprisingly, the researchers also found that RSV pneumonia was associated with low mortality. The reasons for this are unclear, but it may be explained by more consistent use of antiviral therapy, better infection control measures and routine influenza vaccination.

This study is important because it is one of the first outside the industrialized northern hemisphere to document the impact of community respiratory viral infections. While it reports a lower mortality from RVIs, it confirms the ubiquitous and seasonal nature of RVI in all HSCT recipients.

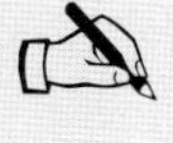

Comparison of PCR, enzyme immunoassay and conventional culture for adenovirus detection in bone marrow transplant patients with hemorrhagic cystitis

Raboni SM, Siqueira MM, Portes SR, Pasquini R. *J Clin Virol* 2003; **27**: 270–5

BACKGROUND. Viral cultures are usually used to diagnose adenovirus-associated haemorrhagic cystitis, which is now a recognized sequel of immunosuppression. In this prospective study various methods for diagnosing adenovirus in bone marrow transplant patients with haemorrhagic cystitis were assessed. Different laboratory techniques, PCR, enzyme immunoassay (EIA) and conventional culture were compared as means of detecting adenovirus in the urine of patients with haematuria in the first 100 days after bone marrow transplantation.

INTERPRETATION. Of the 143 urine samples analysed, 75 were collected in the pre-transplantation period (one from each patient), eight of which had haematuria. Another 68 samples were collected in the post-transplantation phase, all with microscopic or macroscopic haematuria. After transplantation, haematuria occurred in 39% of patients, and was more frequent when the transplant donors were not related to the recipients. Adenovirus was isolated in one pre-transplant patient without symptoms and in three patients with haemorrhagic cystitis grades 3 and 4 (severe), in the second or third month after their transplant. Compared with viral culture, the accuracy, specificity and sensitivity were, respectively, 95, 30 and 100% for EIA and 63, 100 and 60% for PCR. The authors concluded that, despite technical difficulties and the delay before results are obtained, cell culture remains the best method for adenovirus detection in the urine of patients with haemorrhagic cystitis.

Comment

Haemorrhagic cystitis (HC) is a major cause of morbidity following HSCT, occurring as a result of either high-dose cyclophosphamide treatment or viral cystitis |22|. A number of viruses may cause HC, including BK virus, papovavirus, CMV and adenovirus. Adenovirus, like CMV, is likely to result from endogenous viral reactivation rather than *de novo* infection.

The diagnosis of adenovirus infection is usually made by serological tests and viral culture. In the HSCT setting, however, both these tests have serious limitations. Antibody responses are attenuated due to post-transplantation immunosuppression, and viraemia, especially at low levels, can be observed in HSCT recipients in the absence of any symptoms or disease. Viral cultures are also time-consuming and results may not be available for days or weeks, leading to undesirable delays in commencing therapy.

Cell culture in epithelioid cell lines is considered the gold standard method for the diagnosis of adenovirus, although other methods are available, including EIA and PCR |23|.

This study compared PCR, EIA and conventional cell culture for the detection of adenovirus in the urine of patients with HC. The authors found that excretion and duration were directly correlated with the intensity of haematuria in patients with severe HC adenovirus. They also found that, as expected, EIA had low sensitivity but high specificity, and that PCR was associated with high sensitivity but low specificity and a low positive predictive value.

This study provides a salient reminder that, despite the advantages of PCR – speed, sensitivity and the ability to detect non-viable viruses – in certain situations PCR has sufficient limitations, particularly the high number of positive samples and low predictive value, that its routine use in clinical practice cannot be recommended. Indeed, the results of this study would suggest that cell culture, despite its low sensitivity and practical difficulties, would appear to be the best test for clinically significant adenovirus HC.

The results of this study, must, however, be interpreted in the light of our limited understanding of viral HC. Little is known about either the significance of urinary viruses in the post-transplantation setting or the pathogenesis of adenovirus HC. It appears likely, for example, that, like CMV, adenovirus may shed asymptomatically following reactivation after transplantation, and that a positive qualitative adenovirus PCR may simply represent viral reactivation and may not correlate with disease. For these reasons, PCR is unlikely to provide a truly valuable diagnostic tool for adenovirus HC until further research has clarified the levels of viral load that are predictive of disease and the exact role of quantitative PCR.

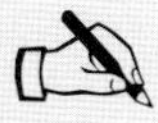

Randomized comparison of oral valacyclovir and intravenous ganciclovir for prevention of cytomegalovirus disease after allogeneic bone marrow transplantation

Winston DJ, Yeager AM, Chandrasekar PH, Snydman DR, Petersen FB, Territo MC; Valacyclovir Cytomegalovirus Study Group. *Clin Infect Dis* 2003; **36**: 749–58; Epub 2003 Mar 03

BACKGROUND. The efficacies of oral valaciclovir and intravenous ganciclovir for prevention of CMV disease after allogeneic bone marrow transplantation were compared in this multicentre randomized study. CMV-seropositive patients who received an allogeneic bone marrow transplant were given high-dose intravenous aciclovir (500 mg/m^2 every 8 h) from the day of transplantation until marrow engraftment. The patients were then randomly assigned to receive either oral valaciclovir, 2 g four times daily ($n = 83$), or intravenous ganciclovir, 5 mg/kg every 12 h for 1 week, and then 6 mg/kg once daily for 5 days per week ($n = 85$), until day 100 after transplantation.

INTERPRETATION. Among patients who received valaciclovir, 12% were infected with CMV and among those who received ganciclovir 19% were infected (HR 1.042; 95% CI 0.391–2.778; $P = 0.934$). Only two patients who received valaciclovir and one who received ganciclovir developed CMV disease (HR 1.943; 95% CI 0.176–21.44; $P = 0.588$). The results suggest that oral valaciclovir may be an effective alternative to intravenous ganciclovir for the prophylaxis of CMV disease after bone marrow transplantation.

Comment

In the past, patients undergoing HSCT were at high risk of CMV infection and CMV disease was a major cause of transplant-related mortality. Intravenous ganciclovir, used as either prophylaxis or as pre-emptive therapy on the basis of diagnosis of CMV antigenaemia or a PCR positive for CMV DNA, has markedly reduced the incidence of CMV disease after transplantation. Unfortunately, ganciclovir requires intravenous access and is also associated with considerable toxicity, including dose-limiting neutropenia, leading to an increased incidence of bacterial and fungal infections and decreased survival rates after transplantation.

Based on previous reports of the effectiveness of high-dose intravenous or oral aciclovir in reducing the risk of CMV infection after transplantation |**24**|, Winston and colleagues investigated the use of valaciclovir, the 1-valvy ester of aciclovir, for prophylaxis of CMV infection after transplantation. This study found that valaciclovir and ganciclovir had similar efficacy for the prevention of CMV infection in allogeneic transplant recipients. Importantly, however, valaciclovir was generally well tolerated, with a low incidence of nephrotoxicity and thrombotic microangiopathy, and was associated with a significantly lower incidence of neutropenia than ganciclovir. This study, the largest of its kind in HSTC recipients, suggests that valaciclovir is a viable alternative to ganciclovir, and may have particular utility in the outpatient setting. Further research is required to define the relative benefits of valaciclovir and valganciclovir, to establish the risk of developing valaciclovir- resistant CMV infection, and to determine whether the dose of valaciclovir can be safely reduced from 2 g four times a day to 1 g three times a day.

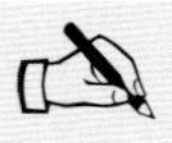

Incidence and outcome of adenovirus disease in transplant recipients after reduced-intensity conditioning with alemtuzumab

Avivi I, Chakrabarti S, Milligan DW, *et al. Biol Blood Marrow Transplant* 2004; **10**: 186–94

BACKGROUND. Among the recipients of allogeneic transplants, adenoviruses are now a major cause of infectious complications. The incidence and outcome of symptomatic adenovirus infection or adenovirus disease after alemtuzumab-based reduced-intensity conditioning were evaluated in 86 consecutive patients.

INTERPRETATION. Adenovirus disease occurred in eleven of the 86 patients (18%), five of whom died of progressive adenovirus disease. This was the most important infectious cause of mortality in this group of patients. The probability of non-relapse mortality was 49% in patients with adenovirus disease compared with 26% in those without ($P = 0.007$). The severity of lymphocytopenia and continuing immunosuppressive therapy were the major risk factors for progressive adenovirus disease and death. Patients who were not receiving immunosuppressive therapy or had had it reduced or withdrawn cleared the virus. The risk of progressive adenovirus disease ($P = 0.05$) was reduced by pre-emptive anti-CMV therapy for CMV reactivation. These results confirm the importance of adenovirus as a post-transplantation pathogen even after reduced-intensity conditioning. The severity of lymphocytopenia, anti-CMV prophylaxis and immunosuppressive therapy all had important influences on the outcome of adenovirus disease.

Comment

As the mortality of CMV and EBV infections following HSCT has declined, mortality and morbidity resulting from other viruses have increased |**25**|. Adenoviruses, in particular, are increasingly being recognized as an important pathogen after stem cell transplantation, occurring in 4.9–20.9% of allograft recipients |**17,26**|. Recent studies have suggested that, like CMV and RVI, adenovirus infections have particularly increased in incidence following reduced-intensity transplantation and in patients who receive alemtuzumab (Campath-1H) for T-cell depletion |**27–29**|.

This study provides further evidence regarding the incidence and outcome of adenovirus infection following T-cell-depleted, reduced-intensity transplantation. The authors found not only that adenovirus infection is increased in patients who have received alemtuzumab conditioning, but that the incidence, severity and outcome of adenovirus infection were greatest in those receiving continued immunosuppression for the prevention or treatment of acute GvHD. Indeed, the findings that reduction of immunosuppression frequently resulted in clinical improvement and clearing of the virus and that those patients who were not severely lymphopenic or receiving continued immunosuppression tended not to develop fatal, disseminated disease suggest that, as is the case for CMV and EBV, the containment of adenovirus is dependent on the development of adenovirus-specific immunity, the kinetics of which are determined by the speed of immune reconstitution and the use of immunosuppressive therapy.

While there is some evidence to suggest that ganciclovir may have a suppressive effect on adenovirus replication and that cidofovir and ribavirin may have some benefit as treatments for established adenovirus infection, the efficacy of any of these agents has not been conclusively proven |**30,31**|. Given the increasing popularity of reduced-intensity transplantation and the trend to more intensive, multi-agent immunosuppression for the management of GvHD, there is an urgent need to develop effective antiviral agents against adenovirus and to establish pre-emptive strategies for initiating antiviral therapy at the onset of adenovirus infection, when the patient is still asymptomatic and disease is limited.

Prompt versus preemptive intervention for EBV lymphoproliferative disease

Wagner HJ, Cheng YC, Huls MH, *et al*. *Blood* 2004; **103**: 3979–81; Epub 2004 Jan 29

BACKGROUND. Uncontrolled expansion of EBV-infected B cells after HSCT causes PTLDs. These disorders can be predicted by an increase in EBV DNA in peripheral blood mononuclear cells. Real-time quantitative PCR analysis was used to determine whether frequent monitoring of EBV DNA, to facilitate pre-emptive treatment, is of value after HSCT. More than 1300 samples from 85 transplant recipients were analysed.

INTERPRETATION. None of the patients whose EBV DNA levels were consistently low developed PTLDs. Nine patients had a high EBV load (more than 4000 EBV copies/μg peripheral blood mononuclear cell DNA) on one occasion, and 16 had high EBV loads detected on two or more occasions. Symptoms consistent with PTLDs developed in only eight of these patients, all of whom were promptly and successfully treated with EBV-specific cytotoxic T cells or CD20 monoclonal antibody. Quantitative measurement of EBV DNA appears to be valuable to facilitate prompt rather than pre-emptive treatment of PTLDs.

Comment

Secondary malignancies are recognized as a major complication of HSCT. The most common neoplastic disease occurring in the first year after HSCT is EBV-induced PTLD |**32**|. The clinical diagnosis of PTLD may be difficult because of the clinical and histological heterogeneity of PTLD. It may present as an infectious mononucleosis-like illness, with fatigue and lymphadenopathy, or as a febrile illness with leucopenia.

Treatment of PTLD may include anti-B-cell monoclonal antibodies, cytotoxic chemotherapy or donor-derived EBV-specific cytotoxic T lymphocytes |**33,34**|. As is the case with CMV infection, pre-emptive therapy of PTLD is feasible because the onset of PTLD is foreshadowed for several weeks by an increase in EBV load in the peripheral blood of patients receiving a transplant from an HLA-mismatched sibling donor or from an unrelated donor |**35**|.

This study used real-time quantitative PCR in HSCT recipients to determine whether it was sufficiently sensitive and specific to support pre-emptive intervention for PTLD. The authors found that EBV viral load varied substantially over time, both between and within patients. While EBV DNA was associated with a diagnosis of PTLD, even high levels of EBV DNA (above 4000 copies/μg) predicted PTLD on only 50% of occasions.

Given the low specificity and positive predictive value of peripheral blood EBV DNA and the availability of safe and effective therapy for PTLD, the results of this study suggest that EBV PCR should be used primarily to confirm a diagnosis of PTLD or to increase the clinical suspicion of PTLD rather than as a basis for pre-emptive therapy. This is in marked contrast to CMV infection after transplantation, for which CMV PCR is highly predictive of CMV disease and may justifiably be used to initiate pre-emptive therapy because the therapy for established CMV disease has a high failure rate and is associated with considerable toxicity.

Conclusion

The increasing trend to reduced intensity and outpatient transplantation and the increasing use of more intensive immunosuppression for the management of GvHD are likely to increase the risk and impact of post-transplantation viral infections over the coming decade. It would seem unlikely that current antiviral therapies will be sufficient to address the potential morbidity and mortality associated with the full range of viral infections, particularly adenovirus, EBV and community respiratory viruses. Rather, it would seem clear that the optimal management of post-HSCT viral infections will require a multidimensional approach based around rigorous scientific, clinical, translational and epidemiological research. Effective management will require:

- the introduction of rapid diagnostic techniques and establishment of pre-emptive therapeutic strategies where appropriate;

- a combination of pharmacological and cellular therapies for the prevention and treatment of viral reactivation and disease after transplantation;

- exploration of means for augmenting immune reconstitution (e.g. vaccination, IL-2, IL-7);

- standardized reporting of infectious outbreaks and nosocomial infections;

- liaison between hospitals and public health units (allowing rapid identification of community outbreaks of RVIs); and

- close collaboration between transplant physicians, nursing staff, virology laboratories, infectious disease physicians and infection control staff.

References

1. Donnelly JP. Bacterial complications of transplantation: diagnosis and treatment. *J Antimicrob Chemother* 1995; **36**: 59–72.

2. Jantunen E, Ruutu P, Niskanen L, Volin L, Parkkali T, Koukila-Kahkola P, Ruutu T. Incidence and risk factors for invasive fungal infection in allogeneic BMT recipients. *Bone Marrow Transplant* 1997; **19**: 801–8.

3. Bostrom L, Ringden O. Viral infections. Clinical bone marrow and blood stem cell transplantation. In: Atkinson K (ed.). *Major Transplant Related Problems, Part VIII*. Cambridge: Cambridge University Press, 2000; pp 758–82.

4. Giralt S. Complications of non-myeloablative stem cell transplantation. In: Giralt S, Slavin S (eds). *Non-myeloablative stem cell transplantation (NST)*. Oxford, UK: Darwin Scientific Publishing Limited, 2000; pp 139–48.

5. Hall C. Respiratory syncytial virus and parainfluenza virus. *N Engl J Med* 2001; **344**: 1917–28.

6. Garcia R, Raad I, Abi-Said D, Bodey G, Champlin R, Tarrand J, Hill LA, Umphrey J, Neumann J, Englund J, Whimbey E. Nosocomial respiratory virus infections. *Infect Control Hosp Epidemiol* 1997; **18**: 412–16.

7. Champlin E, Whimby E. Community respiratory virus infections in bone marrow transplant recipients: the MD Anderson Cancer Centre experience. *Biol Blood Marrow Transplant* 2001; 7: 85–105.

8. Gamadia LE, Rentenaar RJ, Baars PA, Remmerswaal EB, Surachno S, Weel JF, Toebes M, Schumacher TN, ten Berge IJ, van Lier RA. Differentiation of cytomegalovirus-specific CD8(+) T cells in healthy and immunosuppressed virus carriers. *Blood* 2001; **98**: 754–61.

9. Hengel H, Lucin P, Jonjic S, Ruppert T, Koszinowski UH. Restoration of cytomegalovirus antigen presentation by gamma interferon combats viral escape. *J Virol* 1994; **68**: 289–97.

10. Walter EA, Greenberg PD, Gilbert MJ, Finch RJ, Watanabe KS, Thomas ED, Riddell SR. Reconstitution of cellular immunity against cytomegalovirus in recipients of allogeneic

bone marrow by transfer of T-cell clones from the donor. *N Engl J Med* 1995; **333**: 1038–44.

11. Flomenberg P, Babbitt J, Drobyski WR, Ash RC, Carrigan DR, Sedmak GV, McAuliffe T, Camitta B, Horowitz MM, Bunin N. Increasing incidence of adenovirus disease in bone marrow transplant recipients. *J Infect Dis* 1994; **169**: 775–81.

12. Runde V, Ross S, Trenschel R, Lagemann E, Basu O, Renzing-Kohler K, Schaefer UW, Roggendorf M, Holler E. Adenoviral infection after allogeneic stem cell transplantation (SCT): report on 130 patients from a single SCT unit involved in a prospective multi-centre surveillance study. *Bone Marrow Transplant* 2001; **28**: 51–7.

13. Carrigan DR. Adenovirus infections in immunocompromised patients. *Am J Med* 1997; **102**: 71–4.

14. Venard V, Carret A, Corsaro D, Bordigoni P, Le Faou A. Genotyping of adenoviruses isolated in an outbreak in a bone marrow transplant unit shows that diverse strains are involved. *J Hosp Infect* 2000; **44**: 71–4.

15. Broers AE, van Der Holt R, van Esser JW, Gratama JW, Henzen-Logmans S, Kuenen-Boumeester V, Lowenberg B, Cornelissen JJ. Increased transplant-related morbidity and mortality in CMV-seropositive patients despite highly effective prevention of CMV disease after allogeneic T-cell-depleted stem cell transplantation. *Blood* 2000; **95**: 2240–5.

16. Kollman C, Howe CW, Anasetti C, Antin JH, Davies SM, Filipovich AH, Hegland J, Kamani N, Kernan NA, King R, Ratanatharathorn V, Weisdorf D, Confer DL. Donor characteristics as risk factors in recipients after transplantation of bone marrow from unrelated donors: the effect of donor age. *Blood* 2001; **98**: 2043–51.

17. Howard DS, Phillips II GL, Reece DE, Munn RK, Henslee-Downey J, Pittard M, Barker M, Pomeroy C. Adenovirus infections in haematopoietic stem cell transplant recipients. *Clin Infect Dis* 1999; **29**: 1494–501.

18. Baldwin A, Kingman H, Darville M, Foot AB, Grier D, Cornish JM, Goulden N, Oakhill A, Pamphilon DH, Steward CG, Marks DI. Outcome and clinical course of 100 patients with adenovirus infection following bone marrow transplantation. *Bone Marrow Transplant* 2000; **26**: 1333–8.

19. La Rosa AM, Champlin RE, Mirza N, Gajewski J, Giralt S, Rolston KV, Raad I, Jacobson K, Kontoyiannis D, Elting L, Whimbey E. Adenovirus infections in adult recipients of blood and marrow transplants. *Clin Infect Dis* 2001; **32**: 871–6.

20. Legrand F, Berrebi D, Houhou N, Freymuth F, Faye A, Duval M, Mougenot JF, Peuch-maur M, Vilmer E. Early diagnosis of adenovirus infection and treatment with cidofovir after bone marrow transplantation in children. *Bone Marrow Transplant* 2001; **27**: 621–6.

21. Ljungman P, Ward KN, Crooks BN, Parker A, Martino R, Shaw PJ, Brinch L, Brune M, De La Camara R, Dekker A, Pauksen K, Russell N, Schwarer AP, Cordonnier C. Respiratory virus infections after stem cell transplantation: a prospective study from the Infectious Diseases Working Party of the European Group for Blood and Marrow Transplantation. *Bone Marrow Transplant* 2001; **28**: 479–84.

22. Sencer SF, Haake RJ, Weisdorf DJ. Hemorrhagic cystitis after bone marrow transplantation. Risk factors and complications. *Transplantation* 1993; **56**: 875–9.

23. Echavarria MS, Ray SC, Ambinder R, Dumler JS, Charache P. PCR detection of adenovirus in a bone marrow transplant recipient: haemorrhagic cystitis as a presenting manifestation of disseminated disease. *J Clin Microbiol* 1999; **37**: 686–9.

24. Prentice HG, Gluckman E, Powles RL, Ljungman P, Milpied N, Fernandez Ranada JM, Mandelli F, Kho P, Kennedy L, Bell AR. Impact of long-term acyclovir on cytomegalovirus infection and survival after allogeneic bone marrow transplantation. *Lancet* 1994; **343**: 749–53.

25. Li CR, Greenberg PD, Gilbert MJ, Goodrich JM, Riddell SR. Recovery of HLA-restricted (CMV)-specific T-cell responses after allogeneic bone marrow transplant: correlation with CMV disease and effect of ganciclovir prophylaxis. *Blood* 1994; **83**: 1971–9.

26. Blanke C, Clark C, Broun ER, Tricot G, Cunningham I, Cornetta K, Hedderman A, Hromas R. Evolving pathogens in allogeneic bone marrow transplantation: increased fatal adenovirus infections. *Am J Med* 1995; **99**: 326–8.

27. Chakrabarti S, Mautner V, Osman H, Collingham KE, Fegan CD, Klapper PE, Moss PA, Milligan DW. Adenovirus infections following allogeneic stem cell transplantation: the incidence and outcome in relation to graft manipulation, immunosuppression and immune recovery. *Blood* 2002; **100**: 1619–27.

28. Chakrabarti S, Mackinnon S, Chopra R, Kottaridis PD, Peggs K, O'Gorman P, Chakraverty R, Marshall T, Osman H, Mahendra P, Craddock C, Waldmann H, Hale G, Fegan CD, Yong K, Goldstone AH, Linch DC, Milligan DW. High incidence of cytomegalovirus infection after nonmyeloablative stem cell transplantation: potential role of Campath-1H in delaying immune reconstitution. *Blood* 2002; **99**: 4357–63.

29. Chakrabarti S, Avivi I, Mackinnon S, Ward K, Kottaridis PD, Osman H, Waldmann H, Hale G, Fegan CD, Yong K, Goldstone AH, Linch DC, Milligan DW. Respiratory virus infections in transplant recipients after reduced-intensity conditioning with Campath-1H: high incidence but low mortality. *Br J Haematol* 2002; **119**: 1125–32.

30. Chakrabarti S, Collingham KE, Fegan CD, Milligan DW. Fulminant adenovirus hepatitis following unrelated bone marrow transplantation: failure of intravenous ribavirin therapy. *Bone Marrow Transplant* 1999; **23**: 1209–11.

31. Bruno B, Gooley T, Hackman RC, Davis C, Corey L, Boeckh M. Adenovirus infection in hematopoietic stem cell transplantation: effect of ganciclovir and impact on survival. *Biol Blood Marrow Transplant* 2003; **9**: 341–52.

32. Curtis RE, Travis JB, Rowlings PA, Socie G, Kingma DW, Banks PM, Jaffe ES, Sale GE, Horowitz MM, Witherspoon RP, Shriner DA, Weisdorf DJ, Kolb HJ, Sullivan KM, Sobocinski KA, Gale RP, Hoover RN, Fraumeni JF Jr, Deeg HJ. Risk of lymphoproliferative disorders after bone marrow transplantation: a multi-institutional study. *Blood* 1999; **94**: 2208–16.

33. van Esser JW, Niesters HG, van der Holt B, Meijer E, Osterhaus AD, Gratama JW, Verdonck LF, Lowenberg B, Cornelissen JJ. Prevention of Epstein-Barr virus–lymphoproliferative disease by molecular monitoring and pre-emptive rituximab in high-risk patients after allogeneic stem cell transplantation. *Blood* 2002; **99**: 4364–9.

34. Rooney CM, Smith CA, Ng CY, Loftin SK, Sixbey JW, Gan Y, Srivastava DK, Bowman LC, Krance RA, Brenner MK, Heslop HE. Infusion of cytotoxic T cells for the prevention and treatment of Epstein-Barr virus-induced lymphoma in allogeneic transplant recipients. *Blood* 1998; **92**: 1549–55.

35. van Esser JW, van der Holt B, Meijer E, Niesters HG, Trenschel R, Thijsen SF, van Loon AM, Frassoni F, Bacigalupo A, Schaefer UW, Osterhaus AD, Gratama JW, Lowenberg B, Verdonck LF, Cornelissen JJ. Epstein-Barr virus (EBV) reactivation is a frequent event after allogeneic stem cell transplantation (SCT) and quantitatively predicts EBV-lymphoproliferative disease following T-cell-depleted SCT. *Blood* 2001; **98**: 972–8.

12

Clostridium difficile infection

JANE FREEMAN, MARK WILCOX

Introduction

Clostridium difficile has emerged as a major nosocomial pathogen, particularly affecting elderly patients receiving antibiotic treatment. Reports of *C. difficile* infection (CDI) have risen markedly since the disease was first recognized in the late 1970s, and continue to increase. The emergence of epidemic and toxin A-negative, B-positive *C. difficile* strains has led researchers to refocus their investigations of the epidemiology and pathogenesis of *C. difficile*. The following ten studies illustrate the issues associated with the control and prevention of CDI, in addition to current research approaches and novel treatments.

The development and introduction of new antimicrobials into the clinical setting has implications for the prevention of CDI. The significant costs imposed upon institutions and healthcare services by CDI necessitate the re-evaluation of conventionally used treatments against newer therapies. Fluoroquinolones have been described as antibiotics with low risk of predisposing to CDI. However, reports linking the newer fluoroquinolones with CDI are increasing. The low predisposition to CDI of levofloxacin compared with β-lactam therapy was highlighted by Gopal Rao *et al.* in a prospective, randomized trial, which also underlined the well-known association of cephalosporins with CDI. Gaynes *et al.* reported significantly increased rates of CDI associated with formulary change from levofloxacin to gatifloxacin. CDI rates decreased following reversion to levofloxacin use. Fluoroquinolone, cephalosporin or penicillin use was commonly associated with the disease in a prospective study of CDI and unexplained leukocytosis by Wanahita and colleagues. *C. difficile* infection was confirmed in most cases of unexplained leukocytosis, and this emphasizes the need to consider this diagnosis in such cases. The lack of a well-controlled, gut-reflective model has forced *C. difficile* researchers to rely on animal models and human volunteer studies. While both approaches have provided valuable insight into the pathogenesis of *C. difficile*, animal models may not accurately reflect the human gut environment, and studies in human volunteers are limited by ethical considerations. These issues have been addressed in a study of the effects of cefotaxime and its metabolites on the behaviour of *C. difficile* in a gut model. The results obtained closely resemble those seen clinically, and indicate that this is a promising model of *C. difficile* infection, although further validation is necessary.

The emergence of toxin A-negative, toxin B-positive *C. difficile* strains has led to a re-evaluation of the view that toxin B has a lesser role in the pathogenesis of CDI. In an elegant study using a chimaeric mouse model, Savidge *et al.* clearly demonstrate the enterotoxic effects of toxin B. This study sounds a note of caution against reliance on animal models, which, though useful, may not reflect the human environment. The authors state the need to consider both toxins A and B when developing toxin-directed treatments. This is a view echoed by Aboudola *et al.* in their investigation of immunoglobulin (IgG) antibody response to a promising *C. difficile* toxoid vaccine. Further investigations of this vaccine are planned in elderly patients, particularly those mounting a poor IgG response to natural infections. Successful vaccination against CDI would be a welcome preventative measure, particularly given the limited options available for the treatment of the disease. The lack of available therapies for CDI has prompted a search for alternatives. Restoration of colonization resistance by non-pathogenic organisms has been the subject of considerable research. Prior symptomless colonization has previously been shown to reduce the likelihood of subsequent CDI. Merrigan *et al.* demonstrated that colonization of hamsters by a clindamycin-resistant non-toxigenic *C. difficile* strain prevented colonization and infection by a toxigenic strain, both during and after clindamycin treatment. The introduction of organisms carrying antimicrobial resistance genes into the human gut carries with it the potential transfer and dissemination of these genes to a wider pool of organisms. The authors point out the ethical considerations associated with this practice, which may preclude its viability as a treatment for CDI.

Recurrence of CDI is not uncommon, and is similarly frequent following both metronidazole and vancomycin therapy. Fernandez *et al.* found that low albumin levels and stay in an intensive care unit were predictors of metronidazole failure. While there remain unanswered questions, the repeatedly reported association between low albumin and poor outcome in CDI argues for studies to determine the effectiveness of correcting this abnormality in order to improve the therapeutic response. Bowel flora replacement has been described previously as a treatment for recurrent *C. difficile* infection and is revisited by Aas *et al.*, who report a 94% cure rate in 16 patients undergoing nasogastric administration of donor faeces. Environmental contamination is an important factor in nosocomial infections. Eradication of *C. difficile* from the hospital ward environment is particularly difficult since the organism can persist as chemically resistant spores. Wilcox *et al.* report a crossover study of detergent versus hypochlorite cleaning that provides evidence favouring of the use of hypochlorite-based cleaning agents in the hospital environment.

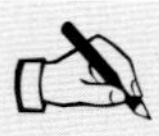

Prevention of fatal *Clostridium difficile*-associated disease during continuous administration of clindamycin in hamsters

Merrigan MM, Sambol SP, Johnson S, Gerding DN. *J Infect Dis* 2003; **188**: 1922–7

BACKGROUND. **Previous studies have shown that most patients colonized by** *C. difficile* **remain asymptomatic, regardless of whether the colonizing strain is**

toxigenic or non-toxigenic. *C. difficile*-associated disease due to toxigenic strains can be prevented in the hamster model by colonization with a non-toxigenic strain following clindamycin administration. In the present study, two non-toxigenic strains, of differing clindamycin susceptibility were investigated for their ability to colonize and prevent CDI in hamsters during clindamycin administration. Strains M13 (clindamycin-resistant, minimum inhibitory concentration [MIC] $\geq$256 mg/l) or M3 (clindamycin-susceptible, MIC 0.5 mg/l) were administered orogastrically (1 $\times$ 10^6 spores/day) on day 3, days 3–5 or days 3–7 during 5 days of clindamycin treatment. Hamsters were challenged with toxigenic strain B1 on days 5, 7 or 9 of clindamycin treatment. M13 (clindamycin-resistant) prevented *C. difficile*-associated diarrhoea (CDAD) in 100% of hamsters. M3 was protective in 0 hamsters on day 5, 20% on day 7 and 100% on day 9. Molecular investigations revealed that strain M13 possesses the *ermB* resistance gene but not the mobilizable genetic element *Tn5398*.

INTERPRETATION. Administration of a non-toxigenic clindamycin-resistant *C. difficile* strain prevents subsequent colonization and disease in clindamycin-treated hamsters, both during and after the treatment course. A clindamycin-susceptible strain was less protective. The risk of transferring clindamycin resistance to other enteric bacteria is highlighted.

Comment

This study builds upon earlier observations that prior symptomless colonization with *C. difficile* strains is associated with a reduced risk of subsequent symptomatic *C. difficile* infection |**1,2**|. A clindamycin-resistant non-toxigenic *C. difficile* strain (M13) colonized hamsters significantly faster than a clindamycin-sensitive strain (M3), and protected 100% of hamsters against colonization and disease when challenged with a toxigenic clindamycin-resistant *C. difficile* strain. Protection was afforded during and after the clindamycin treatment course. By contrast, the clindamycin-sensitive strain afforded protection only after clindamycin administration had ceased. The authors postulate that the patients are at risk of infection by a clindamycin-resistant toxigenic strain during and after clindamycin treatment, whereas clindamycin-sensitive strains are unlikely to colonize during the treatment period. The antimicrobial susceptibility profile of the protecting *C. difficile* strain, as well as the timing of colonization, appeared to be important in generating effective protection against subsequent colonization by a toxigenic strain. It would be interesting to ascertain whether a similar protective effect is observed during treatment with other predisposing antimicrobials.

Administration of organisms containing potentially mobile antimicrobial resistance genes into the human gut microflora is clearly contentious. Although dissemination of *ermB* by the mobile genetic element *Tn5396* was excluded in the protecting strain, the authors rightly point out the possibility that other transfer mechanisms may exist, and the need for further investigation before the possibility of using such strains in humans can be entertained.

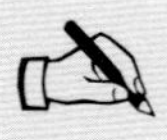

Clostridium difficile toxin B is an inflammatory enterotoxin in human intestine

Savidge TC, Pan W-H, Newman P, O'Brien M, Anton PM, Pothoulakis C.
Gastroenterology 2003; **125**: 413–20

BACKGROUND. *C. difficile* produces two major toxins, toxin A and toxin B, which are structurally similar. Animal experiments have suggested that diarrhoea and colitis occur only as a result of the effects of toxin A. However, toxin A-negative, B-positive *C. difficile* strains have recently been isolated from patients with antibiotic-associated colitis, including fatal cases, suggesting that toxin B may also be important in pathogenesis. A chimaeric animal model of *C. difficile* toxin-induced pathology of the human intestine was developed by transplanting human intestinal xenografts into immunodeficient mice. Intraluminal administration of toxin B, like that of toxin A, induced intestinal epithelial cell damage, increased mucosal permeability, stimulated interleukin (IL)-8 synthesis, and caused an acute inflammatory response. Luminal exposure to both toxins resulted in significantly increased intestinal epithelium cell-specific IL-8 gene expression in quantitative reverse transcription–PCR assays.

INTERPRETATION. Toxin B, like toxin A, is therefore a potent inflammatory enterotoxin for the human intestine. Future therapeutic strategies should target both toxins.

Comment

Despite showing greater cytotoxicity than toxin A in human colonic mucosa, toxin B has not been shown to have any enterotoxic effects in animal models, in contrast to toxin A. There is a growing number of reports of outbreaks of antibiotic-associated diarrhoea due to toxin A-negative, B-positive *C. difficile* strains |3–6|. This important study examined the enterotoxic effects of toxins A and B in human colon *in vivo* using a murine chimaeric model in which human fetal intestine was grafted into immunodeficient mice. The study was very well controlled in terms of toxin purity and activity and of xenograft origin and phenotype. Possible contamination of toxin A and B preparations was excluded as a reason for the observed effects. Acute inflammatory responses, characterized by tissue damage and neutrophil infiltration, epithelial cell damage, increased mucosal permeability and induction of IL-8 expression, were observed in response both to toxin A and toxin B and were similar in the chimaeric model, indicating that toxin B is a potent enterotoxin, like toxin A (Table 12.1). Expression of IL-8 was increased in xenografts exposed to toxin A and toxin B. Increased faecal IL-8 has been demonstrated in patients with *C. difficile* infection |7|, and this study raises the possibility that this may be relevant to the pathophysiology of the disease. In addition, the authors report briefly the presence of human neural crest-derived precursors that are capable of regenerating a functional and humanized enteric nervous system, and suggest the possibility of future studies to determine whether the effects of toxin B depend on enteric neurons.

Table 12.1 Effect of *C. difficile* toxins A and B on histologic severity and myeloperoxidase activity in human intestinal xenografts

	Histologic severity of enterocolitis			
	Epithelial damage	Congestion and oedema	Polymorphonucleocyte infiltration	Myeloperoxidase activity
Buffer control	0.0 ± 0.0	0.5 ± 0.3	0.3 ± 0.3	5401 ± 943
Toxin A treated	0.5 ± 0.3	1.8 ± 0.3	1.1 ± 0.4	16 191 ± 2908*
Toxin B treated	1.1 ± 0.4	2.2 ± 0.2*	1.7 ± 0.4[†]	20 118 ± 5933[†]

Histologic severity of intestinal inflammation was graded by a score of 0–3 (1) epithelial damage, (2) vascular congestion and oedema of the mucosa, and (3) neutrophil margination and infiltration as previously described. Measurement of mucosal myeloperoxidase activity confirmed the histologic findings of polymorphonycleocyte infiltration (number of neutrophils/mg protein). Toxin B significantly induced all parameters compared with buffer-treated grafts. Data are means ± SEM of 6–10 grafts per group.
* $P < 0.05$.
† $P < 0.01$.
Source: Savidge *et al.* (2003).

This study highlights the problems associated with animal models of infection, namely that the pathogenesis of a human disease is not necessarily accurately reflected in animal tissues. The failure of animal tissues to respond to toxin B was demonstrated in mouse ileal loops, in striking comparison to the potent enterotoxic effects seen in the chimaeric model. The ability of toxin A-negative, B-positive strains to cause disease may thus be explained by the enterotoxic activities of toxin B described in this study. In the light of this study, therapeutic approaches such as vaccines, antitoxin immunoglobulins and toxin binding technologies should be directed at both toxin A and toxin B.

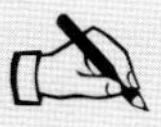

Recurrent *Clostridium difficile* colitis: case series involving 18 patients treated with donor stool administered via a nasogastric tube

Aas J, Gessert CE, Bakken JS. *Clin Infect Dis* 2003; **36**: 580–5

BACKGROUND. **Conventional treatment of CDI is with either metronidazole or vancomycin, but both have a high risk of symptomatic recurrence. Recurrences are also significantly more likely after a single relapse. Bacterial flora replacement therapy has been suggested as a form of probiotic treatment for recurrent *C. difficile* diarrhoea. This report is a retrospective review of 18 subjects who received donor stool by nasogastric tube for recurrent CDI during a 9-year period. The 18 subjects received a total of 64 courses of antimicrobials (range 2–7 courses; median 3 courses). During the 90-day period following donor stool replacement, 15 of 18 patients remained free from *C. difficile* diarrhoea. One patient experienced**

a single recurrence during this period, and two patients died of unrelated illnesses. No adverse effects of donor stool administration were reported.

INTERPRETATION. Donor stool replacement may be of benefit to patients suffering from multiple recurrences of CDI.

Comment

CDI is thought to occur as a result of depletion of gut microflora following antimicrobial exposure. Donor stool administration seeks to reconstitute the depleted gut flora of the recipient by transplanting an intact microflora from the donor. Previous reports of this therapy have usually employed rectal infusion of donor faeces |8–12|. However, this study describes administration of donor stool via a nasogastric tube. The authors cite reduced patient preparation, clinical time, patient inconvenience and cost as reasons for selecting nasogastric as opposed to rectal administration. It should be noted, however, that both approaches involve considerable preparation of both patient (donor selection, consent, preparation for procedure) and donor stool (blood and stool screen for viral, bacterial and protozoal pathogens). In this study, preparation of the patient involved a 4-day course of vancomycin (250 mg q.d.s.), itself a conventional treatment for *C. difficile* diarrhoea. Diarrhoea was reported to have been reduced or even eliminated in most patients by the vancomycin treatment. Although the authors argue that control of diarrhoea *per se* was not the aim of the treatment, and many of the patients enrolled in this study had suffered multiple relapses despite vancomycin treatment, it is nonetheless a confounding factor when interpreting the results of this study. In addition, the preparation of donor faeces is also open to question. The authors do not state that preparation was carried out under anaerobic conditions or with pre-reduced buffers, which would have been desirable in order to preserve the anaerobic components of the donor microflora.

Two patients died from conditions unrelated to stool transplantation. The authors report a 94% cure rate for the 16 patients who survived. One patient experienced a recurrence of symptoms, which were successfully treated with vancomycin. All patients reported that their bowel habits returned to the patterns that had preceded their first episode of CDI. It might be anticipated that patients may find the concept of the procedure unappealing. Surprisingly perhaps, no patient objected to the procedure on the grounds that it lacked aesthetic appeal. This may be a reflection of the debilitation suffered during periods of recurrence, and the frustration at repeated failure of conventional therapy. The number of patients described is understandably small, as this therapy was envisaged as a last resort for patients experiencing multiple relapses. The authors call for a randomized controlled study to assess the therapy as an effective, low-risk and inexpensive alternative to conventional antimicrobial treatment. Despite the high success rate reported in this study, it is difficult to envisage either rectal or, in as this report, nasogastric stool delivery as a viable, practicable alternative to other therapies (antimicrobials, immunoglobulin, probiotics) except in the most recalcitrant of cases.

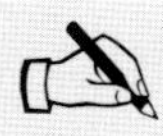

Clostridium difficile vaccine and serum immunoglobulin G antibody response to toxin A

Aboudola A, Kotloff KL, Kyne L, *et al. Infect Immun* 2003; **71**: 1608–10

B ACKGROUND . **Serum antibody responses to toxin A are strongly associated with protection against *C. difficile* diarrhoea. The aim of the study was to determine whether serum concentrations of antitoxin A IgG achieved during vaccination were of similar magnitude to those associated with protection against CDI in clinical studies. Healthy adults received 6.25, 25 or 100 μg parenteral *C. difficile* toxoid vaccine (soluble toxoid or toxoid adsorbed to alum) on days 1, 8, 30 and 60. Serum samples were assayed for antitoxin A IgG on days 1, 8, 15 and 90. In all patients, vaccination produced serum concentrations of antitoxin A IgG that exceeded those associated with protection in previous clinical studies. In the majority of patients the protective level of antibody was exceeded by a factor of 50. These findings support the feasibility of using a vaccine to protect high-risk individuals against *C. difficile* infection.**

I NTERPRETATION . A parenteral toxoid vaccine induced very high-level responses, indicated by high serum concentrations of antitoxin A IgG in all recipients. Serum antitoxin A IgG levels exceeded the levels associated with protection in previous studies. Vaccination may be a feasible preventative measure against *C. difficile* infection in susceptible individuals.

Comment

This study builds on the previous encouraging report on the safety and immunogenicity of a *C. difficile* toxoid vaccine in healthy human volunteers |**13**|. A *C. difficile* toxoid vaccine, containing both toxoid A and toxoid B, was administered parenterally to healthy volunteers and elicited a response resulting in very high levels of antitoxin A IgG in all recipients. High levels of serum antitoxin A IgG have been associated with protection against infection in previous studies |**14,15**|. In this study, the serum antitoxin A IgG levels exceeded concentrations previously associated with protection, by a factor of 50 in most individuals. A good antibody response was therefore observed regardless of the formulation (soluble toxoid or toxoid adsorbed to alum) or the concentration (6.35, 25 or 100 μg) administered. This suggests that the toxoid vaccine is highly immunogenic and more effective than natural infection in eliciting an immune response to *C. difficile* toxin A (Fig. 12.1). However, it remains to be seen whether this vaccine can induce an effective immune response in elderly subjects and in patients suffering from recurrent *C. difficile*-associated diarrhoea, who fail to mount a protective immune response to toxin A during the natural course of *C. difficile* infection |**15**|.

Serum neutralization of toxin A in a cell culture cytotoxicity assay was not significantly elevated in protected individuals, possibly indicating that either toxin A *in vitro* cytotoxicity does not correlate well with *in vivo* enterotoxicity, or that antitoxin A IgG is merely a surrogate marker of a protective immune response. While

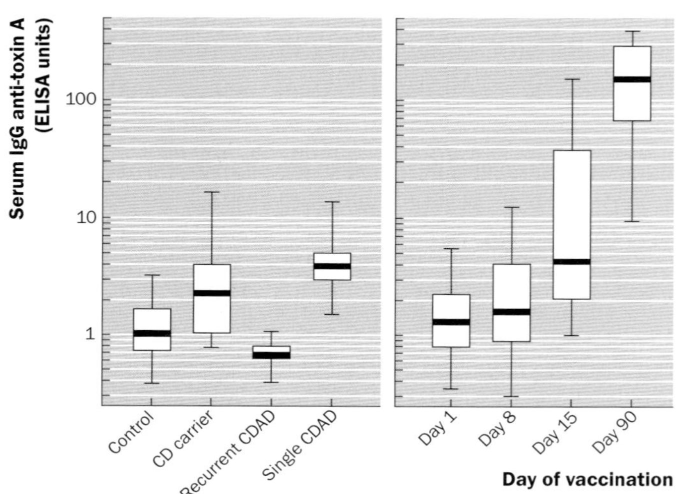

Fig. 12.1 Serum antitoxin A IgG concentrations following natural infection with *C. difficile* (left) or vaccination with *C. difficile* toxoid (right). Results, expressed as ELISA (enzyme-linked immunosorbent assay) units, are shown for control patients not infected with *C. difficile* (Control, *n* = 187), symptom-free carriers of *C. difficile* (CD carrier, *n* = 19), patients with recurrent *C. difficile*-associated diarrhoea (Recurrent CDAD, *n* = 9), patients with a single episode of *C. difficile*-associated diarrhoea (Single CDAD, *n* = 7) and healthy volunteers at various time-points during vaccination with *C. difficile* toxoid (*n* = 30). The median values are shown as bold horizontal lines, the boxes indicate the 25th and 75th percentiles, and the vertical bars indicate the 10th and 90th percentiles. Source: Aboudola *et al.* (2003).

only antitoxin A IgG concentrations were determined as a measure of the vaccine's potential to induce a protective response, the authors emphasize the importance of considering both toxins when directing a therapeutic approach. *C. difficile* toxin A-negative, B-positive strains are increasingly associated with disease, and it is important that any potential vaccine should incorporate both toxins.

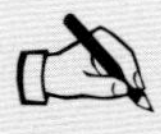

Effects of cefotaxime and desacetylcefotaxime upon *Clostridium difficile* proliferation and toxin production in a triple-stage chemostat model of the human gut

Freeman J, O'Neill FJ, Wilcox MH. *J Antimicrob Chemother* 2003: **52**; 96–102

BACKGROUND. Cefotaxime is well known for its propensity to cause CDI, but the mechanisms behind its predisposition to the disease remain to be elucidated. Previous investigations of *C. difficile* pathogenesis have relied on *in vitro* test tube experiments, animal models or human volunteer studies. A triple-stage chemostat

model of the human gut was used to investigate the behaviour of *C. difficile* and components of the gut microflora in response to exposure to cefotaxime alone and in combination with its active metabolite desacetylcefotaxime. *C. difficile* remained in a steady state with no detectable cytotoxin during non-antibiotic-exposed control periods. During both antibiotic exposure regimens, *C. difficile* germination, proliferation and toxin production were observed. Reductions in viable counts and cytotoxin levels were observed after cessation of antibiotic instillation. Gut bacterial counts, most notably bifidobacteria and bacteroides, decreased in response to both antibiotic exposure regimens. Bacteroides were markedly affected by exposure to the combination cefotaxime–desacetylcefotaxime. This may indicate a possible role for this group of organisms in colonization resistance. The gut model is a promising model for studying pathogenesis in controlled conditions analogous to the *in vivo* situation.

INTERPRETATION. *C. difficile* germination, proliferation and toxin production occurred in response to cefotaxime and desacetylcefotaxime administration, in contrast to non-antibiotic-exposed control periods. Bacteroides were markedly affected by antibiotic treatment, suggesting a role in colonization resistance. The gut model is a promising means of studying *C. difficile* pathogenesis.

Comment

This study describes the use of a triple-stage chemostat model of the human gut as a model of antibiotic-mediated CDI. The model was designed to reproduce the spatial, temporal, nutritional and physicochemical characteristics of the proximal and distal bowel and was validated against the caecal contents of sudden death victims |**16**|. This is a significant step forward in terms of *in vitro* modelling of CDI and as a viable alternative to animal models and human volunteer studies. These approaches are limited either by their ability to reflect the human gut or by ethical issues that preclude the collection of well-controlled data. Following the introduction of *C. difficile* spores to the model, the organism did not proliferate or produce toxin. The authors suggest that this quiescent state is analogous to colonization *in vivo*, particularly in the light of the heavy inoculum used. This study investigated the effects of antibiotic metabolites on *C. difficile*, a subject that has largely been overlooked. The gut model was dosed with cefotaxime alone or in combination with its active metabolite, desacetylcefo-taxime. Antibiotic was instilled at biliary levels to reflect the concentrations seen in the gut. The profound effect of the desacetylcefotaxime treatment on bacteroides and, to a lesser extent, bifidobacteria indicates both that these organisms may be important in colonization resistance and also that antibiotic metabolites may indeed be important in predisposition to CDI. *C. difficile* germination, proliferation and toxin production in response to both antibiotic dosing regimens was clearly observed, and was followed by an equally marked decrease in numbers and cytotoxin titres after cessation of anti-biotic instillation. Further studies using comparator antibiotics are necessary to fully validate this approach to modelling CDI *in vitro*. While the gut model cannot mimic intestinal secretions or immunological events, the advantages of a gut-reflective system that is well controlled in terms of nutrition and antibiotic concentration mean that the gut model promises to be a useful means of studying the pathogenesis of *C. difficile*.

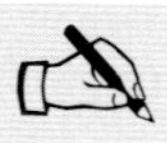

Clostridium difficile infection in patients with unexplained leukocytosis

Wanahita A, Goldsmith EA, Marino BJ, Musher DM. *Am J Med* 2003; **115**: 543–6

BACKGROUND. The present study aimed to determine prospectively what proportion of cases of unexplained leukocytosis in a tertiary care hospital setting is due to unrecognized CDI. Sixty patients who had unexplained leukocytosis (white blood cell [WBC] count $\geq 15 \times 10^9$/l) had faecal specimens tested for *C. difficile* toxin A using an enzyme immunosorbent assay. Fifty-eight per cent of these patients had *C. difficile* toxin in at least one faecal specimen, compared with three (12%) of 26 hospitalized control patients who did not have unexplained leukocytosis ($P <0.001$). Symptoms of colitis were often mild or absent at the time the WBC count was first elevated or, if present, had not been recognized by the attending physicians. Leukocytosis resolved promptly in most patients who were treated with metronidazole. In the 25 patients (42%) who had a negative test for *C. difficile* toxin, leukocytosis also tended to resolve during empirical therapy with metronidazole.

INTERPRETATION. Most patients who had unexplained leukocytosis had CDI. Unexplained leukocytosis in hospitalized patients should prompt a search for evidence of CDI.

Comment

This group first described in an observational study that *C. difficile* infection (CDI) was present in 9% of hospitalized adults whose peripheral WBC count was greater than 15×10^9/l |**17**|. Furthermore, excluding those with haematological malignancy, CDI was found to be present in a quarter of patients with WBC counts greater than 30×10^9/l. However, in that study a diagnosis of CDI could only be considered if the clinician considered the diagnosis and submitted a faecal sample for toxin testing. A review of records established that approximately a fifth of patients with raised WBC counts had clinical features consistent with CDI.

In the present prospective study, most (58%; $P <0.001$) hospitalized patients with unexplained leukocytosis had a positive assay for *C. difficile* toxin (Table 12.2). The actual number of cases associated with CDI may be even greater than this, given the suboptimal sensitivity of the enzyme immunosorbent assay test, particularly for toxin A alone, that was used in this study. Symptoms of colitis eventually appeared in nearly all patients, although in half these were overlooked by clinicians and were noted only in the nursing records. It has been shown previously that medical staff are likely to be unaware of diarrhoea in their patients |**18,19**|. Interestingly, the WBC count normalized in most of the patients after treatment with metronidazole, including nine of 12 symptomatic toxin-negative patients. Rapid symptom improvement in some of these patients suggests spontaneous resolution rather than a response to therapy. Furthermore, the absence of a control treatment group and the fact that approximately a quarter of CDI episodes resolve without specific anti-microbial therapy mean that the significance of this observation is uncertain. The

Table 12.2 Characteristics of the three groups of patients: those with unexplained leukocytosis who were *C. difficile* toxin-positive, those with leukocytosis who were toxin-negative, and controls with leukocytosis

Characteristic	Unexplained leukocytosis		
	Toxin assay positive (*n* = 35)	Toxin assay negative (*n* = 25)	Controls (*n* = 26)
	Number (%) or mean ± SD		
Age (years)	64 ±9.8	64 ± 12	57 ± 11.9
Male sex	35 (100)	25 (100)	24 (92)
Previous *Clostridium difficile* infection	3 (9)	1 (4)	1 (4)
White blood cell count (/mm^3)	23 100 ± 11 000	23 500 ± 7700	12 200 ± 6700
Prior antibiotics	32 (91)	18 (72)	24 (92)
Prior chemotherapy	4 (11)	0	1 (4)
Fever ≥99.8°F	7 (20)	14 (56)*	4 (15)
Days from admission to toxin assay	20 ± 26.3	17 ± 42.5	20 ± 25.2
Positive toxin assays/toxin assays performed	45/61 (74)†	0/49 (0)	4/42 (10)

*Fever was significantly more common in patients with leukocytosis and a negative toxin assay than in patients with leukocytosis and a positive assay or controls (*P* <0.05). Prior antibiotic use was more common in patients with leukocytosis and a positive *C. difficile* toxin assay than in those with leukocytosis and a negative assay (*P* <0.05).
†In 35 patients with at least one positive assay for *C. difficile* toxin, 45 of 61 samples assayed were positive, as compared with 4 of 42 samples in controls (*P* <0.001).
Source: Wanahita *et al.* (2003).

authors briefly discuss the possibility of using empirical therapy with metronidazole in patients with unexplained leukocytosis, but without further investigation of its true effectiveness this approach cannot be supported at this stage. Nevertheless, unexplained leukocytosis, particularly in high-risk individuals, should prompt investigation for CDI.

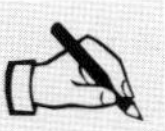

Outbreak of *Clostridium difficile* infection in a long-term care facility: association with gatifloxacin use

Gaynes R, Rimland D, Killum E, *et al. Clin Infect Dis* 2004; **38**: 640–5

BACKGROUND. Fluoroquinolones have been considered to have a low risk of promoting CDI. However, new agents such as moxifloxacin and gatifloxacin have significantly increased anti-anaerobic activity. Investigation of an increased incidence of CDI in a long-term care facility showed that it coincided with a formulary change from levofloxacin to gatifloxacin. This prompted a case–control study. Three control subjects were chosen randomly for each patient with CDI during the endemic

period, yielding 21 cases and 59 controls. Logistic regression analysis only demonstrated associations between CDI and the use of clindamycin (*P* = 0.005) and gatifloxacin, the latter being associated with an increasing risk of CDAD with increasing duration of gatifloxacin therapy (*P* <0.0001).

INTERPRETATION. An outbreak of CDAD in an long-term care facility was associated with a formulary change from levofloxacin to gatifloxacin. The rate of CDAD in this facility decreased after a change back to levofloxacin.

Comment

To date there has been little evidence linking fluoroquinolones with CDI. In a retrospective case–control study of 27 patients over 3 months in a 300-bed tertiary care hospital, prior exposure to cephalosporins and the use of ciprofloxacin were found to be significant risk factors for *C. difficile* infection in a multivariate analysis [20]. Interestingly, in another recent case–control study treatment with fluoroquinolones (odds ratio [OR] 12.7; 95% confidence interval [CI] 2.6–61.6) was the strongest risk factor for CDI [21]. For the patients who received fluoroquinolones, levofloxacin was prescribed by far the most frequently, followed by ciprofloxacin and gatifloxacin. Notably, however, a large prospective study (reviewed in this chapter) recently showed that the incidence of *C. difficile* diarrhoea was significantly lower in patients treated with levofloxacin than in those treated with cefuroxime (2.2 versus 9.2%; *P* <0.0001), and was similar to that in those receiving amoxycillin (1.8%; *P* = 0.7) (see Gopal Rao *et al.*).

In the present study, CDI attack rates in fluoroquinolone recipients were surprisingly high (17 and 34% for levofloxacin and gatifloxacin respectively). This implies that a virulent strain was present and/or a high transmission/cross-infection rate occurred. Unfortunately, *C. difficile* isolates from patients in the long-term care facility in the endemic period were not tested for fluoroquinolone susceptibility and were also not subjected to DNA fingerprinting to establish whether a new clone had been introduced. Some isolates from the separate acute hospital were available for examination, but results for these cannot be extrapolated to the affected unit.

It has been shown that strains belonging to the virulent UK endemic *C. difficile* clone were significantly more fluoroquinolone-resistant than were sporadic strains [22]. Also, individuals with a *C. difficile* strain resistant to the new-generation fluoroquinolone moxifloxacin were significantly more likely to have received a fluoroquinolone in the preceding 3 months than were those who had susceptible strains [23]. The message here is that fluoroquinolones cannot be assumed to be low-risk and that CDI rates should be under surveillance, particularly when new agents are introduced into the formulary for elderly patients. The relative risk of CDI with differing fluoroquinolones remains unclear and is probably affected by the local prevalence of resistant *C. difficile* strains.

In a logistic regression analysis only exposure to clindamycin and the number of days of gatifloxacin were significantly associated with CDI.

Table 12.3 Characteristics of patients in a case–control study of an increased incidence of CDI

Characteristic	Case patients (*n* = 21)	Control subjects (*n* = 59)	*P**
Age, mean years	75.75	71.7	ns
Duration of LTCF stay, median days	38	33	ns
Room-mate with CDAD	5 (24)	7 (12)	ns
Mean no. of comorbidities	3.3	2.9	ns
Mean Horn score	3.08	2.80	ns
Death	9 (43)	19 (32)	ns
GI procedure or surgery	3 (14)	4 (7)	ns
Use of feeding tube	3 (14)	3 (5)	ns
Any antibiotic exposure	21 (100)	32 (54)	0.0001
Clindamycin	5 (24)	2 (3)	0.004
Gatifloxacin	14 (67)	15 (25)	0.0006
Piperacillin–tazobactam	4 (19)	10 (17)	ns
Vancomycin	3 (14)	7 (12)	ns
Duration of gatifloxacin therapy, mean days	14.6	7.45	<0.0002

Data are no. (%) of patients, unless otherwise indicated. ns, not significant.
*The *t* test was used for continuous variables with the exception of length of stay, for which the Wilcoxon rank sum test was used. The χ^2 test was used for non-continuous variables.
Source: Gaynes *et al.* (2004).

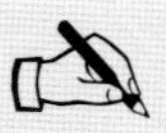

Comparison of the effect of detergent versus hypochlorite cleaning on environmental contamination and incidence of *Clostridium difficile* infection

Wilcox MH, Fawley WN, Wigglesworth N, Parnell P, Verity P, Freeman J. *J Hosp Infect* 2003; **54**: 109–14

BACKGROUND. **C. difficile spores may persist in the hospital environment for many months and are resistant to many commonly used cleaning agents. A ward-based study using a crossover design was performed to determine whether environmental cleaning with a hypochlorite disinfectant compared with a neutral detergent can reduce the incidence of CDI. Thirty-five per cent of 1128 environmental samples collected over 2 years grew C. difficile. There was a significant decrease in the incidence of CDI on one of the two study wards, from 8.9 to 5.3 cases per 100 admissions (P <0.05), using hypochlorite. On the same ward the incidence of CDI was significantly associated with the proportion of culture-positive environmental sites (P <0.05). On the other ward, the only significant correlation between CDI and C. difficile culture-positive environmental sites was in patient side-rooms (P <0.05). Antibiotic use was similar throughout the trial.**

INTERPRETATION. The results provide some evidence that the use of hypochlorite for environmental cleaning may significantly reduce the incidence of CDI, but the potential for confounding factors remains.

Comment

Evidence for an important role for environmental contamination in the aetiology of hospital-acquired infection is poor, and attempts to reduce infection rates by enhancing environmental cleaning have generally proved unsuccessful. However, the environmental persistence of spores and the enhanced endemicity and virulence of particular strains mean that it is possible that reducing the environmental burden may lessen the risk of cross-infection by *C. difficile*. Furthermore, sporulation of *C. difficile* can actually be enhanced when cultured in faeces exposed to non-chlorine-based hospital cleaning agents [24]. Kaatz *et al.* reported that an outbreak of CDI ended following the introduction of disinfection with hypochlorite, and surface contamination decreased to 21% of initial levels [25]. In a recent before-and-after intervention study, Mayfield *et al.* found that the incidence of CDI in patients on a bone marrow transplant unit decreased significantly following substitution of a quaternary ammonium solution by hypochlorite for environmental disinfection [26]. When cleaning based on quaternary ammonium solution was reintroduced, the incidence of CDI increased almost to baseline level.

The present study adds further evidence of the potential of hypochlorite-based disinfection to reduce the incidence of CDI. The significant decrease in CDI incidence during hypochlorite cleaning on one of the two study wards (Fig. 12.2) represented 17 fewer cases of cytotoxin-positive diarrhoea than during detergent-based cleaning. As found by Samore and colleagues [27], the frequency of positive personnel hand culture was strongly correlated with the intensity of environmental contamination, at least on one study ward. It is unknown why the results differed markedly between the two study wards, which were very similar. Major confounding factors

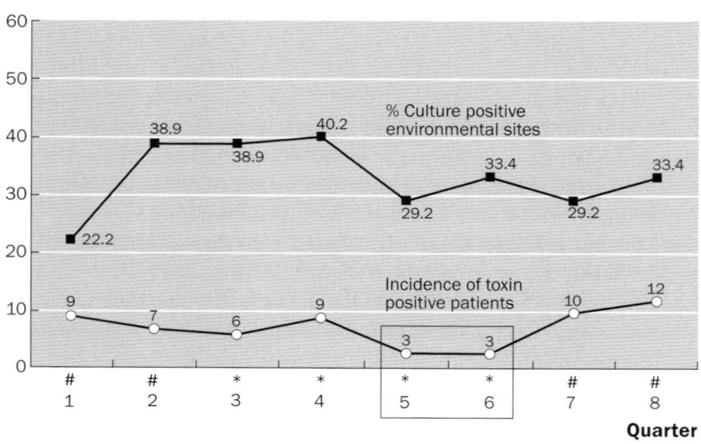

Fig. 12.2 Quarterly incidence of *C. difficile* infection and ward contamination during detergent (#) and chlorine (*) cleaning. Source: Wilcox *et al.* (2003).

were not obvious (antibiotic use was similar during each cleaning period), but variations in prescribing, patient type or cleaning efficiency may have influenced either the incidence of CDI or environmental contamination.

However, while hypochlorite-based cleaning may be more effective in reducing levels of environmental *C. difficile* spores, it is uncertain whether such long-term use, particularly at high concentrations, is sustainable, given its corrosive nature. Another potential drawback of hypochlorite-based disinfection is its reduced effectiveness on soiled surfaces, although products are available that combine detergent and hypochlorite components. It has been estimated that each CDI case costs more than £4000, primarily because of hotel costs associated with prolonged length of stay |28|. This high figure can be used to justify expenditure on improved standards of hospital cleanliness, possibly including the use of hypochlorite-based products, particularly in CDI endemic units.

Clostridium difficile-associated diarrhoea in patients with community-acquired lower respiratory infection being treated with levofloxacin compared with beta-lactam-based therapy

Gopal Rao G, Mahankali Rao CS, Starke IL. *J Antimicrob Chemother* 2003; **51**: 697–701

BACKGROUND. Fluoroquinolones have been considered to have a low risk of promoting CDI. Newer fluoroquinolones such as moxifloxacin and gatifloxacin have increased anti-anaerobic activity in comparison with older agents such as ciprofloxacin and levofloxacin. Levofloxacin is used in some centres to treat patients hospitalized with lower respiratory tract infection (LRTI), but its relative risk compared with generally favoured β-lactam-based therapy is unclear. In a prospective open-label trial, 490 hospitalized patients were treated for LRTI with levofloxacin and 448 with β-lactams such as cefuroxime or amoxycillin. The overall incidence of CDI (toxin A-positive diarrhoea) was 3.8%, and there was a lower incidence in levofloxacin recipients versus patients treated with β-lactams (2.2 versus 5.6%; *P* <0.01), particularly cefuroxime (9.2%; *P* <0.0001). There was no significant difference in the incidence of CDI between patients treated with levofloxacin or amoxycillin (2.2 versus 1.8%; *P* = 0.6). Cefuroxime and amoxycillin recipients had a significantly longer duration of treatment than patients in the levofloxacin group. Levofloxacin patients had a significantly shorter duration of hospitalization compared with the β-lactam group (mean 11.7 versus 13.3 days; *P* <0.01), especially compared with cefuroxime recipients (mean 16 days; *P* <0.0000001). Patients with CDI had a longer duration of hospital stay than those without CDI (25.8 versus 11.9 days; *P* <0.0000001).

INTERPRETATION. Levofloxacin was less likely to induce CDI and was associated with a shorter duration of hospital stay compared with LRTI therapy based on β-lactams (primarily cefuroxime).

Comment

Comment on this study area has been made earlier in this chapter (see Gaynes *et al.*).

The present study is unusual in two main respects: first its prospective nature, and secondly its much larger size than other studies in this area. For these reasons, the main finding that hospitalized patients treated with levofloxacin for LRTI were significantly less likely to develop CDI than those receiving β-lactam therapy is potentially important. However, care needs to be taken when interpreting the data. The main differences seen are between levofloxacin and cefuroxime (not amoxycillin) recipients. This is not that surprising, given the known relatively high propensity of cefuroxime to induce CDI. No information is provided about the power of the study to detect a true difference in CDI between amoxycillin and levofloxacin recipients. Also, we are not told what, if any, follow-on oral therapy was used for intravenous cefuroxime recipients. The secondary finding that levofloxacin patients had a shorter hospital stay is of interest, but the data analysis carried out does not inform as to whether or not this reduced duration of stay was related to the reduction in CDI.

Other caveats in this study include the use of a *C. difficile* toxin A-only detection method. Hence, CDI caused by toxin A-negative, toxin B-positive strains (estimated to account for approximately 8% of cases in the study hospital) would have been missed. It was assumed by the authors that such cases should have been evenly distributed between the different antibiotic treatment groups. Lastly, there was a potential for allocation bias in the study, as randomization was according to specific clinicians. Clinicians were assigned to prescribe β-lactam- or levofloxacin-based therapy. We are not told whether such allocation was successful, and this was switched after 12 months of a 17-month study. While a fifth of amoxycillin patients also received erythromycin, comparable data are not provided for the other antibiotic groups.

Factors associated with failure of metronidazole in *Clostridium difficile*-associated disease

Fernandez A, Anand G, Friedenberg F. *J Clin Gastroenterol* 2004; **38**: 414–18

BACKGROUND. Approximately 10% of patients fail to respond to first-line therapy for CDI (usually oral metronidazole). Vancomycin is considered as second-line therapy (i.e. it is for metronidazole non-responders) but it is unclear which patients could benefit from vancomycin treatment. This retrospective review of patients treated for CDI while hospitalized during a 21-month period aimed to determine factors associated with failure to respond (improvement in symptoms, including reduction of diarrhoea to two or fewer episodes per day) within 5 days to metronidazole therapy. Of 119 CDI patients, 99 had sufficient data available to include them in the analysis; of these, 61 (62%) responded to metronidazole and 38 (38%) were treatment failures. Albumin less than 2.5 g/l (OR 11.7; 95% CI 4.0–31.6) and intensive care unit stay at or before diagnosis (OR 4.1; 95% CI 1.3–12.2) were the only variables associated with treatment failure.

When considering these two variables together (low albumin, intensive care unit care), the area under the receiver operating characteristic curve was 0.80 for predicting treatment failure.

INTERPRETATION. An albumin level below 2.5 g/l and intensive care unit stay are predictors of failure of metronidazole therapy for CDI.

Comment

Low albumin has been reported previously as a risk factor in CDI. Kyne *et al.* found that low serum albumin and continuation of systemic antibiotic treatment were associated with symptom recurrence after the end of therapy |**29**|. Also, low serum albumin was reported as an independent predictor of a poor outcome in patients with CDI |**30**|. A low albumin concentration may be secondary to protein-losing enteropathy and/or decreased protein intake. Notably, Rybolt *et al.* found evidence of protein-losing enteropathy in all cases of pseudomembranous colitis, 43% of patients with *C. difficile* diarrhoea, and half of nursing home residents who were *C. difficile* culture-positive (but *C. difficile* cytotoxin-negative); none of 15 healthy elderly control subjects had such evidence |**31**|. No explanation is available for the high prevalence of protein loss in culture-positive but symptom-free patients.

There are several anomalies in this study. First, the authors do not comment on the very high primary rate of failure of metronidazole (38%). While up to 37% of patients have symptomatic recurrences following treatment of CDI |**28**|, it is generally considered that at least 90% of cases respond at least initially to either metronidazole or to vancomycin |**32**|. An analysis is performed to determine the predictive value for metronidazole treatment failure of having both a low albumin level and intensive care unit care. While this predictive value was calculated as 80%, very few patients will in practice have both of these; unfortunately, we are not told what proportion of patients this applied to in the present study. This leads to another issue; almost one-third of the patients reviewed had an intensive care unit stay at or before diagnosis. This is a bizarrely high proportion and is atypical of CDI patient cohorts. Also, why were some (we are not told how many) patients treated with 250 mg oral metronidazole four times daily (as opposed to 500 mg t.d.s.)? No analysis is presented to determine whether the choice of dosage influenced the outcome.

The authors state in their introduction that identification of risk factors for metronidazole treatment failure (Table 12.4) is important 'because some patients may benefit from receiving vancomycin as initial treatment of CDAD'. However, they conclude that this study does not provide enough information to advocate a switch to vancomycin in patients with risk factors for metronidazole treatment failure. Therefore, the abstract should not conclude 'These patients may benefit from oral vancomycin therapy at outset'. The retrospective design of the study was never going to answer such a possibility, and indeed it is eminently plausible that factors associated with metronidazole failure may be true also for vancomycin. Prospective studies are needed to define the relative roles of metronidazole and vancomycin in

Table 12.4 Percentage of study group who improved on metronidazole by day 5

Patient variables	Improved n = 61(%)	Not improved n = 38(%)	P
Mean age (range)	65.4 (38–92)	67.5 (23–96)	0.566
Gender			
Female	35 (57.4)	16 (42.1)	0.154
Male	26 (42.6)	22 (57.9)	
Diabetes	16 (26.2)	13 (34.2)	0.266
Nursing home*	30 (49.2)	22 (57.9)	0.262
Antibiotics†	33 (54.1)	21 (55.3)	0.573
Haemodialysis	7 (11.4)	5 (13.5)	0.519
Albumin ≤2.5	16 (26.2)	29 (76.3)	<0.001
ICU‡	12 (19.7)	15 (39.5)	0.028

* This includes patients admitted from a nursing home, skilled nursing facility, or rehabilitation hospital.
† Indicates receiving antibiotics during the treatment of *C. difficile*.
‡ Patient resided in the ICU during hospitalization prior to or at time of CDAD treatment.
Source: Fernandez *et al*. (2004).

patients in whom CDI treatment fails. The repeatedly reported association between low albumin and poor outcome in CDI argues for studies to determine the effectiveness of correcting this abnormality to improve the therapeutic response.

Conclusion

These reviews highlight several clinically important advances in the understanding of CDI. Unexplained leukocytosis should prompt investigation for CDI in hospitalized patients, particularly those with recent antimicrobial exposure. Recurrence of CDI frequently affects the frail elderly; the observation that a low albumin level is a predictor of metronidazole failure in CDI suggests that correction of poor nutritional status may influence the likelihood of symptomatic recurrence. Fluoroquinolones cannot be considered to be risk-free in terms of propensity to cause CDI, and further studies are needed to characterize this risk, particularly in the susceptible elderly. One way forward, and an alternative to clinical studies, is the use of models that simulate CDI. The availability of a human gut model that is predictive of the clinical setting has obvious advantages over animal experiments. It is clear that toxin A-negative, toxin B-positive *C. difficile* strains are pathogenic; the chimaeric mouse model study discussed here underpins these observations by demonstrating the enterotoxic effects of toxin B.

Several advances have been made in the quest to find effective preventative strategies for CDI. Successful infection control strategies should ideally include attempts to control environmental contamination by *C. difficile*. The available evidence suggests that hypochlorite-based cleaning may be more efficacious than alternatives. Three potential therapeutic approaches to the prevention of CDI have been reviewed. First, the amelioration of gut flora using healthy donor faeces; while this has been claimed to reliably cure patients with recurrent CDI, it lacks widespread applicability. Secondly, administration of a non-toxigenic, antibiotic-resistant *C. difficile* strain was effective in an animal model; again, there are concerns here about the clinical viability of such an approach. Lastly, and most promisingly, the search for an effective vaccine continues; the latest studies using a toxoid vaccine highlight a tangible intervention strategy for the future.

References

1. Shim JK, Johnson S, Samore MH, Bliss DZ, Gerding DN. Primary symptomless colonisation by *Clostridium difficile* and decreased risk of subsequent diarrhoea. *Lancet* 1998; **351**: 633–6.

2. Sambol SP, Merrigan MM, Tang JK, Johnson S, Gerding DN. Colonization for the prevention of *Clostridium difficile* disease in hamsters. *J Infect Dis* 2002; **186**: 1781–9.

3. Embil J, Al-Barrak A, Dyck B, Olekson K, Nicoll D, Giercke S, Degagne P, Kennedy J, Kabani A, Harding G, Alfa M. The one-year experience following an outbreak of toxin A (–) toxin B (+) *Clostridium difficile* associated disease in a Canadian tertiary care hospital. *Clin Infect Dis* 1999; **29**: Abstract 451, p 1041.

4. Sambol SP, Merrigan MM, Lyerly D, Gerding DN, Johnson S. Toxin gene analysis of a variant strain of *Clostridium difficile* that causes human clinical disease. *Infect Immun* 2000; **68**: 5480–7.

5. Lyerly DM, Neville LM, Evans DT, Fill J, Allen S, Greene W, Sautter R, Hnatuck P, Torpey DJ, Schwalbe R. Multicenter evaluation of the *Clostridium difficile* TOX A/B test. *J Clin Microbiol* 1998; **36**: 184–90.

6. Limaye AP, Turgeon DK, Cookson BT, Fritscher TR. Pseudomembranous colitis caused by a toxin A(–) B(+) strain of *Clostridium difficile*. *J Clin Microbiol* 2000; **38**: 1696–7.

7. Steiner TS, Flores CA, Pizarro TT, Guerrant RL. Fecal lactoferrin, interleukin-1 beta, and interleukin-8 are elevated in patients with severe *Clostridium difficile* colitis. *Clin Diagn Lab Immunol* 1997; **4**: 719–22.

8. Bowden TA, Mansberger AR, Lykins LE. Pseudomembraneous enterocolitis: mechanism of restoring floral homeostasis. *Am Surg* 1981; **47**: 178–83.

9. Schwan A, Sjolin S, Trottestam U, Aronsson B. Relapsing *Clostridium difficile* enterocolitis cured by rectal infusion of normal faeces. *Scand J Infect Dis* 1984; **16**: 211–15.

10. Tvede M, Rask-Madsen J. Bacteriotherapy for chronic relapsing *Clostridium difficile* diarrhoea in six patients. *Lancet* 1989; **i**: 1156–60.

11. Persky SE, Brandt LJ. Treatment of recurrent *Clostridium difficile*-associated diarrhea by administration of donated stool directly through a colonoscope. *Am J Gastroenterol* 2000; **95**: 3283–5.

12. Apisarnthanarak A, Razavi B, Mundy LM. Adjunctive intracolonic vancomycin for severe *Clostridium difficile* colitis: case series and review of the literature. *Clin Infect Dis* 2002; **35**: 690–6.

13. Kotloff KL, Wasserman SS, Losonsky GA, Thomas W Jr, Nichols R, Edelman R, Bridwell M, Monath TP. Safety and immunogenicity of increasing doses of a *Clostridium difficile* toxoid vaccine administered to healthy adults. *Infect Immun* 2001; **69**: 988–95.

14. Kyne L, Warny M, Qamar A, Kelly CP. Asymptomatic carriage of *Clostridium difficile* and serum levels of IgG antibody against toxin A. *N Engl J Med* 2000; **342**: 390–7.

15. Kyne L, Warny M, Qamar A, Kelly CP. Association between antibody response to toxin A and protection against recurrent *Clostridium difficile* diarrhoea. *Lancet* 2001; **357**: 189–93.

16. Macfarlane GT, Macfarlane S, Gibson GR. Validation of a three-stage compound continuous culture system for investigating the effect of retention time on the ecology and metabolism of bacteria in the human colon. *Microb Ecol* 1998; **35**: 180–7.

17. Wanahita A, Goldsmith E, Musher D. Leukocytosis in a tertiary care hospital with particular attention to the role of infection caused by *Clostridium difficile*. *Clin Infect Dis* 2002; **34**: 1585–92.

18. Kyne L, Moran A, Keane C, O'Neill D. Hospital-acquired diarrhoea in elderly patients: epidemiology and staff awareness. *Age Ageing* 1998; **27**: 339–43.

19. Bennett RG, Greenough III WB. *Clostridium difficile* diarrhea: a common—and over-looked—nursing home infection. *Geriatrics* 1990; **45**: 77–87.

20. Yip C, Loeb M, Salama S, Moss L, Olde J. Quinolone use as a risk factor for nosocomial *Clostridium difficile*-associated diarrhea. *Infect Control Hosp Epidemiol* 2001; **22**: 572–5.

21. McCusker ME, Harris AD, Perencevich E, Roghmann MC. Fluoroquinolone use and *Clostridium difficile*–associated diarrhea. *Emerg Infect Dis* 2003; **9**: 730–3.

22. Wilcox MH, Fawley WN, Freeman J, Brayson J. In vitro activity of new generation fluoroquinolones against genotypically distinct and indistinguishable *Clostridium difficile* isolates. *J Antimicrob Chemother* 2000; **46**: 551–6.

23. Ackermann G, Tang-Feldman YJ, Schaumann R, Henderson JP, Rodloff AC, Silva J, Cohen SH. Antecedent use of fluoroquinolones is associated with resistance to moxifloxacin in *Clostridium difficile*. *Clin Microbiol Infect* 2003; **9**: 526–30.

24. Wilcox MH, Fawley WN. Hospital disinfectants and spore formation by *Clostridium difficile*. *Lancet* 2000; **356**: 1324.

25. Kaatz GW, Gitlin SD, Schaberg DR, Wilson KH, Kauffman CA, Seo SM, Fekety R. Acquisition of *Clostridium difficile* from the hospital environment. *Am J Epidemiol* 1988; **127**: 1289–94.

26. Mayfield JL, Leet T, Miller J, Mundy LM. Environmental control to reduce transmission of *Clostridium difficile*. *Clin Infect Dis* 2000; **31**: 995–1000.

27. Samore MH, Venkataraman L, DeGirolami PC, Arbeit RD, Karchmer AW. Clinical and molecular epidemiology of sporadic and clustered cases of nosocomial *Clostridium difficile* diarrhoea. *Am J Med* 1996; **100**: 32–40.

28. Wilcox MH, Cunnliffe JG, Trundle C, Redpath C. Financial burden of hospital acquired *Clostridium difficile* infection. *J Hosp Infect* 1996; **34**: 23–30.

29. Kyne L, Farrell RJ, Kelly CP. *Clostridium difficile*. *Gastro Clin North Am* 2001; **30**: 753–77.

30. Ramaswamy R, Grover H, Corpuz M. Prognostic criteria in *Clostridium difficile* colitis. *Am J Gastroenterol* 1996; **91**: 460–4.

31. Rybolt AH, Bennett RG, Laughon BE, Thomas DR, Greenough WB 3rd, Bartlett JG. Protein-losing enteropathy associated with *Clostridium difficile* infection. *Lancet* 1989; i: 1353–5.

32. Wilcox MH, Spencer RC. *Clostridium difficile* infection: responses, relapses and re-infections. *J Hosp Infect* 1992; **22**: 85–92.

13

Meningitis

JEREMY DAY

Introduction

Meningitis remains a disease that continues to cause significant morbidity and mortality in both industrialized and developing countries [1,2]. For example, last year more than 21 000 people suffered with meningitis in the African 'meningitis belt' and there were over 2300 deaths [3]. There are between 1800 and 2500 cases of bacterial meningitis notified in England and Wales each year. Despite the availability of penicillin for 60 years, mortality rates remain high, at around 12%, for the common causes of bacterial meningitis. Death is often not due to the failure of antimicrobial therapy as such, but to the inflammatory consequences of infection. Over the years there has been great interest in the potential benefit of adjunctive treatments in bacterial meningitis. In the past 18 months there have been two major trials published investigating the role of treatment with steroids in children and adults with bacterial meningitis. They arrived at different conclusions, and underline the importance of applying the findings of research to the population from whom the conclusions were drawn.

There has been a marked reduction in illness due to *Haemophilus influenzae* in the industrialized countries as a result of effective vaccination. It appears that pneumococcal vaccination may be similarly effective through the establishment of herd immunity and perhaps through the limitation of the spread of antibiotic-resistant strains.

The necessary minimum duration of treatment with antibiotics remains undetermined for many infections. Evidence is accumulating that short-course therapy may be sufficient in meningococcal disease, although there remains a need for controlled trials.

Neurological sequelae, in particular deafness, remain a significant problem after meningitis. Koomen *et al.* describe a simple five-point rule that can be used to predict infants who are at risk of this side effect so that timely intervention can be provided.

The aetiology of meningitis varies according to geographical location and patient subgroup. While in the past it has been pneumococcus, *Mycobacterium tuberculae* and *Neisseria meningitidis* that have accounted for the main burden of disease, the advent of the HIV epidemic has brought the fungal pathogen *Cryptococcus neoformans* to the fore. Cryptococcal meningitis is now the second leading cause of death in HIV patients in sub-Saharan Africa. When the scale of the HIV epidemic is considered, it is clear that this illness will be a major world public health burden in the ensuing years in the absence of readily available antiretroviral therapy. Where antiretroviral therapy is available, it appears that the subsequent immune reconstitution is likely to offer meaningful protection against relapse. Questions about the best management of raised intracranial pressure in this illness remain unanswered.

Finally, O'Sullivan and colleagues consolidate the knowledge of the differing clinical syndromes caused by the herpes simplex viruses through their large retrospective study of cases diagnosed at their centre.

Dexamethasone treatment in childhood bacterial meningitis in Malawi: a randomised controlled trial

Molyneux EM, Walsh AL, Forsyth H, *et al. Lancet* 2002; **360**: 211–18

BACKGROUND. This was a double-blind, randomized, placebo-controlled trial to assess the impact of adjunctive treatment with dexamethasone in children with bacterial meningitis in a developing country. Five hundred and ninety-eight children admitted to the Queen Elizabeth Central Hospital, Blantyre, Malawi, were recruited. The primary outcome was any death. Secondary outcomes included sequelae, in-hospital deaths and death after discharge. Physical, neurological, developmental and hearing assessments were performed 1 and 6 months after discharge. Analysis was done by intention to treat. Three hundred and seven patients (51%) were assigned to dexamethasone and 295 (49%) to placebo. Three hundred and thirty-eight (40%) patients had *Streptococcus pneumoniae*, 170 (28%) *Haemophilus influenzae* type b, 66 (11%) *Neisseria meningitidis* and 29 (5%) *Salmonella* spp. Seventy-eight (13%) patients had no growth on culture. The number of overall deaths was the same in the two treatment groups (relative risk [RR] 1.00; 95% confidence interval [CI] 0.8–1.25; $P = 0.93$). At the final outcome, sequelae were identified in 84 (28%) children on steroids and in 81 (28%) on placebo (RR 0.99; 95% CI 0.78–1.27; $P = 0.7$). The number of children dying in hospital did not differ between groups.

INTERPRETATION. This trial was designed to determine the value of adjunctive steroids in the treatment of bacterial meningitis in children in Malawi. Antibiotics were prescribed according to the Malawi national guidelines. The authors found that adjuvant steroids do not improve outcome in children with acute bacterial meningitis in Malawi.

Comment

Animal studies have revealed that inflammation in the subarachnoid space is a major contributor to morbidity and mortality in bacterial meningitis, an effect that is mediated by pro-inflammatory cytokines such as tumour necrosis factor |4|. This provides a rationale for the use of corticosteroids in bacterial meningitis, and indeed animal models of the disease demonstrate a benefit, although this depends upon various factors, including the timing of administration of steroids in relation to antibiotic therapy. Previous randomized double-blind placebo-controlled trials with smaller numbers of patients (up to 200) with bacterial meningitis in the developed world have demonstrated a reduced risk, or a trend towards a reduced risk, of neurological sequelae (in particular sensorineural hearing loss in *Haemophilus influenzae* type b infection) in children receiving steroids before or with their antibiotics.

This study is by far the largest double-blind placebo-controlled trial of the use of adjuvant steroids in children with bacterial meningitis. The results need to be considered in the context of a developing country, where antibiotic choice is limited, presentation to hospital is relatively late, facilities for intensive nursing and monitoring are limited, and where there is a high rate of HIV infection and malnutrition. In addition, initial treatment was with penicillin and chloramphenicol—antibiotics that are ineffective for 20% of the *Haemophilus* or pneumococcal isolates by *in vitro* susceptibility testing. Moreover, the beneficial anti-inflammatory effect of steroids may be less marked when benzyl penicillin or chloramphenicol is used than when third-generation cephalosporins or amoxycillin are used, because there is more rapid initial cell lysis with these latter agents and subsequently more robust secondary meningeal inflammation |**5**|. The trial data demonstrate a trend to support this, with a lower death rate in the small number of children initially treated with ceftriaxone, and less hearing loss in the patients on ceftriaxone receiving steroids than in those not receiving steroids, although the numbers were too small for definitive conclusions to be drawn.

The trial was criticized for three reasons |**6**|. First, some correspondents felt that the primary outcome measure should have been death and neurological sequelae rather than death alone. However, there remains no significant difference between treatment groups when the data are analysed this way. Secondly, the authors were criticized for recommending that there is no place for the use of steroids in bacterial meningitis within this patient population when in fact *H. influenzae* type b is likely to be a common infecting agent in sub-Saharan Africa, where there is poor vaccination coverage. Adjuvant steroids have been shown to be useful in the developed world in meningitis due to this organism. However, this trial clearly demonstrated no benefit in the patient population studied and therefore the investigators' conclusions remain valid. Thirdly, critics noted that the results suggested that in patients receiving ceftriaxone there was a trend towards a better outcome in the patients who were receiving steroids rather than placebo. Some patients received ceftriaxone as their initial antibiotic treatment because during the course of the trial it became apparent that there was increasing resistance to chloramphenicol developing among the *H. influenzae* isolates. The trial protocol was amended such that if the Gram stain was available at admission and showed Gram negative rods the child could initially be treated with ceftriaxone. Thirty-one patients met this criterion throughout the course of the trial and had *H. influenzae* infection. These patients had an overall better outcome than patients treated with chloramphenicol and penicillin, but the group was too small for conclusions to be drawn regarding the value of dexamethasone. The authors are currently undertaking a larger study of the use of ceftriaxone with this patient population. In the developed world, where *H. influenzae* type b meningitis has become extremely rare due to successful vaccination campaigns, it is now pertinent to ask whether children with presumed bacterial meningitis should still receive adjuvant steroids along with the initial empirical antibiotics.

This trial admirably answered the question posed—whether there is a place for the use of adjunctive steroids in the treatment of bacterial meningitis according to current national guidelines in Malawi. The answer is no. It also serves to demonstrate the importance of treatment guidelines being locally relevant, due to differences in resources, patterns of disease, and host and pathogen characteristics.

Dexamethasone in adults with bacterial meningitis

de Gans J, van de Beek D, for the European Dexamethasone in Adulthood Bacterial Meningitis Study Investigators. *N Engl J Med* 2002; **347**: 1549–56

BACKGROUND. This was a prospective, randomized, double-blind, multicentre trial of adjuvant treatment with dexamethasone, compared with placebo, in adults with acute bacterial meningitis. Dexamethasone (10 mg) or placebo was administered 15–20 min before or with the first dose of antibiotic and was given every 6 h for 4 days. The primary outcome measure was the score on the Glasgow Outcome Scale at 8 weeks (a score of 5, indicating a favourable outcome, versus a score of 1–4, indicating an unfavourable outcome). A subgroup analysis according to the causative organism was performed. Analyses were performed on an intention-to-treat basis. One hundred and fifty-seven patients were randomly assigned to the dexamethasone group and 144 to the placebo group. Dexamethasone treatment was associated with a reduction in the risk of an unfavourable outcome (RR 0.59; 95% CI 0.37–0.94; $P = 0.03$) and was also associated with a reduction in mortality (RR of death 0.48; 95% CI 0.24–0.96; $P = 0.04$). Among the patients with pneumococcal meningitis, there were unfavourable outcomes in 26% of the dexamethasone group, compared with 52% of the placebo group (RR 0.50; 95% CI 0.30–0.83; $P = 0.006$). Gastrointestinal bleeding occurred in two patients in the dexamethasone group and in five patients in the placebo group. The authors conclude that early treatment with dexamethasone improves the outcome in adults with acute bacterial meningitis and does not increase the risk of gastrointestinal bleeding.

INTERPRETATION. This was a well-designed, prospective, randomized, double-blind, placebo-controlled trial that demonstrates a benefit of adjuvant treatment with steroids in bacterial meningitis in adults in Western Europe, and the safety of steroids used in this group of patients at this dosage and duration.

Comment

As in children, mortality and morbidity rates are high among adults with acute bacterial meningitis, especially those with pneumococcal meningitis. The poor outcome in adult bacterial meningitis does not seem to be due to microbiological failure, since cerebrospinal fluid (CSF) cultures are usually sterile 24–48 h after starting treatment. In studies of bacterial meningitis in animals, adjuvant treatment with corticosteroids has beneficial effects. However, until this trial it has been much less clear whether there is a benefit to be gained from combining steroids with antibiotics to treat adults with bacterial meningitis. One prospective trial, neither placebo-controlled nor blinded, showed dexamethasone treatment to be of benefit in a subgroup of patients with pneumococcal meningitis, but the lack of other data has meant that it has been difficult to recommend routine steroid administration in adults.

The timescale of this trial illustrates some of the difficulties in trying to perform research on meningitis in the industrialized world—it took 9 years to recruit 301 patients. Baseline characteristics between the two treatment groups were similar, suggesting that the randomization process was working well, although there were more patients with seizure history in the dexamethasone group. However, it is surprising that no data are presented regarding blood pressure for each group, since, along with coma on admission and *Streptococcus pneumoniae* infection, hypotension was found to be a predictor of poor outcome. The number of patients with coma or *S. pneumoniae* infection was similar between groups.

The two most commonly isolated organisms were *S. pneumoniae* (36%) and *Neisseria meningitidis* (32%). The most frequently prescribed initial antibiotics were amoxycillin and penicillin (77% of patients), a third-generation cephalosporin (8%) and penicillin or amoxycillin combined with a cephalosporin (8%). Seventy-two per cent of *S. pneumoniae* isolates underwent antibiotic susceptibility testing at a reference laboratory; all were penicillin-sensitive. Eighty-two per cent of the *N. meningitidis* isolates underwent susceptibility testing; just one isolate had intermediate resistance. Ninety-seven per cent of patients received an initial antibiotic regimen that provided adequate antimicrobial coverage (no difference between groups).

This trial found a significant benefit from adjuvant steroid treatment in bacterial meningitis. The benefit was predominantly one of reduction in the number of deaths; there was no significant difference in neurological sequelae between the groups. Importantly, there was no increase in neurological sequelae in survivors in the treatment group. However, it is difficult to draw firm conclusions about the effect of dexamethasone on neurological sequelae because of the small numbers. Moreover, outcome was analysed at 8 weeks, which is insufficient time to document recovery from neurological sequelae, and so longer-term follow-up of these patients is important.

Subgroup analysis by infecting organism revealed that there was a highly significant effect for unfavourable outcome or death for steroid treatment with *S. pneumoniae*, but no significant difference with *N. meningitidis* infections (Table 13.1).

Reassuringly there were no significant differences in the incidence of adverse events between the two groups, in particular gastrointestinal bleeding and hyperglycaemia.

The authors conclude that dexamethasone (10 mg/day for 4 days) should be given to all adults with suspected bacterial meningitis, since they demonstrated a reduction in unfavourable outcome and death, with no evidence of increased risk of serious adverse events.

The study population differs from many around the world in that the incidence of penicillin resistance among isolates was extremely low. Where penicillin resistance is

Table 13.1 Outcomes 8 weeks after admission, according to culture results*

Outcome and culture results	Dexamethasone group	Placebo group	Relative risk (95% CI)†	P value
	no./total no. (%)			
Unfavourable outcome				
All patients	23/157 (15)	36/144 (25)	0.59 (0.37–0.94)	0.03
Streptococcus pneumoniae	15/58 (26)	26/50 (52)	0.50 (0.30–0.83)	0.006
Neisseria meningitidis	4/50 (8)	5/47 (11)	0.75 (0.21–2.63)	0.74
Other bacteria	2/12 (17)	1/17 (6)	2.83 (0.29–27.8)	0.55
Negative bacterial culture‡	2/37 (5)	4/30 (13)	0.41 (0.08–2.06)	0.40
Death				
All patients	11/157 (7)	21/144 (15)	0.48 (0.24–0.96)	0.04
S. pneumoniae	8/58 (14)	17/50 (34)	0.41 (0.19–0.86)	0.02
N. meningitidis	2/50 (4)	1/47 (2)	1.88 (0.76–20.1)	1.00
Other bacteria	1/12 (8)	1/17 (6)	1.42 (0.10–20.5)	1.00
Negative bacterial culture	0/37	2/30 (7)	–	0.20
Focal neurologic abnormalities				
All patients	18/143 (13)	24/119 (20)	0.62 (0.36–1.09)	0.13
S. pneumoniae	11/49 (22)	11/33 (33)	0.67 (0.33–1.37)	0.32
N. meningitidis	3/46 (7)	5/44 (11)	0.57 (0.15–2.26)	0.48
Other bacteria	3/11 (27)	3/16 (19)	1.45 (0.36–5.92)	0.66
Negative bacterial culture	1/37 (3)	5/26 (19)	0.14 (0.02–1.13)	0.07
Hearing loss				
All patients	13/143 (9)	14/119 (12)	0.77 (0.38–1.58)	0.54
S. pneumoniae	7/49 (14)	7/33 (21)	0.67 (0.25–1.69)	0.55
N. meningitidis	3/46 (7)	5/44 (11)	0.57 (0.15–2.26)	0.48
Other bacteria	2/11 (18)	1/16 (6)	2.91 (0.30–28.3)	0.55
Negative bacterial culture	1/37 (3)	1/26 (4)	0.70 (0.05–10.7)	1.00

* The analyses of unfavourable outcome and death included all patients and were performed with a last-observation-carried-forward procedure. The analyses of neurologic abnormalities and hearing loss included all surviving patients who underwent neurologic examination at eight weeks.
† CI, confidence interval.
‡ Included in this category are two patients in whom cerebrospinal fluid culture was not performed.
Source: de Gans *et al.* (2002).

more common, vancomycin may be among the antibiotics of first choice. Steroids do seem to impair the passage of vancomycin across the blood–brain barrier in animal models of bacterial meningitis, and therefore it may not be appropriate to use steroids when this antibiotic is used, since successful outcome in meningitis is related to the prompt delivery of effective antimicrobial therapy.

Since entry to this trial also depended upon CSF findings consistent with bacterial meningitis, the trial was criticized for potentially introducing a delay in treatment for patients (since steroids had to be given before or with the first antibiotic dose after CSF examination). If the authors' recommendation is accepted, then patients who have conditions other than bacterial meningitis will receive steroids along with empirical antibiotic therapy. A concern was expressed that this might result in an increased rate of steroid-related adverse events. However, patients without bacterial meningitis are unlikely to get more than one dose of dexamethasone before the CSF findings are known, adverse events were low in any case and therefore the effect of giving steroids to patients without bacterial meningitis is analogous to giving antibiotics to these patients.

It seems likely that, in the future, guidelines for treatment of suspected adult meningitis will include dexamethasone along with empirical antibiotics until the diagnosis is confirmed.

Does dexamethasone affect ceftriaxone penetration into cerebrospinal fluid in adult bacterial meningitis

Buke AC, Cavusoglu C, Karasulu E, Karakartal G. *Int J Antimicrob Agents* 2003; **21**: 452–6

BACKGROUND. Trough CSF ceftriaxone concentrations were measured daily to investigate the effect of dexamethasone on ceftriaxone penetration into CSF in adult patients with acute bacterial meningitis. Patients were divided into two groups in this double-blind randomized study. In Group 1 ($n = 6$) patients were given ceftriaxone with dexamethasone whereas in Group 2 ($n = 6$) patients were only administered ceftriaxone. Plasma and CSF samples were collected 24, 48, 72, 96 and 264 h after the study treatments. The trough CSF ceftriaxone concentrations were measured using high-performance liquid chromatography (HPLC) and microbiological assay. CSF ceftriaxone concentrations were 3.21 mg/l at 24 h in Group 1 and 4.85 mg/l at the same time in Group 2 by HPLC. Although microbiological assay results were lower than the HPLC results, the trough CSF ceftriaxone concentrations in the dexamethasone group were at least 10^3 times higher than the minimum inhibitory concentrations of the susceptible strains. It was concluded that the ceftriaxone concentration in CSF was adequate and ceftriaxone penetration was not significantly affected by concomitant dexamethasone use in adult patients with acute bacterial meningitis.

INTERPRETATION. There are few published data on the pharmacokinetics of antibiotics combined with steroids in the treatment of meningitis in adults. There have been concerns that the use of adjuvant steroids in bacterial meningitis may reduce antibiotic penetration into the CSF due to a reduction in blood–brain barrier permeability which has been increased as a result of inflammation [7]. This paper provides reassuring evidence that, despite evidence of decreased CSF penetration by ceftriaxone when administered with dexamethasone, the minimum inhibitory concentrations attained should still be sufficient for effective bacterial killing.

Comment

Despite relatively small numbers of patients, this paper is strengthened by the frequent sampling rate. Patients received intravenous dexamethasone 15 min before the first dose of ceftriaxone at a dose of 8 mg t.i.d. Two methods were used to access the trough concentrations of ceftriaxone in the CSF: HPLC and a microbiological assay. In general, HPLC is considered the preferred method for measuring drug concentrations in different body compartments, since it delivers more consistent results. CSF/plasma ceftriaxone concentration ratios ranged from 7 to 9% in Group 1 and from 7 to 11% in Group 2. There was no significant difference between the area under the curve for ceftriaxone concentrations between the two groups when measured by HPLC, but there was a statistical difference between CSF trough concentrations for the two groups when the microbiological assay was used. However, CSF concentrations by the microbiological assay remained at least 10^3 times higher than the minimum inhibitory concentration of susceptible strains in the steroid group. These data suggest that, in the treatment of bacterial meningitis and in the absence of antibiotic resistance, adequate levels of ceftriaxone are achieved when it is co-administered with steroids. It should be remembered that there is evidence from animal models that steroids reduce the CSF levels of vancomycin, the antibiotic of choice when there is β-lactamase resistance |8|. There is a pressing need for more data on the effect of steroids on the pharmacokinetics of antibiotics in humans, although ultimately the treatment policy should be based on data from trials using clinical end-points.

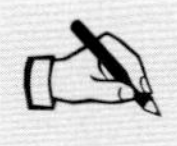

Three days of intravenous benzyl penicillin treatment of meningococcal disease in adults

Ellis-Pegler R, Galler L, Roberts S, Thomas M, Woodhouse A. *Clin Infect Dis* 2003; **37**: 658–62

BACKGROUND. In this paper from New Zealand, the investigators treated adults (aged over 15 years) with meningococcal disease with intravenous benzyl penicillin (12 MU [megaunit] [7.2 g] per day) for 3 days. Sixty-one adults with suspected meningococcal disease were consecutively admitted during the 33-month period; three patients were excluded. The 58 patients had a mean age (± standard deviation [SD]) of 27.9 ± 14.5 years (median 21 years; range 15–70 years). Forty-four patients had confirmed and 14 patients had probable meningococcal disease. Fifty-seven patients received 12 MU (7.2 g) and one received 8 MU (4.8 g) of benzyl penicillin per day. Thirteen patients received additional antibiotics within the first 24 h because of diagnostic uncertainties. Patients received a mean (± SD) of 3.0 ± 0.5 days of treatment. No patients relapsed. Five patients died. All but one death occurred during benzyl penicillin treatment, and the only post-treatment death was not due to meningococcal disease.

INTERPRETATION. This paper provides evidence that 3 days of treatment with benzyl penicillin for meningococcal disease may be sufficient therapy, and that current recommendations regarding duration of treatment are excessive.

Comment

The necessary duration of treatment is undetermined for many common infectious diseases. Shortening antibiotic treatment courses may offer benefits, both clinical (reduced risk of side effects and length of hospital stay) and financial. Most authorities recommend 7–10 days' treatment with antibiotics for meningococcal disease, although the rationale for this is unclear. In the developing world it has been common to use shorter courses of therapy, usually of the order of 5 days |**9,10**|, and there is some experience from uncontrolled studies in the use of shorter-course (4 or 5 days) antibiotic therapy compared with longer (7 days or more) treatment in meningococcal disease. This paper offers tantalizing evidence that 3 days of therapy with benzyl penicillin may be sufficient treatment for meningococcal disease. The administered dose was 1.2 g at 4-h intervals for 3 days. Fifty-eight patients admitted met the diagnostic criteria for confirmed or probable meningococcal disease. Forty-four patients had confirmed (by blood or CSF culture or polymerase chain reaction [PCR]) and 14 patients had probable disease. Thirty-five of these patients had CSF examination; 27 had abnormal CSF results. Fourteen patients had received antibiotics before arriving at the hospital (nine benzyl penicillin and five amoxycillin). All 58 patients received benzyl penicillin but 13 received additional antibiotics within the first 24 h. Of the five deaths, three occurred on the day of presentation, one occurred on day 3 due to septic shock, and one occurred on day 15 of multiple organ failure without reculture of *N. meningitidis* from any site. Follow-up appears to have been performed on an informal basis, either through the patient's general practitioner or the hospital service, and there were no follow-up details for seven patients. There were no microbiological relapses. The prevalence of β-lactam resistance in the local population also needs to be considered when making decisions about duration of treatment and initial antibiotic choice. While a randomized controlled trial to demonstrate the equivalence of short-course with longer-course therapy for the different meningococcal syndromes is desirable, it would be incredibly difficult to complete a trial of this nature, since the sample size needed would be enormous, running into thousands of patients. This work provides some reassurance about the use of shorter-course therapy for meningococcal disease.

Effect of a nonavalent conjugate vaccine on carriage of antibiotic-resistant *Streptococcus pneumoniae* in day-care centres

Dagan R, Givon-Lavi N, Zamir O, Fraser D. *Pediatr Infect Dis J* 2003; **22**: 532–40

BACKGROUND. In industrialized societies, day-care centres (DCCs) play an important role in the spread of antibiotic-resistant pneumococci, both within the facility and from the facility to the community. This study was conducted to determine the effect of a nonavalent pneumococcal conjugate vaccine (PCV-9) on the carriage of antibiotic-resistant pneumococci in the DCC. Healthy DCC attendees aged 12–35 months were randomized to receive either PCV-9 or a control vaccine (conjugate meningococcus C vaccine) in a double-blinded manner. Nasopharyngeal swabs were obtained from each subject before vaccination, and regularly over the

2 years of follow-up. The serotype and antibiotic susceptibility of each isolate were determined. A total of 132 and 130 evaluable subjects received either PCV-9 or the control vaccine, respectively. Of the 3748 specimens obtained, 2450 (65%) were positive for S. pneumoniae. The resistance rates to penicillin, trimethoprim–sulphamethoxazole and erythromycin were 36, 35 and 16% respectively. Resistance rates to one or more and three or more antibiotic categories were 52 and 9% respectively. Antibiotic resistance was found mainly in the five serotypes included in the pneumococcal conjugate vaccines (6B, 9V, 14, 19F and 23F) and in two related serotypes (6A and 19A). In the vaccinated group the authors observed a clear and significant reduction of the carriage rate of the serotypes included in the vaccine and the related serotype 6A, and an increase in the carriage rate of the serotypes not included in the vaccine. In parallel, a significant decrease in the carriage rate of antibiotic-resistant pneumococci was observed. The reduction in the carriage of antibiotic-resistant pneumococci was seen in all age windows but was greater in the age window <36 months.

INTERPRETATION. This study from Israel found high rates of antibiotic-resistant S. pneumoniae in children attending DCCs. Pneumococcal vaccination against nine common invasive serotypes decreased the rate of carriage of antibiotic-resistant isolates, and of the isolates covered by the vaccine. Overall carriage rates of pneumococcus were similar for vaccinated and control subjects.

Comment

Nasal carriage of pneumococci is important because of its relationship to both invasive disease and spread of the pathogen. Pneumococcus causes significant disease and mortality in all age groups and remains an important worldwide health problem. The development of antibiotic resistance since the 1960s underlines the importance of developing preventive strategies alongside effective treatments. DCCs have been associated with outbreaks of antibiotic-resistant pneumococcal disease, probably because there are frequent close person-to-person contacts and a high rate of anti-microbial use, leading to pressure to select resistance. The same authors have previously shown the use of this vaccine to lead to a significant reduction in the carriage of vaccine-type (VT) serotypes in day-care attendees |**11**|. Overall carriage rates of pneumococcal serotypes remain the same in vaccinated attendees because of replacement with strains that do not occur or cross-react with VT serotypes. Most antibiotic-resistant pneumococcal strains belong to a limited number of serotypes that commonly cause human infection. This led the investigators to hypothesize that vaccination of day-care attendees might reduce the carriage of antibiotic-resistant strains.

The S. pneumoniae carriage rate before vaccination was 80 and 81% in the pneumococcal vaccination and control groups respectively. Antibiotic susceptibility testing was carried out for oxacillin, trimethoprim–sulphamethoxazole, clindamycin, erythromycin, tetracycline and chloramphenicol. The strains most likely to have antibiotic resistance were serotypes 6B, 9V, 14, 19F and 23F—all serotypes included in the vaccine. Penicillin resistance was most commonly found within these serotypes and the related serotypes 6A and 19A. A significant reduction was seen in the carriage rate of the serotypes included in the nonavalent vaccine and the related serotype 6A in the vaccinated subjects, but not in the other serotypes. There was a significant increase in the carriage rate of the non-VT pneumococci. This replacement phenomenon resulted in similar overall carriage rates of pneumococci between vaccinated and control groups, but in a significantly lower rate of carriage of antibiotic-resistant strains for vaccinated subjects, this finding being significant for all the tested antibiotic resistance patterns. The effect of vaccination was most marked in the younger age group (24–29 months); there was also an independent reduction in the carriage of antibiotic-resistant strains as age and the time since vaccination increased. This latter effect may have been due to boosting specific immunity in vaccinated subjects through contact with the highly circulating VT in the DCC. There was no reduction in the carriage of the 19A strain, which is immunologically related to the 19F strain contained within the vaccine and is one of the most antibiotic-resistant serotypes. It has recently been demonstrated that children less than 6 years old attending DCCs are a strong independent risk factor for the development of invasive pneumococcal disease in adult household members age 18–64 years. Thus, the reduction in the carriage of antibiotic-resistant strains in DCC attenders may have beneficial effects for the wider community. There needs to be careful surveillance to determine whether the VT serotypes will eventually be replaced by antibiotic-resistant non-VT serotypes. While these data are undoubtedly interesting, it is the effect on the vaccine recipient's health that is most important, and it would be most useful to determine whether there is any clinical benefit in terms of reduced episodes or severity of pneumococcal disease in these subjects.

Vaccination of day-care centre attendees reduces carriage of *Streptococcus pneumoniae* among their younger siblings

Givon-Lavi N, Fraser D, Dagan R. *Pediatr Infect Dis J* 2003; **22**: 524–32

B A C K G R O U N D . The investigators conducted a study to determine whether administration of a pneumococcal conjugate vaccine to toddlers attending DCCs could prevent the acquisition of S. *pneumoniae* of the VT serotypes by their younger siblings. These data result from a spin-off trial from the cohort studied in the previous paper. Forty-six younger siblings of the children described above (23 siblings of the PnCRM9 recipients and 23 of the controls), aged less then 18 months, were enrolled, and nasopharyngeal cultures were obtained monthly until the children reached the age of 18 months or started to attend the DCC, if before the age of 18 months. Pneumococcal isolates were serotyped and tested for antibiotic susceptibility. Of 306 cultures obtained from the younger siblings, 151 (49%) were positive. In the PnCRM9 recipients, cultures were significantly less frequently positive for the VT S. *pneumoniae* than in the controls (13 and 21% respectively; *P* <0.001). The same pattern was seen in the younger siblings of PnCRM9 recipients compared with the siblings of controls (21 and 34% respectively; *P* = 0.017). The reverse trend was seen for non-VT strains in both the DCC attendees (44 and 34% respectively; *P* <0.001) and their younger siblings (19 and 13% respectively; *P* = 0.15). There was a significant decrease in the carriage rate of antibiotic-resistant *S. pneumoniae* in both the PnCRM9 recipients and their younger siblings. The relative risks (and 95% CIs) of carrying *S. pneumoniae* that was not susceptible to penicillin and resistant to one or more, two or more and three or more antibiotic categories among younger siblings of PnCRM9 recipients versus siblings of controls were 0.47 (0.31–0.70), 0.49 (0.33–0.71), 0.46 (0.30–0.73) and 0.49 (0.21–1.17) respectively. When acquired, VT and antibiotic-resistant *S. pneumoniae* were carried for a significantly shorter period by siblings of PnCRM9 recipients than by siblings of controls.

INTERPRETATION. The marked effect of PnCRM9 administration to DCC attendees on the carriage of VT and antibiotic-resistant *S. pneumoniae* among their younger household close contacts demonstrates a herd effect of the vaccine.

Comment

These data demonstrate a probable community benefit from the vaccination of DCC attendees. There were significantly fewer VT-positive cultures from the siblings of vaccinated DCCs compared with controls, although again there was no difference overall in the number of *S. pneumoniae*-positive cultures from either group. Interestingly, the effect of vaccination for the non-VT serotype 6A seen in DCCs was not demonstrated in the younger siblings (although the numbers of isolates of this serotype were small). Again, the reduction in the number of antibiotic-resistant isolates from siblings of vaccinated DCCs was significantly lower than the number from the siblings of controls. There was also a trend for shorter duration of carriage of VT strains in siblings of vaccinated patients compared with siblings of controls. Because of the small numbers, it was not possible to determine whether the lower rate of carriage in the siblings of vaccine recipients was due to a lower rate of acquisition or this lower duration of carriage. Again, the impact of a lower carriage rate on the patients' risk of clinical disease was not determined in this study.

Discontinuation of secondary prophylaxis for cryptococcal meningitis in human immunodeficiency virus-infected patients treated with highly active antiretroviral therapy: a prospective, multicentre, randomised study

Vibhagool A, Sungkanuparph S, Mootsikapun P, *et al. Clin Infect Dis* 2003; **36**: 1329–31

BACKGROUND. A prospective, multicentre, randomized study was conducted with HIV-infected patients who were treated successfully for acute cryptococcal meningitis, were receiving secondary prophylaxis with fluconazole, and were naive for antiretroviral therapy. Culture-proven cryptococcal meningitis was treated in accordance with international guidelines. Successful treatment (defined by sterilization of CSF) was followed by secondary prophylaxis with fluconazole at the dose of 200 mg daily. Antiretroviral treatment was initiated with zidovudine, lamivudine and efavirenz. Alternative treatment was available for drug intolerances. Once the HIV viral load was undetectable and CD4 count had risen above 100 cells/μl for 3 months, the patients were randomized in a 1:1 ratio to continue or discontinue fluconazole secondary prophylaxis. Twenty-two patients were randomized to the former group and 20 to the latter. The median CD4 count was 11 and 6 cells/μl respectively at the time of initiation of highly active antiretroviral therapy (HAART) and 170 and 167 cells/μl in each group at randomization. The median duration of follow-up was 48 weeks. There were no relapses of cryptococcal meningitis in either group. No data are presented for median CD4 count after 48 weeks of follow-up.

INTERPRETATION. The trial suggests that there is meaningful anticryptococcal immune reconstitution with HAART, and that it is probably safe to discontinue secondary prophylaxis, although the duration of follow-up is short.

Comment

Worldwide, cryptococcal meningitis is second only to tuberculosis as the commonest cause of death in HIV-infected patients, accounting for up to 20% of all AIDS deaths. The advent of HAART has had a huge impact on the morbidity and mortality of HIV patients. However, many trials of HAART use surrogate markers, such as rise in CD4 count or the suppression of viral load, as primary end-points. There remains a pressing need for trials demonstrating the effectiveness of treatment using clinical end-points. While there is evidence of the safety of discontinuing secondary prophylaxis in *Pneumocystis carinii* pneumonia, the evidence for other opportunistic infections is less clear, decisions often being based on anecdote or published series of case reports |12,13|. This is the first randomized controlled trial of the discontinuation of fluconazole prophylaxis following treatment for cryptococcal meningitis in the post-HAART era. It is difficult to draw any firm conclusions from any comparison between the two groups as there were no events in either arm, and the trial was underpowered to demonstrate equivalence between the two 'interventions'. However, before the introduction of HAART the relapse rate for cryptococcal meningitis in HIV patients without fluconazole secondary prophylaxis was between 37 and 60%, compared with 4% in those taking secondary prophylaxis. There is an obvious danger in comparing results over time from unrelated patient groups, but the trial provides some reassurance that the rise in CD4 count seen in HAART is a meaningful immune reconstitution as far as relapse from cryptococcal disease is concerned. Long-term follow-up would be desirable.

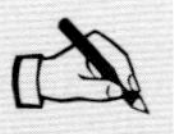

A randomised, double-blind, placebo-controlled trial of acetazolamide for the treatment of elevated intracranial pressure in cryptococcal meningitis

Newton PN, Thai Le H, Tip NQ, *et al*. *Clin Infect Dis* 2002; **35**: 769–72

BACKGROUND. A trial of oral acetazolamide for the treatment of raised intracranial pressure in Thai adults with cryptococcal meningitis, headache and an opening CSF pressure of at least 200 mm CSF. Acetazolamide was given at a dose of 750–1000 mg/day in divided doses. The primary outcome measures were CSF opening pressure, headache, and serum potassium and bicarbonate levels 14 days after starting treatment. The trial was stopped early after the recruitment of 22 patients because those who received acetazolamide developed significantly lower venous bicarbonate levels and higher chloride levels and had serious adverse events more frequently than subjects who received placebo. At 14 days headache was improved in both groups, but there was no improvement in intracranial pressure or Karnofsky score in either group.

INTERPRETATION. The study investigators concluded that acetazolamide should not be used in combination with amphotericin B because of an increased rate of adverse events in the active drug arm (5 of 12 patients versus 0 of 10 patients). Reported adverse events were two deaths (one after developing blindness, one after developing acidosis), peripheral neuropathy, severe symptomatic acidosis and blindness.

Comment

Raised intracranial pressure is a frequent finding in cryptococcal meningitis, and is believed to be a major factor in determining outcome. The exact mechanism of raised intracranial pressure is not determined, nor is the optimum therapy, but suggested treatments have included repeated lumbar puncture, lumbar drains, ventriculo-peritoneal shunts, steroids, mannitol and acetazolamide. Acetazolamide reduces the rate of CSF production from the choroid plexus and thus may be a useful therapy for raised intracranial pressure in cryptococcal meningitis. It is cheap, readily available and well tolerated when used in other conditions, such as acute mountain sickness or idiopathic intracranial hypertension. However, it can cause hypokalaemia and metabolic acidosis, particularly in patients with renal impairment. Transient renal impairment and hypokalaemia are common in patients receiving amphotericin, the mainstay of treatment in cryptococcal disease.

This trial was stopped early because of a difference in reported adverse events in the on-treatment group. However, these complications occur frequently in crypto-coccal meningitis, on-treatment death rates approaching 40% in some series. It would seem reasonable from the data presented to conclude that three of the adverse events (neuropathy, blindness and one of the deaths) were not related to acetazol-amide. There are then only two adverse events in the treatment group compared with none in the placebo group; given the small number of patients recruited by the time

the trial was stopped, it is not possible to comment on the significance of this. Moreover, the drug dosages used in this trial (750–1000 mg per day) were relatively high,
especially given the likely weight of the patients. There is evidence that in acute
mountain sickness doses of 250–500 mg per day of acetazolamide give the same
benefit as higher doses in trekkers and mountaineers, who are considerably better
nourished than patients with AIDS. The trial needs to be repeated, perhaps with a
lower dose of acetazolamide. Cryptococcal meningitis remains a disease for which
there is a pressing need to develop better antifungal and adjunctive treatment.

Clinical spectrum and laboratory characteristics associated with detection of herpes simplex virus DNA in cerebrospinal fluid

O'Sullivan CE, Aksamit AJ, Harrington JR, Harmsen WS, Mitchell PS, Patel R.
Mayo Clin Proc 2003; **78**: 1347–52

BACKGROUND. The authors describe the clinical, neurological and laboratory
characteristics of patients with herpes simplex virus (HSV) type 1 (HSV-1) or HSV
type 2 (HSV-2) DNA detected in CSF using the PCR. Clinical, laboratory and
demographic data were determined from 249 CSF specimens (collected from
247 patients over 10 years of age) that tested positive for HSV-1 or HSV-2 DNA at a
tertiary diagnostic and treatment centre over a 20-month period. The median age of
the 200 patients whose age was available was 70 years versus 40 years for those
with HSV-1 or HSV-2 DNA in CSF respectively. Detailed data were available for
39 and 78 patients with positive PCR results for HSV-1 and HSV-2 respectively. Of
those with HSV-1 DNA detected in CSF, 89% had encephalitis, whereas most patients
with HSV-2 DNA detected in CSF had findings compatible with meningitis. Only five
(7%) of 69 patients in whom HSV-2 was detected in CSF had genital lesions at
presentation, and none of the assessable patients with HSV-2 who had recurrent
meningitis had active genital lesions at presentation.

INTERPRETATION. The authors attempted to clinically characterize the syndromes caused
by herpes simplex virus infections of the central nervous system. In this series HSV-1 appears
to cause a predominantly encephalitic syndrome, while HSV-2 appears to cause a
predominantly meningitic syndrome.

Comment

HSV-1 infection usually occurs in childhood and more than 60% of the population
will be seropositive by the age of 40 years. Twenty per cent of the US population older
than 12 years are infected with HSV-2 |**14**|. A wide variety of neurological complica-
tions have been described, including encephalitis, meningitis, radiculitis and myelitis.
These are thought to occur as a result of reactivation of latent infection rather
than primary infection. HSV-1 is the commonest cause of encephalitis in the
Western world. HSV-2 has more commonly been described as causing an illness at

the meningitic end of the spectrum, although hard evidence for this has been sparse. The development of type-specific molecular techniques enables the determination of the HSV type associated with the particular syndromes. Of note, these investigators found that there was a difference in the age distribution of illness caused by the herpes subtypes (and, by inference, a shorter incubation period for neurological syndrome development in HSV-2 infections compared with HSV-1), and that patients with meningitis (headache, neck stiffness, photophobia and vomiting) were more likely to have positive HSV-2 PCR reactions than HSV-1 reactions. Patients with HSV-2 infection were also likely to have higher CSF lymphocyte counts and protein levels than those with HSV-1. This may be related to the ages of the patient groups, or be due to the predominant anatomical site affected by the virus. All the patients with HSV-2 infection survived, although approximately 20% received no antiviral treatment, and all made a complete recovery. The survival rate for HSV-1 infection was 82%, and almost a third of patients had some residual deficit. The study was limited in that it was retrospective, but also in the fact that the questionnaire used to extract data from the clinical notes by the referring doctor depended upon the virus type isolated from CSF. This would have introduced a bias into the study that meant that the incidence of encephalitis in patients with HSV-2 infection may have been underestimated. Distinguishing between HSV-1 and HSV-2 infection has some merit in that the prognosis appears different for these two infections— information that is helpful for the attending physicians and the patient. In the future, resources need to be allocated to finding more effective treatments for HSV-1 infections.

Hearing loss at school age in survivors of bacterial meningitis: assessment, incidence, and prediction

Koomen I, Grobbee DE, Roord JJ, Donders R, Jennekens-Schinkel A, van Furth AM. *Pediatrics* 2003; **112**: 1049–53

BACKGROUND. The investigators aimed to establish the incidence of sensorineural hearing loss in children who survived non-*Haemophilus influenzae type B* (Hib) bacterial meningitis, in order to develop a prediction rule to identify those who are at risk of hearing loss. This was a retrospective examination of a cohort of 628 school-aged children who were born between January 1986 and December 1994 and had survived non-Hib bacterial meningitis between January 1990 and December 1995. The presence of sensorineural hearing loss (>25 dB) was determined, based on information from questionnaires and medical records. Potential risk factors for hearing loss were obtained from medical records; independent predictors were identified using multivariate logistic regression analysis, leading to the formulation of a prediction rule. The incidence of hearing loss was 7%. The hearing of 68% of the children was evaluated as part of their routine follow-up after bacterial meningitis, resulting in the detection of 75% of the cases of hearing loss. The remaining 25% were detected after this follow-up had ended. Using a prediction rule based on five factors (duration of symptoms before

admission for more than 2 days, absence of petechiae, CSF glucose level ≤0.6 mmol/l, *S. pneumoniae*, and ataxia) 62% of the post-meningitic children were selected as being at risk. All cases of hearing loss were in this at-risk group.

INTERPRETATION. It should be possible to predict which children with meningitis are most at risk of deafness, such that it can be identified early and the impact on the child's development can be minimized.

Comment

Sensorineural hearing loss is the commonest severe complication of bacterial meningitis, and bacterial meningitis is the commonest cause of acquired hearing loss in young children |15|. Hearing loss can be difficult to diagnose in young infants, and late diagnosis can have serious consequences for the child's development, resulting in language delay and impaired integration and social development. Previously proposed risk factors for deafness have not resulted in reliable prediction |2|. Delayed diagnosis may also have consequences for treatment, since the development of ossification of the cochlear can result in technical difficulties when inserting cochlear implants. It is recommended that all children who have had bacterial meningitis should undergo hearing tests as part of the routine follow-up. Difficulties with resource allocation mean that up to 25% of children do not have formal hearing tests after bacterial meningitis; the ability to reliably predict which children will develop this complication may help health services to deliver appropriate care more effectively. Children included in the trial suffered meningitis due to infection with *S. pneumoniae*, *S. agalactiae*, *Escherichia coli*, *Neisseria meningitidis* or *Listeria monocytogenes*. Patients infected with *Haemophilus influenzae* type b were excluded. Children who had cognitive or behavioural problems before their disease were excluded. Twenty-nine parameters were examined as potential risk factors for deafness. Seven per cent of children in the cohort had deafness following their disease, and there was considered to be late detection in 25% of these cases. The five-point rule developed had a high rate of predicting false positives, but was extremely sensitive in detecting at-risk children, and would still result in fewer children undergoing formal hearing evaluation than currently receive it (Fig. 13.1, Table 13.2). However, it needs to be evaluated in a prospective trial before it can be implemented in current practice. Because of the exclusion criteria used in this trial, it may not be applicable to those patients who have pre-existing cognitive or behavioural problems.

Conclusion

Research findings need to be interpreted in their appropriate context. Thus, Molyneux *et al.*, through their large, well-designed trial, precisely answered their question regarding the benefit of adjunctive steroids in bacterial meningitis in children in Malawi. It might seem that this is at odds with previous research regarding the benefit of steroids in *Haemophilus influenzae* type b disease in children, but when

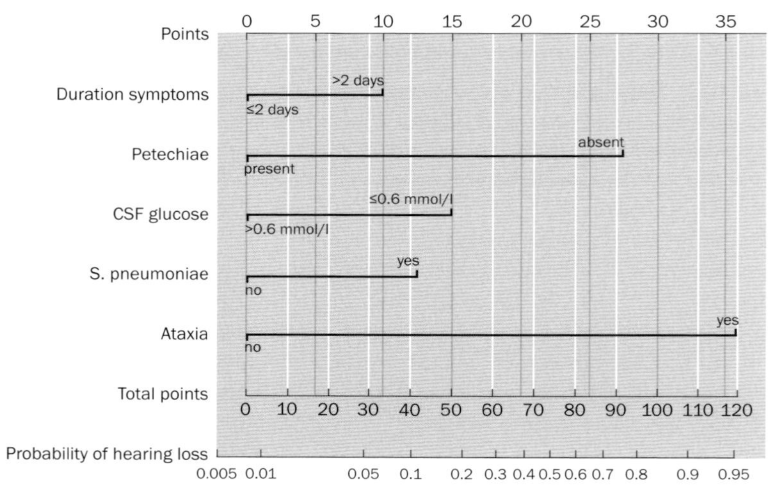

Fig. 13.1 Nomogram for predicting probability of hearing loss in survivors of non-haemophilus influenzae type b childhood bacterial meningitis. Source: Koomen *et al.* (2003).

Table 13.2 Number of patients with and without hearing loss across categories of the risk score

Risk score	Patients in the cohort (*n* = 628)	Patients with hearing loss (*n* = 43)	Patients without hearing loss (*n* = 585)
0	236 (38)	0	236 (40)
1–24	86 (14)	2 (5)	84 (14)
25–36	87 (14)	5 (11)	82 (14)
37–63	197 (31)	24 (56)	173 (30)
≥64	22 (3)	12 (28)	10 (2)

Values represent numbers (percentages).
Source: Koomen *et al.* (2003).

the particular circumstances of the children receiving treatment in Malawi are considered it is not surprising. Moreover, the investigators have used the results of their subanalysis to develop further hypotheses, which they are now testing, rather than to draw further conclusions.

In developed countries where there is little penicillin resistance, it is likely that guidelines for the treatment of bacterial meningitis in adults will be revised to include intravenous dexamethasone along with empirical antibiotics.

Regarding cryptococcal meningitis, the immune reconstitution seen with HAART appears to offer meaningful protection against relapse from cryptococcal disease, but longer follow-up is needed. Further efforts are needed to determine the best management of raised intracranial pressure.

Questions remain to be answered regarding the optimal duration of antimicrobial therapy in bacterial and cryptococcal meningitis, the optimal treatment of complications such as raised intracranial pressure, the place of steroids in areas where the prevalence of *Haemophilus influenzae* infection is low, and on the pharmacokinetics of antibiotics in the CSF of adults with bacterial meningitis.

References

1. Quagliarello VJ, Scheld WM. Treatment of bacterial meningitis. *N Engl J Med* 1997; **336**: 708–16.

2. Arditi M, Mason EO Jr, Bradley JS, Tan TQ, Barson WJ, Schutze GE, Wald ER, Givner LB, Kim KS, Yogev R, Kaplan SL. Three-year multicenter surveillance of pneumococcal meningitis in children: clinical characteristics, and outcome related to penicillin susceptibility and dexamethasone use. *Pediatrics* 1998; **102**: 1087–97.

3. http://www.dfid.gov.uk/News/PressReleases/files/pr04december03.html.

4. Tunkel AR, Scheld WM. Corticosteroids for everyone with meningitis? *N Engl J Med* 2002; **347**: 1613–15.

5. McCracken GH Jr. Rich nations, poor nations, and bacterial meningitis. *Lancet* 2002; **360**: 183.

6. Principi N, Esposito S. Dexamethasone in acute bacterial meningitis. *Lancet* 2002; **360**: 1610; author reply 1610–11.

7. Coyle PK. Glucocorticoids in central nervous system bacterial infection. *Arch Neurol* 1999; **56**: 796–801.

8. Paris MM, Hickey SM, Uscher MI, Shelton S, Olsen KD, McCracken GH Jr. Effect of dexamethasone on therapy of experimental penicillin- and cephalosporin-resistant pneumococcal meningitis. *Antimicrob Agents Chemother* 1994; **38**: 1320–4.

9. Puddicombe JB, Wali SS, Greenwood BM. A field trial of a single intramuscular injection of long-acting chloramphenicol in the treatment of meningococcal meningitis. *Trans R Soc Trop Med Hyg* 1984; **78**: 399–403.

10. Marhoum el Filali K, Noun M, Chakib A, Zahraoui M, Himmich H. Ceftriaxone versus penicillin G in the short-term treatment of meningococcal meningitis in adults. *Eur J Clin Microbiol Infect Dis* 1993; **12**: 766–8.

11. Dagan R, Givon-Lavi N, Zamir O, Sikuler-Cohen M, Guy L, Janco J, Yagupsky P, Fraser D. Reduction of nasopharyngeal carriage of Streptococcus pneumoniae after administration of a 9-valent pneumococcal conjugate vaccine to toddlers attending day-care centers. *J Infect Dis* 2002; **185**: 927–36.

12. Furrer H, Egger M, Opravil M, Bernasconi E, Hirschel B, Battegay M, Telenti A, Vernazza PL, Rickenbach M, Flepp M, Malinverni R. Discontinuation of primary prophylaxis against Pneumocystis carinii pneumonia in HIV-1-infected adults treated with combination antiretroviral therapy. Swiss HIV Cohort Study. *N Engl J Med* 1999; **340**: 1301–6.

13. Weverling GJ, Mocroft A, Ledergerber B, Kirk O, Gonzales-Lahoz J, d'Arminio Monforte A, Proenca R, Phillips AN, Lundgren JD, Reiss P. Discontinuation of Pneumocystis carinii pneumonia prophylaxis after start of highly active antiretroviral therapy in HIV-1 infection. EuroSIDA Study Group. *Lancet* 1999; **353**: 1293–8.

14. Fleming DT, McQuillan GM, Johnson RE, Nahmias AJ, Aral SO, Lee FK, St Louis ME. Herpes simplex virus type 2 in the United States, 1976 to 1994. *N Engl J Med* 1997; **337**: 1105–11.

15. Woolley AL, Kirk KA, Neumann AM Jr, McWilliams SM, Murray J, Freind D, Wiatrak BJ. Risk factors for hearing loss from meningitis in children: the Children's Hospital experience. *Arch Otolaryngol Head Neck Surg* 1999; **125**: 509–14.

14

Rickettsial infection

PHILIPPE PAROLA, DIDIER RAOULT, FRÉDÉRIQUE GOURIET

Introduction

Rickettsiae were not discovered until the twentieth century. These organisms were first described as short Gram-negative rods that retained fuchsine when stained by the method of Gimenez. They are obligate intracellular bacteria. The taxonomic classification of the genera of rickettsias has been subject to constant modification and recent developments in molecular taxonomic methods have resulted in reclassification within the Rickettsiales. However, there are two groups of diseases that are still usually called 'rickettsioses'. These include scrub typhus, due to *Orientia tsutsugamushi*, and disease due to bacteria of the genus *Rickettsia*, including the spotted fever group and the typhus group. The spotted fever group comprises more than 30 species and the typhus group consists of the two species *R. prowazekii* and *R. typhi*. These agents are associated with arthropods such as ticks, mites, fleas and lice, which may act as the vector and/or reservoir of the organism. These vectors play an important role in the transmission of rickettsial micro-organisms. They require specific optimal environmental conditions, and this determines the geographical distribution of the vector and consequently the areas where there is a risk of rickettsiosis. The reservoir (flying squirrels, for example) can play an important role in the spread of the disease and is responsible for sporadic cases of *R. prowazekii* in the US.

The diagnosis of rickettsioses was based on serological testing, and the reference technique is the indirect immunofluorescence assay. However, cross-reactions are common and this technique cannot discriminate among rickettsioses. Other techniques were developed subsequently, and serological tests, including cross-adsorption assays, and Western blotting tests are able to detect antibodies to suspected antigens. Immunodetection in a skin biopsy has also been proposed for diagnosis. The spectrum of the rickettsioses has increased dramatically with the introduction of cell and molecular biological methods. Since 1991, eight new species or new diseases have been described: *R. japonica* in Japan, *R. honei* on Flinders Island (between Australia and Tasmania), *R. africae* in Africa and the West Indies, *R. slovaca* in Europe, *R. aeschlimannii* in Africa and Europe, *R. helvetica* in Europe and Asia, *R. heilongjanghensis* in Asia and *R. parkeri* in the US. Two new subspecies have also been reported: *R conorii astrakhan* in Russia, Africa and Kosovo and *R. sibirica mongolotimonae* in China, Europe and Africa.

Recently, the number of reported cases of travel-associated tick-borne rickettsioses has risen significantly worldwide. This may be explained by increasing international travel to endemic areas and better recognition of rickettsial diseases by physicians. African tick bite fever, Mediterranean spotted fever, Indian tick typhus, Astrakhan fever, Rocky Mountain spotted fever, Queensland tick typhus and *R. aeschlimannii* infection are examples of rickettsioses that have been reported in international travellers.

This review provides an outline of our current knowledge of the microbiological diagnosis, treatment and possible prevention of the rickettsioses, and also considers future prospects.

African tick bite fever

Jensenius M, Fournier PE, Kelly P, Myrvang B, Raoult D. *Lancet Infect Dis* 2003; **3**: 557–64

BACKGROUND. **African tick bite fever is a rickettsiosis of the spotted fever group that has emerged recently as one of the most common causes of acute febrile illness in international travellers. The disease is associated with headache, prominent neck muscle myalgia, inoculation eschars, and regional lymphadenitis (Table 14.1). The causative agent is a *Rickettsia africae*, the reservoir and vector of which are ungulate ticks of the genus *Amblyomma*. This rickettsial disease occurs in sub-Saharan Africa and the French West Indies. Indigenous population reports on African tick bite fever are scarce, but the number of reported cases in travellers from Europe and elsewhere has recently increased significantly. The treatment is doxycycline, which is associated with rapid recovery in most patients. For microbiological diagnosis the immunofluorescence assay is recommended, but seroconversion is commonly delayed and this limits the usefulness of the test.**

Table 14.1 Signs and symptoms of African tick bite fever

Characteristic		Frequency (%)
Fever		59–100
Headache		62–83
Myalgia		63–87
	Neck muscle myalgia	81
Inoculation eschar		53–100
	Multiple eschars	21–54
Regional lymphadenitis		43–100
Cutaneous rash		15–46
	Maculopapular	15–26
	Vesicular	0–21
Aphthous stomatitis		11

Source: Data compiled from references |**1–4**|.

INTERPRETATION. This rickettsiosis is recognized as an international travel-associated disease, and is becoming more important with the expansion of international safari tourism to southern Africa. It emerged in Europe and elsewhere. Travellers to endemic areas should be informed of the risk of contracting African tick bite fever and be encouraged to take personal protective measures against tick bites.

Comment

The authors review and describe the biology, epidemiology, pathophysiology, clinical presentation, diagnosis and treatment of African tick bite fever. They provide interesting data on the role of emerging bacteria encountered in tropical and sub-tropical regions in the world, where malaria, hepatitis A and other uncommon diseases such as dengue, Japanese encephalitis and parasitic infections occur.

Rickettsia parkeri: a newly recognized cause of spotted fever rickettsiosis in the United States

Paddock CD, Sumner JW, Comer JA, *et al*. *Clin Infect Dis* 2004; **38**: 805–11

BACKGROUND. Rickettsiae of the spotted fever group are obligate intracellular bacteria of the genus *Rickettsia*. They are transmitted by ticks, including many that bite humans. Only 15 species of *Rickettsia* are recognized as human pathogens. *R. rickettsi* was thought to be the only agent of Rocky Mountain spotted fever in humans in the US. *R. parkeri* was first identified more than 60 years ago in the Gulf Coast in *Amblyomma maculatum* ticks collected from the southern US. The authors describe the first human case caused by *R. parkeri* infection. The disease was confirmed by serological testing, immunohistochemical staining, cell culture isolation, and molecular methods. In febrile patients with eschar (Fig. 14.1) following a tick bite, application of specific laboratory assays may identify additional cases of *R. parkeri* rickettsiosis or possibly other novel rickettsioses of the spotted fever group in the US.

INTERPRETATION. The clinical manifestation was relatively mild: febrile illness accompanied by inoculation eschar and maculopapular rash. Laboratory abnormalities included mild leucopenia and elevated hepatic enzyme levels, and rapid clinical response to therapy with doxycycline, which are also features of other rickettsioses of the spotted fever group. Cross-reactivity was observed with other rickettsias of the spotted fever group and patient serum specimens showed an antibody titre not significantly different from the titres obtained for *R. akarii* and *R. rickettsii*. Immunohistochemical staining revealed rickettsias of the spotted fever group in the cytoplasm of a few cells in foci of perivascular infiltrates. Seven days after inoculation of Vero cells with triturated biopsy specimens, staining and electronic microscopy demonstrated infected cells with intracellular bacteria. Use of a polymerase chain reaction (PCR) assay targeting the *gltA* and *rompA* genes allowed the identification of *R. parkeri*.

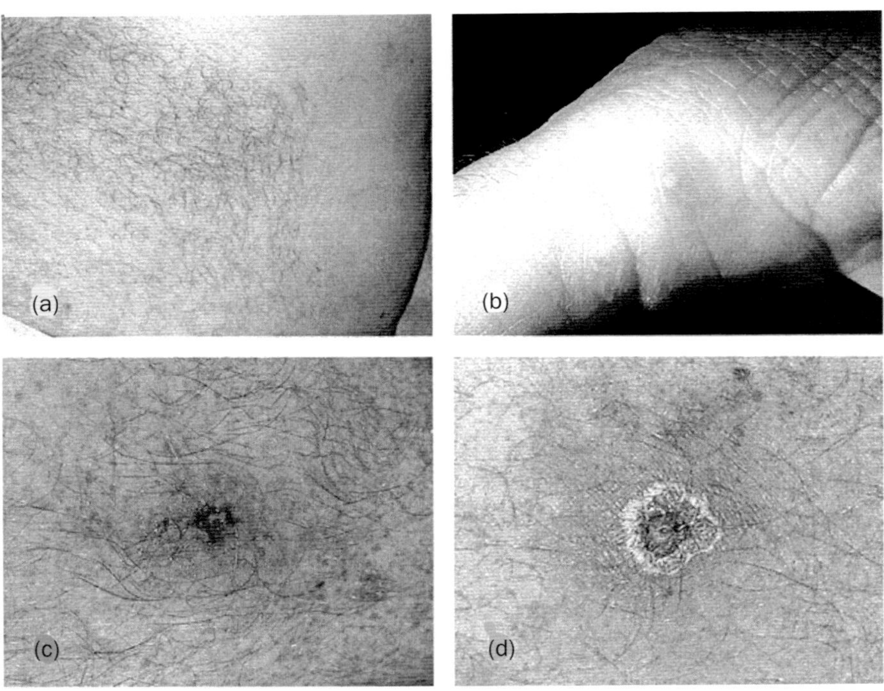

Fig. 14.1 Cutaneous lesions in a patient infected with *Rickettsia parkeri*. (a) A diffuse, pink macular rash involving the abdomen. (b) A small pustule on the medial aspect of the first digit. (c and d) Eschars on the pretibial aspects of the right and left lower legs, respectively. Source: Paddock *et al*. (2004).

Comment

In the first part of the twentieth century, *R. rickettsi* was considered the only agent of tick-borne rickettsial diseases in all the Americas. Any other rickettsia obtained from a tick was considered to be non-pathogenic; among these were *R. parkeri* (first identified in 1939), *R. bellii*, *R. rhipicephali* and *R. montanensis*. In the rest of the world, three pathogenic species of tick-borne rickettsioses were established: *R. conorii* in Europe, Africa and Asia, *R. sibirica* in Siberia and *R. australis* in Australia. A single species was considered the agent of all tick-borne rickettsioses in a specific geographical area. In 1991, the spectrum of rickettsioses increased dramatically with the advent of cell culture and molecular biological testing methods, and this challenged older ideas about rickettsial diseases. This report shows that any tick isolate is a potential pathogen as soon as the infected tick bites a human being, and atypical cases of febrile rash should be investigated properly by cell culture and/or molecular biological testing. Basic serological testing using only the already suspected antigens gives only confirmatory information. Therefore, the results of serological testing are presumptive and should be interpreted with caution. In this case, only cell culture allowed the identification of the causative agent properly, and this is the first report of an infection with this agent.

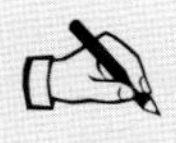

Flying squirrel-associated typhus, United States

Reynolds MG, Krebs JS, Comer JA, *et al. Emerg Infect Dis* 2003; **9**: 1341–3

BACKGROUND. Infections with *R. prowazekii* are rarely described in the US. Other than man, the flying squirrel acts as a reservoir. This is the only known vertebrate reservoir and is linked to most sporadic cases of typhus in the US. In March 2002, typhus fever was diagnosed in two patients resident in West Virginia and Georgia. They were both hospitalized with febrile illness and both had recently been in contact with flying squirrels or their nests. The diagnosis was made by serological testing (indirect immunofluorescence assay).

INTERPRETATION. The authors describe two cases of typhus associated with the flying squirrel and provide a review of Centers for Disease Control (CDC) records, which identified two additional cases between 1985 and 2002. The disease can be severe, resulting in protracted hospital stays, particularly when diagnosis and appropriated treatment are delayed. In these two cases, when tetracycline antibiotics were given the clinical response was rapid. These cases show how important it is that physicians should remain alert to signs and symptoms of epidemic typhus, be aware of any history of animal contact, and know about appropriate diagnosis methods and antibiotic treatments.

Comment

Cases of sporadic epidemic typhus (*R. prowazekii*) affect humans when conditions are favourable for the person-to-person spread of body lice. No epidemic surveillance is performed for epidemic typhus in the US. Cases of non-epidemic typhus in the US are rarely described and documented. They are not associated with the classical man–louse–man–cycle of epidemic typhus. These infections occur in the eastern US, and in one-third of cases there is contact with flying squirrels or their nests. Diagnosis of *R. prowazekii* infection was done by serological immunofluorescence testing, but this test lacks specificity because of the cross-reaction with *R. typhi*. The PCR and organism culture are specific diagnosis tools, but their sensitivity depends on the clinical specimen. CDC provides this test when specimens are submitted from health laboratories.

Rickettsioses in Swedish travellers, 1997–2001

Rahman A, Tegnell A, Vene S, Giesecke J. *Scand J Infect Dis* 2003; **35**: 247–50

BACKGROUND. Several European countries and the US report occasional imported cases of rickettsioses. This disease is often considered a minor problem in travellers and underestimation may occur. In Sweden, this disease is rarely diagnosed. During 1997–2001, 77 cases of rickettsioses were diagnosed; 14 cases were diagnosed as belonging to the typhus group and 63 to the spotted fever group. In the typhus group, signs of hepatic involvement occurred more frequently. The estimated risk of rickettsioses in destinations outside Europe varied from 1 case in 140 000 travellers to Southeast Asia to 1 in 1600 travellers to southern Africa. Over the 5-year period, in southern Africa, the risk of infection increased, and is now four to five times higher than the risk of acquiring malaria in the same region. In travellers with febrile illness, rickettsiosis is an important differential diagnosis to consider, especially in those who had visited South Africa. In addition, the serological response may be considerably delayed; in patients with a negative first serology, serological testing should be repeated. If there is a strong suspicion of rickettsiosis, antibiotic treatment may be introduced before the diagnosis is confirmed.

INTERPRETATION. Most (54%) patients diagnosed with rickettsioses had visited South Africa. Most of the cases in this group were 50- to 59-year-old males, but the database does not give enough details to perform a proper analysis on gender and age. Exposure is linked to the type of travel; it may be very high on safaris in wildlife parks, where the risk of tick bites is high. There was an increasing number of cases in individuals returning from South Africa. During the first 4 years of the study, the incidence was between 30 and 40 per 100 000 travellers, but by 2001 it had risen to 100. The number of travellers remained stable. The national surveillance data collected at the Swedish Institute for Infectious Disease Control (SMI) showed that the risk to a Swedish traveller of acquiring a rickettsiosis in South Africa is four to five times higher than that of contracting malaria.

Comment

Rickettsiose are emerging diseases. This study made a descriptive analysis of the group of patients diagnosed with rickettsiosis in Sweden during a 5-year period and tried to define risk areas for rickettsial infections in travellers. In Swedish travellers, an increase in the number of cases was observed. This emerging disease should be considered by physicians as an important differential diagnosis in febrile travellers, especially those who have recently visited South Africa. It is important to remember that they should also be aware that both the onset and the serological response may be considerably delayed. In addition, in patients with a suggestive epidemiology and clinical symptoms antibiotic treatment may have to be started before confirmatory laboratory results are available.

Increased detection of rickettsialpox in a New York City hospital following the anthrax outbreak of 2001: use of immunohistochemistry for the rapid confirmation of cases in an era of bioterrorism

Koss T, Carter EL, Grossman ME, *et al. Arch Dermatol* 2003; **139**: 1545–52

BACKGROUND. Rickettsialpox is an acute self-limited febrile illness caused by *Rickettsia akarii* and is transmitted by a haematophagous mite, *Liponyssoides* *sanguineus*. Rickettsialpox begins with skin lesions that form black eschars that may be mistaken for signs of potentially more serious diseases, such as cutaneous anthrax or chickenpox. The cluster of cutaneous anthrax cases associated with bioterrorism in October 2001 probably heightened awareness of and concern about cutaneous eschars. For the period from 23 February 2001 to 31 October 2002, the authors report 18 cases of rickettsialpox seen in a large tertiary care hospital in New York city. To confirm the clinical diagnosis, skin biopsy specimens, serological tests and immunohistochemical (IHC) tests were performed. They applied immunohistochemistry to paraffin-embedded skin biopsy specimens and compared the reported incidence of rickettsialpox before, during and after the cluster of cutaneous anthrax cases. Immunohistochemistry revealed rickettsias of the spotted fever group in all 16 eschars and in five of the nine papulovesicles tested. Serological testing revealed a four-fold or greater increase in immunoglobulin G antibody titres reactive with *R. akarii* in all nine patients for whom acute and convalescent phase samples were available; six patients had single titres indicative of rickettsialpox infection ($\geq$1.64). Of the 18 patients, nine (50%) presented in the 5 months following the bioterrorism attacks. The bioterrorism attacks of October 2001 may have led to increased awareness and detection of this disease.

INTERPRETATION. The clinical presentation of the patients was similar to that in historical reports, most patients presenting with the classical triad of fever, necrotic eschar and papulovesicular rash. This presentation alerts the clinician, but the disease is commonly confused with more serious diseases, such as cutareous anthrax and chickenpox. General routine laboratory tests do not contribute to the diagnosis of rickettsialpox. In the series, the most frequent laboratory abnormalities were elevated blood cell count and elevated erythrocyte sedimentation rate, in the youngest patient. Immunohistochemical staining of skin biopsy specimens, particularly from eschars, is a sensitive technique for confirming the clinical diagnosis. For all 16 eschars the histopathological features were characterized by variable degrees of epidermal necrosis, and immunohistochemical staining revealed spotted fever. Serological testing can be useful in confirming the diagnosis of rickettsialpox; seroconversion may not occur for several weeks and at least two patient visits are necessary for the collection of serum samples. All 16 patients received doxycycline for 7 days. Early recognition of the rickettsialpox clinical presentation and immunohistochemistry should lead to more rapid diagnosis.

Comment

Rickettsialpox remains endemic in New York city. The 18 cases seen in a 20-month period represent a three-fold increase in the annual number of cases. In cases of natural exposure or acts of bioterrorism, cutaneous anthrax is the differential diagnosis of rickettsialpox. This underlines the importance of the clinician's ability to diagnose patients presenting with fever, eschar and a papulovesicular rash eruption, especially in an endemic area. During the acute phase, the rickettsialpox infection should be confirmed using serological testing and immunohistochemical staining, but also cell culture and molecular methods; the last two methods were not performed in this study.

Physician knowledge of the diagnosis and management of Rocky Mountain spotted fever: Mississippi, 2002

O'Reilly M, Paddock C, Elchos B, Goddard J, Childs J, Currie M. *Ann NY Acad Sci* 2003; **990**: 295–301

BACKGROUND. Rocky Mountain spotted fever (RMSF), is a tick-borne illness caused by *R. rickettsi*. It is endemic in the US, with the highest incidence in the south central and south-eastern parts of the country. Diagnosis of RMSF is often a challenge because patients frequently present with non-specific symptoms during the early stages of illness. RMSF has a high case fatality rate without treatment. The median time from onset of symptoms to death is only 8 days. Early recognition and treatment of RMSF is crucial. This study of physician's knowledge was performed in two public health districts in Mississippi. One hundred and forty-eight primary care physicians were selected at random and were mailed surveys regarding RMSF diagnosis, treatment and prevention. Eighty-four of the 148 (57%) physicians responded from different specialities and different health districts, and responses were compared using the χ^2 test. The findings included almost universal (99%) recognition of doxycycline as the antibiotic agent of choice for treating adults and adolescents. Only 21% of family practice physicians and 25% of emergency medicine physicians correctly identified doxycycline as the antibiotic of choice for treating children with RMSF. Twenty-three per cent of the physicians' responses indicated that waiting for the development of a rash before prescribing antibiotics was an appropriate treatment strategy. Continuing education efforts should focus on antibiotic selection in paediatric patients and the initiation of therapy before the onset of rash in appropriate patients.

INTERPRETATION. RMSF can be difficult to diagnose and treat appropriately. In this study, physicians were evaluating the treatment of patients with RMSF in two districts. Despite the different rates of RMSF between the two districts, no difference in correct response rates for RMSF diagnosis, treatment and prevention was observed. In addition, a statistically significant difference was observed for the paediatricians who correctly identified doxycycline as the antibiotic treatment of choice, despite the low total number of responses for paediatricians. The gaps in knowledge identified in this survey should be used as the starting point for education programmes designed to increase physicians' knowledge of RMSF and to improve their management of the illness.

Comment

Ingrained resistance to prescribing tetracycline in paediatric patients may be the biggest obstacle to appropriate therapeutic practice. Recommendations about the safety of a short course of doxycycline should be targeted at physicians whose speciality includes but is not limited to paediatrics. In treating children 8 years of age or younger who are suspected of having RMSF, doxycycline is the agent of choice, but this has not been communicated effectively to all physicians caring for children. In addition, many physicians are not familiar with the initiation of antibiotic therapy before the development of rash in patients with suspected RMSF. High mortality rates in untreated patients and the rapid progression of illness to death in fatal cases highlight the need for a rapid treatment decision.

Rickettsia aeschlimannii in Spain: molecular evidence in *Hyalomma marginatum* and five other tick species that feed on humans

Fernandez-Soto P, Encinas-Grandes A, Perez-Sanchez R. *Emerg Infect Dis* 2003; **9**: 889–90

BACKGROUND. First isolated in *Hyalomma marginatum* in Morocco in 1997, *R. aeschlimanii* belongs to the spotted fever group of rickettsias. It was later found in other tick species, suggesting that other vectors may also be suitable for this rickettsia. This rickettsia is a human pathogen; two cases have been described in the literature. Over the past 6 years, 3059 ticks attached to persons were collected from Castilla León in north-western Spain. The ticks belonged to 16 species. They were analysed systematically by a PCR method to detect *Borrelia burgdorferi*, *Anaplasma phagocytophila* and *Rickettsia* species. In the search for rickettsias, all DNA samples were tested for a fragment of the rickettsial *gltA* gene, and in the samples in which *gltA* was found a fragment of the rickettsial *ompA* gene was amplified and sequenced for identification. This procedure allowed the identification of *R. aeschlimanii* for the first time in Spain. *R. aeschlimanii* was found in 35 tick specimens belonging to *Hyalomma* species and in five other species.

INTERPRETATION. The high number of rickettsias isolated in ticks was unexpected; there were six species belonging to four genera. Of these six species, *H. marginatum* was the fourth most anthropophilic species in this study and showed the highest infection rate, making it the main vector of *R. aeschlimanii* in Spain. The next most important vectors are *Rhipicephalus* species, in particular *R. bursa*. Mediterranean spotted fever is endemic in the region. Among the ticks analysed, only one specimen of *R. conorii* was found; *R. aeschlimanii* was more prevalent in these same ticks.

Comment

This observation expands the geographical distribution of *R. aeschlimanii* and the range of its potential tick vectors. *R. aeschlimanii* is present in Castilla León, the largest region in Spain, and is present in six species of ticks that feed on humans. Moreover, some cases of rickettsia infection diagnosed as Mediterranean spotted fever in Spain could be *R. aeschlimanii* infection. This explains why, in southern Spain, patients with Mediterranean spotted fever have several *tâche noire*. Systematic identification of rickettsial species in human infections will be helpful in order to increase the number of recognized human infections. Several rickettsial species may be prevalent in the same area, as observed, for example, with *R. slovaca*, *R. mongolotimonae* and *R. conorii* in southern France, *R. africae* and *R. conorii* in sub-Saharan Africa and *R. conorii* and Israeli spotted fever rickettsia in Sicily and Portugal.

Scrub typhus re-emergence in the Maldives

Lewis MD, Yousuf AA, Lerdthusnee K, Razee A, Chandranoi K, Jones JW. *Emerg Infect Dis* 2003; **9**: 1638–41

BACKGROUND. Scrub typhus due to *Orientia tsutsugamushi* is an acute febrile rural zoonosis endemic in the Asia-Pacific region. About one million cases of scrub typhus have been estimated to occur each year and a billion people may be exposed. In the Republic of Maldives, consisting of 26 coral atolls in the Indian Ocean, an outbreak of febrile illness which began in the summer of 2002 was investigated by the local Ministry of Health and the Armed Forces Research Institute of Medical Sciences in Bangkok. Up to April 2003, officials recorded 168 cases linked to this outbreak (they were identified in several of the islands constituting the Maldives), and ten deaths were recorded. A total of 38 cases were confirmed in the laboratory to be scrub typhus. Diagnosis was made by serology, including an enzyme-linked immunoabsorbent assay (ELISA) test, indirect immunoperoxidase and/or indirect immunofluorescence. Furthermore, *O. tsutsugamushi* DNA was identified by PCR in two of four whole blood samples studied.

INTERPRETATION. Before this study, the last cases of scrub typhus in the Republic of Maldives had been recorded as long ago as during World War II by British troops. The reappearance of the disease in the Maldives 58 years after the last reported cases was confirmed by serology and molecular methods, providing direct evidence of the pathogen in human samples.

Comment

Scrub typhus may have been unrecognized, misdiagnosed or not reported in the Maldives for decades because of a lack of surveillance and laboratory facilities. The death of three adolescents on Gadhoo Island brought the disease to the attention of the health authorities, which began educating healthcare providers and alerted the public. The disease is transmitted by the bites of the larvae of several species of trombiculid mites (*Leptotrombidium* spp., commonly called 'chiggers'), which usually feed on rats but may readily bite humans on any part of the body. Chiggers are known as vectors but also as reservoirs of the disease because of the transovarian and trans-stadial transmission of the bacteria in mites. Thus, although re-emerging in 2003, *O. tsutsugamushi* has probably always been present in the Maldives. Occupational diseases among rural residents engaged in agricultural or gathering activities were identified in this study, as were rodent habitats close to humans. Several hypothesis have been made to explain the highest number of cases, which occurred on one of the islands, Gadhoo Island. There, a large die-off of wild and domestic cats occurred in 2000, leading to a large increase in the population of rodents in contact with humans. The rodents' habitats may have been disturbed after an aggressive campaign to clean up trash sites and yards. Also, climatic factors may influence the vectors' life cycles and thus the epidemiology of the diseases they transmit. A discussion of any climatic changes that had occurred in recent years in the Maldives would have been interesting. Numbers of cases on the different atolls of the Maldives between 28 May 2002 and 27 April 2003 are shown in Fig. 14.2.

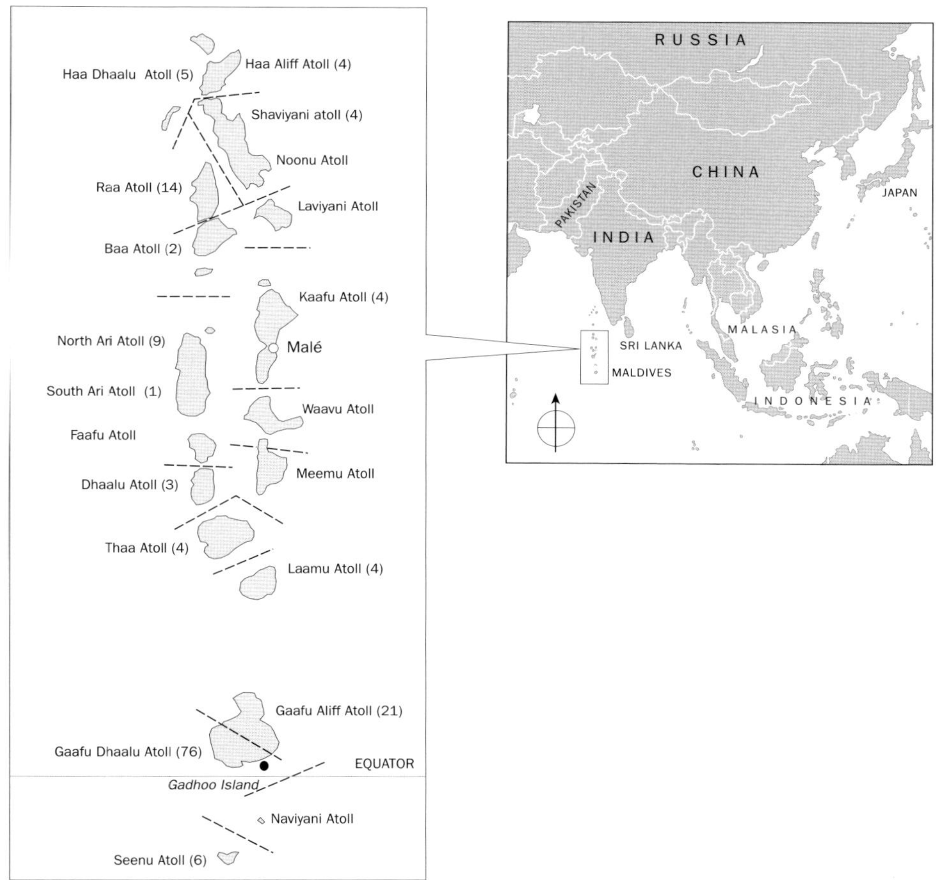

Fig. 14.2 Atolls in the Republic of Maldives. The total numbers of cases between 28 May 2002 and 27 April 2003 are shown in parentheses next to the name of the atoll.
Source: Lewis *et al.* (2003).

Differentiating dengue virus infection from scrub typhus in Thai adults with fever

Watt G, Jongsakul K, Chouriyagune C, Paris R. *Am J Trop Med Hyg* 2003; **68**: 536–8

BACKGROUND. Typical clinical features of scrub typhus due to *O. tsutsugamushi* include a papule at the bite site that later ulcerates, forming an eschar that is typically associated with fever, drainage lymphadenopathy, a macular or maculopapular rash, headache and myalgia. However, eschars and rashes may be absent or unnoticed. Thus, scrub typhus may be misdiagnosed as one of several other diseases that may also present as acute undifferentiated illness in the same area, such as dengue fever. In this prospective study, the authors aimed to identify characteristics that would distinguish between scrub typhus and dengue in HIV-negative patients from northern Thailand presenting with fever of unclear aetiology. Clinical and laboratory features of 54 patients with scrub typhus (confirmed by an immunoperoxidase assay) and 35 with dengue (confirmed by an ELISA assay) were evaluated during a 4-month study in the rainy season. Haemorrhagic manifestations were more common with dengue fever, particularly bleeding from the gums, which was reported only by dengue fever patients (27%; *P* <0.001). Furthermore, a low platelet count (<140 000/mm^3) and a low white blood cell count (<5000/mm^3) were strongly associated with dengue infection.

INTERPRETATION. Three features that could help to distinguish scrub typhus from dengue were identified: bleeding from the gums, the platelet count and the blood cell count. These results were supported by significant statistical comparisons.

Comment

Providing simple clues to aid in diagnosis or in the determination of a diagnosis score is helpful when a disease is most frequently diagnosed by serological assays, because of the delay needed for seroconversion, particularly in areas lacking laboratory facilities. Differentiating dengue from scrub typhus is important in the field. Supportive therapy and monitoring dengue patients closely in hospital for digestive bleeding are important. On the other hand, scrub typhus requires prompt antibiotic treatment (doxycycline being the reference drug) as the case fatality rate is high (up to 30%). As suggested by the authors, the simple criteria shown here to be helpful should be tested in other areas of Asia where both infections are endemic. However, treating undifferentiated fever illnesses in remote areas of Asia with doxycycline could also be considered as the treatment of life-threatening susceptible pathogens such as *O. tsutsugamushi* but also agents of leptospirosis. Indeed, the mortality of scrub typhus remains high (it is still around 15% in northern Thailand) because of multiple factors, including late presentation, delayed diagnosis or misdiagnosis, inappropriate presumptive treatment with β-lactams and a lower level of drug susceptibility.

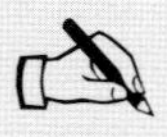

In vitro reactivation of human immunodeficiency virus-1 upon stimulation with scrub typhus rickettsial infection

Moriuchi M, Tamura A, Moriuchi H. *Am J Trop Med Hyg* 2003; **68**: 557–61

BACKGROUND. In recent years it has been shown that HIV-1 infection does not affect the clinical severity of scrub typhus. Furthermore, although a transient increase in the HIV-1 load is usually seen in patients with AIDS presenting a concomitant infection, several reports have shown that *O. tsutsugamushi* infection suppresses HIV-1 replication both *in vivo* and *in vitro*. In this study, *in vitro* HIV-1 infection was conducted using (i) peripheral blood mononuclear cells (PBMC) acutely infected with HIV-1 and (ii) PBMC derived from HIV-1-infected patients who were receiving highly active antiretroviral therapy (HAART) and whose plasma viral load was undetectable. Interestingly, pretreatment with *O. tsutsugamushi* rendered PBMC resistant to HIV-1, but it otherwise increased HIV-1 replication. Furthermore, stimulation by *O. tsutsugamushi* led to HIV-1 replication in PBMC from patients receiving HAART.

INTERPRETATION. These results suggest that *O. tsutsugamushi* does not necessarily suppress HIV-1 replication, as shown in recent years, but has the potential to increase it.

Comment

Numerous host factors may be involved in the variability of the effect of *O. tsutsugamushi* infection. For example, it was shown in this study that upregulation of the activity of the HIV-1 long terminal repeat secondary to pro-inflammatory cytokine production would increase viral replication. On the other hand, downregulation of the chemokine receptor used to infect the cell would inhibit the entry of HIV-1. However, more studies are needed to increase our understanding of interactions between *O. tsutsugamushi* and HIV-1 in co-infected patients.

Conclusion

In recent years, rickettsial diseases have been re-emerging and they have become an important field in today's medicine. New agents have been described: some are non-pathogenic agents but others are associated with characteristic clinical patterns. In addition, different species of rickettsia are found in different areas of the world. Some of the agents can be defined as variants of older diseases, whereas others are new and represent distinct entities with unique epidemiological and clinical features—mostly in the group of spotted fevers.

The curiosity of physicians and molecular biology-based identification methods have been important in recognizing these new infections. It is important to study new rickettsial agents or differences in the pathogenicity of rickettsial strains in specific areas, and in countries where a rickettsial agent had already been identified. Active identification procedures have led to the discovery of other agents; for example, acquired tick-borne agents have been described recently in France (*R. conorii, R. helvetica, R. mongolotimonae, R. aeschlimannii* and *R. slovaca*), South Africa (*R. conorii, R. africae, R. aeschlimannii* and *R. mongolotimonae*) and Australia (*R. australis* and *R. honei*). In these cases, the use of systematic specific diagnostic techniques, such as serological testing, PCR and culture, has made it possible to identify these unexpected agents. In places where no tick-borne rickettsioses had been observed previously, such as Japan, Flinders Island and Astrakhan (in Russia), the use of specific and systematic diagnostic tools has allowed the identification of new rickettsial diseases.

In addition, knowledge of the interrelationships between hosts and vectors may contribute to better understanding of how pathogens circulate in nature. Some potential pathogenic strains of rickettsia that are associated with arthropods have been found in human specimens, allowing the description of new infectious diseases. Any tick isolate of a rickettsia species is a potential pathogen as soon as the infected tick bites a human. For *R. parkeri* it took 60 years to demonstrate this.

An additional new aspect is linked to the health of travellers and tourists. The geographical origins of patients must be taken into account in our routine medical work. For example, travellers to endemic areas should be informed about the risk of contracting African tick bite fever, and tourists should protect themselves against ticks.

There should be continuing efforts to improve physicians' knowledge about the diagnosis and management of rickettsioses, and when there is a strong suspicion of rickettsiosis treatment may have to be started without confirmation of the diagnosis. Microbiological investigations, such as culture and PCR, make it possible to identify the causative agent, but a presumptive diagnosis obtained by serological testing should be interpreted with caution. Through the combination of clinical with microbiological investigations it is possible to diagnose classical rickettsial disease and to discover new rickettsial diseases.

References

1. Fournier PE, Roux V, Caumes E, Donzel M, Raoult D. Outbreak of *Rickettsia africae* infections in participants of an adventure race in South Africa. *Clin Infect Dis* 1998; **27**; 316–23.

2. Raoult D, Fournier PE, Fenollar F, Jensenius M, Prioe T, de Pina JJ, Caruso G, Jones N, Laferl H, Rosenblatt JE, Marrie TJ. *Rickettsia africae*, a tick-borne pathogen in travelers to sub-Saharan Africa. *N Engl J Med* 2001; **344**; 1504–10.

3. Smoak BL, McClain JB, Brundage JF, Broadhurst L, Kelly DJ, Dasch GA, Miller RN. An outbreak of spotted fever rickettsiosis in US Army troops deployed to Botswana. *Emerg Infect Dis* 1996; **2**: 217–21.

4. Jensenius M, Fournier PE, Vene S, Hoel T, Hasle G, Henriksen AZ, Hellum KB, Raoult D, Myrvang B; Norwegian African Tick Bite Fever Study Group. African tick bite fever in travellers to rural sub-Equatorial Africa. *Clin Infect Dis* 2003; **36**: 1411–17.

List of abbreviations

AFLP	amplified fragment length polymorphism		ELISPOT	enzyme-linked immunospot
AGV	accessory gene regulator		EORTC	European Organisation for Research and Treatment of Cancer
AS	aggregation substance			
ATP	adenosine triphosphate		ESP	enterococcal surface protein
BAL	bronchoalveolar lavage		FEV1	forced expiratory volume in one second
BCESM	*Burkholderia cepacia* Epidemic Strain Marker			
			FVC	forced vital capacity
BCSA	*Burkholderia cepacia*-selective agar		GISA	glycopeptide intermediately resistant *S. aureus*
BHI	brain heart infusion		GM-CSF	granulocyte-macrophage colony-stimulating factor
BL	bronchoalveolar lavage			
BT	bismuth–thiol		GvHD	graft-versus-host disease
CA	community-acquired		HA	hospital-acquired
CbpA	choline-binding protein A		HAART	highly active antiretroviral therapy
CDAD	*Clostridium difficile*-associated diarrhoea			
			HC	haemorrhagic cystitis
CDC	Centers for Disease Control		HEPA	high efficiency particulate airflow
CDI	*Clostridium difficile* infection			
CF	cystic fibrosis		hGISA	heterogeneously resistant to glycopeptides
CFU	colony-forming unit			
CI	confidence interval		Hib	*Haemophilus influenzae type B*
CMI	cell-mediated immune			
CMV	cytomegalovirus		HLA-DR	human leukocyte antigen-D related
CSF	cerebrospinal fluid			
CSF	colony-stimulating factor		HPLC	high-performance liquid chromatography
CT	computed tomography			
CTL	cytotoxic T lymphocyte		HR	hazard ratio
DCC	day-care centre		HSCT	haematopoietic stem cell transplantation
DosR	dormancy survival regulator			
DOTS	directly observed therapy, short-course		HSV	herpes simplex virus
			hVISA	heterogeneous vancomycin-intermediate *Staphylococcus aureus*
EBA	early bactericidal activity			
EBMT	European Group for Blood and Marrow Transplantation		IA	invasive aspergillosis
			ICU	intensive care unit
EBS	enterococcal binding substance		ID	identification
EBV	Epstein–Barr virus		IFI	invasive fungal infection
EIA	enzyme immunoassay		IFN-γ	interferon-γ
ELISA	enzyme-linked immunosorbent assay		Ig	immunoglobulin
			IgG	immunoglobulin G

IHC	immunohistochemical
IL	interleukin
IPA	invasive pulmonary aspergillosis
IRM	infection-related mortality
ISPPD	International Symposium on Pneumococci and Pneumococcal Disease
ITS2	internal transcribed spacer 2
LPS	lipopolysaccharide
LRTI	lower respiratory tract infection
MBC	minimum bacteriocidal concentration
MDR	multidrug-resistant
MDRTB	multidrug-resistant tuberculosis
MDS	
MIC	minimum inhibitory concentration
MLST	multilocus sequence typing
MRSA	methicillin-resistant *Staphylococcus aureus*
MSSA	methicillin-sensitive *Staphylococcus aureus*
MSSA	methicillin-susceptible *Staphylococcus aureus*
MU	megaunit
NAC	non-albicans Candida
NCCLS	National Committee for Clinical Laboratory Standards
NO	nitric oxide
OR	odds ratio
ORF	open reading frames
PAP-AUC	population analysis profile × area under the curve
PBMC	peripheral blood mononuclear cells
PBP	penicillin-binding protein
PCAT	*Pseudomonas cepacia* azelaic acid medium
PCR	polymerase chain reaction
PCV	pneumococcal conjugate vaccine
PFGE	pulsed-field gel electrophoresis
PPNMT	perioperative prophylaxis with nasal mupirocin or triclosan
PspA	pneumococcal surface protein A
PTLD	post-transplant lymphoproliferative disorder
PVL	Panton–Valentine leukocidin
RAPD	random amplification of polymorphic DNA
rDNA	ribosomal deoxyribonucleic acid
RFLP	restriction fragment length polymorphism
RMSF	Rocky Mountain spotted fever
RR	relative risk
RSV	respiratory syncytial virus
RVI	respiratory virus infection
SAB	*Staphylococcus aureus* bacteraemia
SA-RVS	*Staphylococcus aureus* with reduced susceptibility to vancomycin
SCCmec	staphylococcal chromosomal cassette mec
SD	standard deviation
SFC	spot-forming cells
SMI	Swedish Institute for Infectious Disease Control
SSI	surgical site infection
TB	tuberculosis
TST	tuberculin skin test
UTI	urinary tract infection
VAP	ventilator-acquired pneumonia
VISA	vancomycin-intermediate *Staphylococcus aureus*
VRE	vancomycin-resistant enterococci
VREF	vancomycin-resistant *Enterococcus faecium*
VRSA	vancomycin-resistant *Staphylococcus aureus*
VS-MRSA	vancomycin-sensitive MRSA
VT	vaccine-type (serotype)
WBC	white blood cell
WHO	World Health Organization

Index of papers reviewed

Aarestrup FM, Wiuff C, Molbak K, Threlfall EJ. Is it time to change fluoroquinolone breakpoints for *Salmonella* spp.? *Antimicrob Agents Chemother* 2003; 47(2): 827–9. **168**

Aas J, Gessert CE, Bakken JS. Recurrent *Clostridium difficile* colitis: case series involving 18 patients treated with donor stool administered via a nasogastric tube. *Clin Infect Dis* 2003; 36(5): 580–5. **223**

Aboudola S, Kotloff KL, Kyne L, Warny M, Kelly EC, Sougioultzis S, Giannasca PJ, Monath TP, Kelly CP. *Clostridium difficile* vaccine and serum immunoglobulin G antibody response to toxin A. *Infect Immun* 2003; 71(3): 1608–10. **225**

Anderson DJ, Murdoch DR, Sexton DJ, Reller LB, Stout JE, Cabell CH, Corey GR. Risk factors for infective endocarditis in patients with enterococcal bacteremia: a case–control study. *Infection* 2004; 32(2): 72–7. **86**

Avivi I, Chakrabarti S, Milligan DW, Waldmann H, Hale G, Osman H, Ward KN, Fegan CD, Yong K, Goldstone AH, Linch DC, Mackinnon S. Incidence and outcome of adenovirus disease in transplant recipients after reduced-intensity conditioning with alemtuzumab. *Biol Blood Marrow Transplant* 2004; 10(3): 186–94. **212**

Baddley JW, Pappas PG, Smith AC, Moser SA. Epidemiology of *Aspergillus terreus* at a University Hospital. *J Clin Micro* 2003; 41(12): 5525–9. **4**

Barenfanger J, Arakere P, Dela Cruz R, Imran A, Drake C, Lawthron J, Verhulst SJ, Khardori N. Improved outcomes associated with limiting identification of *Candida* spp. in respiratory secretions. *J Clin Microbiol* 2003; 41(12): 5645–9. **15**

Bert F, Clarissou J, Durand F, Delefosse D, Chauvet C, Lefebvre P, Lambert N, Branger C. Prevalence, molecular epidemiology, and clinical significance of heterogeneous glycopeptide-intermediate *Staphylococcus aureus* in liver transplant recipients. *J Clin Microbiol* 2003; 41(11): 5147–52. **138**

Bethell D, Hall G, Goodman TR, Klein N, Pollard AJ. Resolution of orbitocerebral aspergillosis during combination treatment with voriconazole and amphotericin plus adjunctive cytokine therapy. *J Paediatr Hematol Oncol* 2004; 26: 304–7. **52**

Bhan MK, Bahl R, Sazawal S, Sinha A, Kumar R, Mahalanabis D, Clemens JD. Association between *Helicobacter pylori* infection and increased risk of typhoid fever. *J Infect Dis* 2002; 186(12): 1857–60. **173**

Boshoff HI, Reed MB, Barry CE 3rd, Mizrahi V. DnaE2 polymerase contributes to *in vivo* survival and the emergence of drug resistance in *Mycobacterium tuberculosis*. *Cell* 2003; 113(2): 183–93. **198**

Brouwer AE, Rajanuwong A, Chierakul W, Griffin GE, Larsen RA, White NJ, Harrison TS. Combination antifungal therapies in HIV-associated cryptococcal meningitis: a randomised trial. *Lancet* 2004; 363(9423): 1764–7. **42**

Buchheidt D, Hummel M, Schleiermacher D, Spiess B, Schwerdtfeger R, Cornely OA, Wilhelm S, Reuter S, Kern W, Sudhoff T, Morz H, Hehlmann R. Prospective clinical evaluation of a LightCycler-mediated polymerase chain reaction assay, a nested-PCR assay and a galactomannan enzyme-linked immunosorbent assay for detection of invasive aspergillosis in neutropenic cancer patients and haematological stem cell transplant recipients. *Br J Haematol*; 125(2): 196–202. **34**

Buke AC, Cavusoglu C, Karasulu E, Karakartal G. Does dexamethasone affect ceftriazone penetration into cerebrospinal fluid in adult bacterial meningitis. *Int J Antimicrob Agents* 2003; 21(5): 452–6. **247**

Centers for Disease Control and Prevention (CDC). Vancomycin-resistant *Staphylococcus aureus*, New York, 2004. *MMWR Morb Mortal Wkly Rep* 2004; 53(15): 322–3. **129**

Cesaro S, Toffolutti T, Messina C, Calore E, Alaggio R, Cusinato R, Pillon M, Zanesco L. Safety and efficacy of caspofungin and liposomal amphotericin B, followed by voriconazole in young patients affected by refractory invasive mycosis. *Eur J Haematol* 2004; 73: 50–5. **48**

Chang S, Sievert DM, Hageman JC, Boulton ML, Tenover FC, Downes FP, Shah S, Rudrik JT, Pupp GR, Brown WJ, Cardo D, Fridkin SK; Vancomycin-Resistant *Staphylococcus aureus* Investigative Team. Infection with vancomycin-resistant *Staphylococcus aureus* containing the vanA resistance gene. *N Engl J Med* 2003; 348(14): 1342–7. **125**

Charles PG, Ward PB, Johnson PD, Howden BP, Grayson ML. Clinical features associated with bacteremia due to heterogeneous vancomycin-intermediate *Staphylococcus aureus*. *Clin Infect Dis* 2004; 38: 448–51. **136**

Cooper BS, Stone SP, Kibbler CC, Cookson BD, Roberts JA, Medley GF, Duckworth GJ, Lai R, Ebrahim S. Systematic review of isolation policies in the hospital management of methicillin-resistant *Staphylococcus aureus*: a review of the literature with epidemiological and economic modelling. *Health Technol Assess* 2003; 7(39): 1–194. **79**

Creti R, Imperi M, Bertuccini L, Fabretti F, Orefici G, Di Rosa R, Baldassarri L. Survey for virulence determinants among *Enterococcus faecalis* isolated from different sources. *J Med Microbiol* 2004; 53(1): 13–20. **97**

Crump JA, Barrett TJ, Nelson JT, Angulo FJ. Re-evaluating fluoroquinolone breakpoints for *Salmonella enterica* serotype Typhi and for non-Typhi salmonellae. *Clin Infect Dis* 2003; 37(1): 75–81. **167**

Crump JA, Luby SP, Mintz ED. The global burden of typhoid fever. *Bull World Health Organ* 2004; 82: 346–53. **176**

Crump JA, Youssef FG, Luby SP, Wasfy MO, Rangel JM, Taalat M, Oun SA, Mahoney FJ. Estimating the incidence of typhoid fever and other febrile illnesses in developing countries. *Emerg Infect Dis* 2003; 9(5): 539–44. **174**

Cui L, Ma X, Sato K, Okuma K, Tenover FC, Mamizuka EM, Gemmell CG, Kim MN, Ploy MC, El-Solh N, Ferraz V, Hiramatsu K. Cell wall thickening is a common feature of vancomycin resistance in *Staphylococcus aureus*. *J Clin Microbiol* 2003; 41(1): 5–14. **130**

Cunha MV, Leitao JH, Mahenthiralingam E, Vandamme P, Lito L, Barreto C, Salgado MJ, Sa-Correia I. Molecular analysis of *Burkholderia cepacia* complex strains from a Portuguese cystic fibrosis center: a 7-year study. *J Clin Microbiol* 2003; 41: 4113–20. **149**

Dagan R, Givon-Lavi N, Zamir O, Fraser D. Effect of a nonavalent conjugate vaccine on carriage of antibiotic-resistant *Streptococcus pneumoniae* in day-care centres. *Pediatr Infect Dis* 2003; 22(6): 532–40. **116 249**

Danaher PJ, Walter EA. Successful treatment of chronic meningitis caused by

Djokomoeljanto R, Van Der Meer JW.
Persistence of *Salmonellae* in blood and
bone marrow: randomized controlled trial
comparing ciprofloxacin and
chloramphenicol treatments against enteric
fever. *Antimicrob Agents Chemother* 2003;
47(5): 1727–31.   **166**

**Gaynes R, Rimland D, Killum E,
Lowery HK, Johnson TM 2nd, Killgore G,
Tenover FC.** Outbreak of *Clostridium
difficile* infection in a long-term care facility:
association with gatifloxacin use. *Clin Infect
Dis* 2004; 38(5): 640–5.   **229**

Givon-Lavi N, Fraser D, Dagan R.
Vaccination of day-care centre attendees
reduces carriage of *Streptococcus pneumoniae*
among their younger siblings. *Pediatr Infect
Dis* 2003; 22(6): 524–32.   **251**

Gopal Rao G, Mahankali Rao CS, Starke I.
Clostridium difficile-associated diarrhoea
in patients with community-acquired lower
respiratory infection being treated
with levofloxacin compared with
beta-lactam-based therapy. *J Antimicrob
Chemother* 2003; 51(3); 697–701.   **233**

**Gosling RD, Uiso LO, Sam NE, Bongard E,
Kanduma EG, Nyindo M, Morris RW,
Gillespie SH.** The bactericidal activity of
moxifloxacin in patients with pulmonary
tuberculosis. *Am J Respir Crit Care Med*
2003; 168(11): 1342–5.   **192**

**Guimerá M, García-Bustín D,
Noda-Cabrera A, Sánchez-González R,
Montelongo RG.** Cutaneous infection by
Fusarium: successful treatment with
voriconazole. *Br J Dermatol* 2004; 150:
770–95.   **49**

**Hajjeh RA, Sofair AN, Harrison LH,
Lyon GM, Arthington-Skaggs BA,
Mirza SA, Phelan M, Morgan J,
Lee-Yang W, Ciblak MA, Benjamin LE,
Sanza LT, Huie S, Yeo SF, Brandt ME,
Warnock DW.** Incidence of bloodstream
infections due to *Candida* species and *in
vitro* susceptibilities of isolates collected
from 1998 to 2000 in a population-based

active surveillance program. *J Clin Micro*
2004; 42(4): 1519–27.   **9**

**Herrero IA, Fernandez-Garayzabal JF,
Moreno MA, Dominguez L.** Dogs should be
included in surveillance programs for
vancomycin-resistant enterococci. *J Clin
Microbiol* 2004; 42(3): 1384–5.   **95**

**Horvath LL, Hospenthal DR, Murray CK,
Dooley DP.** Direct isolation of *Candida* spp
from blood cultures on the chromogenic
medium CHROMagar candida. *J Clin
Microbiol* 2003; 41: 2629–32.   **12**

**Howe RA, Monk A, Wootton M, Walsh TR,
Enright MC.** Vancomycin susceptibility
within methicillin-resistant *Staphylococcus
aureus* lineages. *Emerg Infect Dis* 2004;
10(5): 855–7.   **133**

**Husain S, Alexander BD, Munoz P,
Avery RK, Houston S, Pruett T, Jacobs R,
Dominguez EA, Tollemar JG,
Baumgarten K, Yu CM, Wagener MM,
Linden P, Kusne S, Singh N.** Opportunistic
mycelial fungal infection in organ
transplant recipients: emerging importance
of non-*Aspergillus* mycelial fungi.
Clin Infect Dis 2003; 37(2): 221–9.   **7**

**Husain S, Kwak EJ, Obman A,
Wagener MM, Kusne S, Stout JE,
McCurry KR, Singh N.** Prospective
assessment of Platelia *Aspergillus*
galactomannan antigen for the diagnosis of
invasive aspergillosis in lung transplant
recipients. *Am J Transplant* 2004; 4(5):
796–802.   **28**

**Jackson LA, Neuzil KM, Yu O, Benson P,
Barlow WE, Adams AL, Hanson CA,
Mahoney LD, Shay DK, Thompson WW,
for the Vaccine Safety Datalink.**
Effectiveness of pneumococcal
polysaccharide vaccine in older adults.
N Engl J Med 2003; 348(18): 1747–55.   **106**

**Jensenius M, Fournier PE, Kelly P,
Myrvang B, Raoult D.** African tick bite
fever. *Lancet Infect Dis* 2003; 3(9):
557–64.   **262**

Jódar L, Carlone G, Dagan R, Goldblatt D, Käyhty H, Klugman K, Plikaytis B, Siber G, Kohberger R, Chang I, Cherian T. Serological criteria for evaluation and licensure of new pneumococcal conjugate vaccine formulations for use in infants. *Vaccine* 2003; 21: 3265–72.   **110**

Johnson JR, Clabots C, Hirt H, Waters C, Dunny G. Enterococcal aggregation substance and binding substance are not major contributors to urinary tract colonization by *Enterococcus faecalis* in a mouse model of ascending unobstructed urinary tract infection. *Infect Immun* 2004; 72(4): 2445–8.   **98**

Klugman KP, Madhi SA, Huebner RE, Kohberger R, Mbelle N, Pierce N, for the Vaccine Trialists Group. A trial of 9-valent pneumococcal conjugate vaccine in children with and those without HIV infection. *N Engl J Med* 2003; 349(14): 1341–8.   **117**

Koomen I, Grobbee DE, Roord JJ, Donders R, Jennekens-Schinkel A, van Furth AM. Hearing loss at school age in survivors of bacterial meningitis: assessment, incidence, and prediction. *Pediatrics* 2003; 112(5): 1049–53.   **256**

Koss T, Carter EL, Grossman ME, Silvers DN, Rabinowitz AD, Singleton J Jr, Zaki SR, Paddock CD. Increased detection of rickettsialpox in a New York City hospital following the anthrax outbreak of 2001: use of immunohistochemistry for the rapid confirmation of cases in an era of bioterrorism. *Arch Dermatol* 2003; 139(12): 1545–52.   **266**

Kristich CJ, Li YH, Cvitkovitch DG, Dunny GM. Esp-independent biofilm formation by *Enterococcus faecalis.* *J Bacteriol* 2004; 186(1): 154–63.   **99**

Kumar D, Rotstein C, Miyata G, Arlen D, Humar A. Randomized, double-blind, controlled trial of pneumococcal vaccination in renal transplant recipients. *J Infect Dis* 2003; 187(10): 1639–45.   **113**

Lass-Florl C, Speth C, Mayr A, Wurzner R, Dierich MP, Ulmer H, Dietrich H. Diagnosing and monitoring of invasive aspergillosis during antifungal therapy by polymerase chain reaction: an experimental study in mice. *Diagn Microbiol Infect Dis* 47(4): 569–72.   **38**

Lewis MD, Yousuf AA, Lerdthusnee K, Razee A, Chandranoi K, Jones JW. Scrub typhus re-emergence in the Maldives. *Emerg Infect Dis* 2003; 9(12): 1638–4.   **270**

Lion T, Baumgartinger R, Watzinger F, Matthes-Martin S, Suda M, Preuner S, Futterknecht B, Lawitschka A, Peters C, Potschger U, Gadner H. Molecular monitoring of adenovirus in peripheral blood after allogeneic bone marrow transplantation permits early diagnosis of disseminated disease. *Blood* 2003; 102(3): 1114–20.   **204**

Ljungman P, Brand R, Einsele H, Frassoni F, Niederwieser D, Cordonnier C. Donor CMV serologic status and outcome of CMV-seropositive recipients after unrelated donor stem cell transplantation: an EBMT megafile analysis. *Blood* 2003; 102(13): 4255–60.   **206**

Ljungman P, Ribaud P, Eyrich M, Matthes-Martin S, Einsele H, Bleakley M, Machaczka M, Bierings M, Bosi A, Gratecos N, Cordonnier C; Infectious Diseases Working Party of the European Group for Blood and Marrow Transplantation. Cidofovir for adenovirus infections after allogeneic hematopoietic stem cell transplantation: a survey by the Infectious Diseases Working Party of the European Group for Blood and Marrow Transplantation. *Bone Marrow Transplant* 2003; 31(6): 481–6.   **207**

Lodise TP, McKinnon PS, Swiderski L, Rybak MJ. Outcomes analysis of delayed antibiotic treatment for hospital-acquired *Staphylococcus aureus* bacteraemia . *Clin Infect Dis* 2003; 36(11): 1418–23.   **75**

Lucet JC, Chevret S, Durand-Zaleski I, Chastang C, Regnier B; Multicenter Study Group. Prevalence and risk factors for carriage of methicillin-resistant *Staphylococcus aureus* at admission to the intensive care unit. *Arch Intern Med* 2003; 163(2): 181–8. **78**

Machado CM, Boas LS, Mendes AV, Santos MF, da Rocha IF, Sturaro D, Dulley FL, Pannuti CS. Low mortality rates related to respiratory virus infections after bone marrow transplantation. *Bone Marrow Transplant* 2003; 31(8): 695–700. **208**

Mai NL, Phan VB, Vo AH, Tran CT, Lin FY, Bryla DA, Chu C, Schiloach J, Robbins JB, Schneerson R, Szu SC. Persistent efficacy of Vi conjugate vaccine against typhoid fever in young children. *N Engl J Med* 2003; 349(14): 1390–1. **182**

Marr KA, Crippa F, Leisenring W, Hoyle M, Boeckh M, Balajee SA, Nichols WG, Musher B, Corey L. Itraconazole versus fluconazole for prevention of fungal infections in patients receiving allogenenic stem cell transplants. *Blood* 2004; 103: 1527–33. **44**

Martinez JA, Ruthazer R, Hansjosten K, Barefoot L, Snydman DR. Role of environmental contamination as a risk factor for acquisition of vancomycin-resistant enterococci in patients treated in a medical intensive care unit. *Arch Intern Med* 2003; 163(16): 1905–12. **89**

McCann S, Byrne JL, Rovira M, Shaw P, Ribaud P, Sica S, Volin L, Olavarria E, Mackinnon S, Trabasso P, VanLint MT, Ljungman P, Ward K, Browne P, Gratwohl A, Widmer AF, Cordonnier C; Infectious Diseases Working Party of the EBMT. Outbreaks of infectious diseases in stem cell transplant units: a silent cause of death for patients and transplant programmes. *Bone Marrow Transplant* 2004; 33(5): 519–29. **202**

McCool TL, Cate TR, Tuomanen EI, Adrian P, Mitchell TJ, Weiser JN. Serum immunoglobulin G response to candidate vaccine antigens during experimental human pneumococcal colonization. *Infect Immun* 2003; 71(10): 5724–32. **118**

McDowell A, Mahenthiralingam E, Dunbar KE, Moore JE, Crowe M, Elborn JS. Epidemiology of *Burkholderia cepacia* complex species recovered from cystic fibrosis patients: issues related to patient segregation. *J Med Microbiol* 2004; 53: 663–8. **149**

Merrigan MM, Sambol SP, Johnson S, Gerding DN. Prevention of fatal *Clostridium difficile*-associated disease during continuous administration of clindamyin in hamsters. *J Infect Dis* 2003; 188(12): 1922–7. **220**

Millar BC, Jiru X, Walker MJ, Evans JP, Moore JE. False identification of *Coccidioides immitis*: do molecular methods always get it right? *J Clin Microbiol* 2003; 41(12): 5778–80. **17**

Mitnick C, Bayona J, Palacios E, Shin S, Furin J, Alcantara F, Sanchez E, Sarria M, Becerra M, Fawzi MC, Kapiga S, Neuberg D, Maguire JH, Kim JY, Farmer P. Community-based therapy for multidrug-resistant tuberculosis in Lima, Peru. *N Engl J Med* 2003; 348(2): 119–28. **191**

Moise-Broder PA, Sakoulas G, Eliopoulos GM, Schentag JJ, Forrest A, Moellering RC Jr. Accessory gene regulator group II polymorphism in methicillin-resistant *Staphylococcus aureus* is predictive of failure of vancomycin therapy. *Clin Infect Dis* 2004; 38(12): 1700–5. **132**

Molrine DC, Antin JH, Guinan EC, Soiffer RJ, MacDonald K, Malley R, Malinoski F, Trocciola S, Wilson M, Ambrosino DM. Donor immunization with pneumococcal conjugate vaccine and early protective antibody responses following allogeneic hematopoietic cell transplantation. *Blood* 2003; 101(3): 831–6. **107**

O'Sullivan CE, Aksamit AJ, Harrington JR, Harmsen WS, Mitchell PS, Patel R. Clinical spectrum and laboratory characteristics associated with detection of herpes simplex virus DNA in cerebrospinal fluid. *Mayo Clin Proc* 2003; 78(11): 1347–52. **255**

Paddock CD, Sumner JW, Comer JA, Zaki SR, Goldsmith CS, Goddard J, McLellan SL, Tamminga CL, Ohl CA. *Rickettsia parkeri*: a newly recognized cause of spotted fever rickettsiosis in the United States. *Clin Infect Dis* 2004; 38(6): 805–11. **263**

Pappas PG, Rex JH, Lee J, Hamill RJ, Larsen RA, Powderly W, Kauffman CA, Hyslop N, Mangino JE, Chapman S, Horowitz HW, Edwards JE, Dismukes WE; NIAID Mycoses Study Group. A prospective observational study of candidemia: epidemiology, therapy and influences on mortality in hospitalised adult and pediatric patients. *Clin Infect Dis* 2003; 37(5): 634–43. **10**

Parry CM, Hien TT, Dougan G, White NJ, Farrar JJ. Typhoid fever. *N Engl J Med* 2002; 347: 1770–82 [review]. **164**

Price CS, Paule S, Noskin GA, Peterson LR. Active surveillance reduces the incidence of vancomycin-resistant enterococcal bacteremia. *Clin Infect Dis* 2003; 37: 921–8. **90**

Raad I, Hachem R, Hanna H, Afif C, Escalante C, Kantarjian H, Rolston K. Prospective, randomized study comparing quinupristin–dalfopristin with linezolid in the treatment of vancomycin-resistant *Enterococcus faecium* infections. *J Antimicrob Chemother* 2004; 53(4): 646–9. **92**

Raboni SM, Siqueira MM, Portes SR, Pasquini R. Comparison of PCR, enzyme immunoassay and conventional culture for adenovirus detection in bone marrow transplant patients with hemorrhagic cystitis. *J Clin Virol* 2003; 27(3): 270–5. **209**

Rahman A, Tegnell A, Vene S, Giesecke J. Rickettsioses in Swedish travellers, 1997–2001. *Scand J Infect Dis* 2003; 35(4): 247–50. **265**

Reynolds MG, Krebs JS, Comer JA, Sumner JW, Rushton TC, Lopez CE, Nicholson WL, Rooney JA, Lance-Parker SE, McQuiston JH, Paddock CD, Childs JE. Flying squirrel-associated typhus, United States. *Emerg Infect Dis* 2003; 9(10): 1341–3. **265**

Richter MY, Jakobsen H, Birgisdottir A, Haeuw JF, Power UF, Del Giudice G, Bartolini A, Jonsdottir I. Immunization of female mice with glycoconjugates protects their offspring against encapsulated bacteria. *Infect Immun* 2004; 71(1): 187–95. **108**

Rovira M, Jimenez M, De La Bellacasa JP, Mensa J, Rafel M, Ortega M, Almela M, Martinez C, Fernandez-Aviles F, Martinez JA, Urbano-Ispizua A, Carreras E, Montserrat E. Detection of *Aspergillus* galactomannan by enzyme immunoabsorbent assay in recipients of allogeneic hematopoietic stem cell transplantation: a prospective study. *Transplantation* 2004; 77(8): 1260–4. **26**

Salerno-Goncalves R, Wyant TL, Pasetti MF, Fernandez-Vina M, Tacket CO, Levine MM, Sztein MB. Concomitant induction of CD4+ and CD8+ T-cell responses in volunteers immunized with *Salmonella enterica* serovar typhi strain CVD 908-htrA. *J Immunol* 2003; 170(5): 2734–41. **181**

Sanguinetti M, Posteraro B, Pagano L, Pagliari G, Fianchi L, Mele L, La Sorda M, Franco A, Fadda G. Comparison of real-time PCR, conventional PCR, and galactomannan antigen detection by enzyme-linked immunosorbent assay using bronchoalveolar lavage fluid samples from hematology patients for diagnosis of invasive pulmonary aspergillosis. *J Clin Microbiol* 2003; 41(8): 3922–5. **16 36**

Savidge TC, Pan WH, Newman P, O'Brien M, Anton PM, Pothoulakis C. *Clostridium difficile* toxin B is an inflammatory enterotoxin in human intestine. *Gastroenterology* 2003; 125(2): 413–20. **222**

Schnappinger D, Ehrt S, Voskuil MI, Liu Y, Mangan JA, Monahan IM, Dolganov G, Efron B, Butcher PD, Nathan C, Schoolnik GK. Transcriptional adaptation of *Mycobacterium tuberculosis* within macrophages: insights into the phagosomal environment. *J Exp Med* 2003; 198(5): 693–704. **195**

Sendid B, Caillot D, Baccouch-Humbert B, Klingspor L, Grandjean M, Bonnin A, Poulain D. Contribution of the Platelia *Candida*-specific antibody and antigen tests to early diagnosis of systemic *Candida tropicalis* infection in neutropenic adults. *J Clin Microbiol* 2003; 41(10): 4551–8. **13 24**

Shigeru K, Toru M, Hideyo Y, Takeshi M, Akio U, Akira I, Yoshihito N, Hideo I. A multicenter open-label clinical study of Micafungin in the treatment of deep-seated mycosis in Japan. *Scand J Infect Dis* 2004; 36(5): 372–9. **48**

Sieradzki K, Tomasz A. Alterations of cell wall structure and metabolism accompany reduced susceptibility to vancomycin in an isogenic series of clinical isolates of *Staphylococcus aureus. J Bacteriol* 2003; 185(24): 7103–10. **131**

Spiess B, Buchheidt D, Baust C, Skladny H, Seifarth W, Zeilfelder U, Leib-Mosch C, Morz H, Hehlmann R. Development of a LightCycler PCR assay for detection and quantification of *Aspergillus fumigatus* DNA in clinical samples from neutropenic patients. *J Clin Microbiol* 2003; 41(5): 1811–18. **31**

Sterling TR, Lehmann HP, Frieden TR. Impact of DOTS compared with DOTS-plus on multidrug resistant tuberculosis and tuberculosis deaths: decision analysis. *Br Med J* 2003; 326(7389): 574. **188**

Suzuki Y, Kamigaki T, Fujino Y, Tominaga M, Ku Y, Kuroda Y. Randomized clinical trial of pre-operative intranasal mupirocin to reduce surgical-site infection after digestive surgery. *Br J Surg* 2003; 90(9): 1072–5. **77**

Tazume K, Hagihara M, Gansuvd B, Higuchi A, Ueda Y, Hirabayashi K, Hojo M, Tanabe A, Okamoto A, Kato S, Hotta T. Induction of cytomegalovirus-specific CD4+ cytotoxic T lymphocytes from seropositive or negative healthy subjects or stem cell transplant recipients. *Exp Hematol* 2004; 32(1): 95–103. **203**

Tenover FC, Weigel LM, Appelbaum PC, McDougal LK, Chaitram J, McAllister S, Clark N, Killgore G, O'Hara CM, Jevitt L, Patel JB, Bozdogan B. Vancomycin-resistant *Staphylococcus aureus* isolate from a patient in Pennsylvania. *Antimicrob Agents Chemother* 2004: 48(1): 275–80. **127**

Thomas KE, Owens CM, Veys PA, Novelli V, Costoli V. The radiological spectrum of invasive aspergillosis in children: a 10-year review. *Pediatr Radiol* 2003; 33: 453–60. **22**

Vandenesch F, Naimi T, Enright MC, Lina G, Nimmo GR, Heffernan H, Liassine N, Bes M, Greenland T, Reverdy ME, Etienne J. Community-acquired methicillin-resistant *Staphylococcus aureus* carrying Panton-Valentine leukocidin genes: worldwide emergence. *Emerg Infect Dis* 2003; 9: 978–84. **69**

Van Griethuysen A, Van 't Veen A, Buiting A, Walsh T, Kluytmans J. High percentage of methicillin-resistant *Staphylococcus aureus* isolates with reduced susceptibility to glycopeptides in The Netherlands. *J Clin Microbiol* 2003; 41: 2487–91. **70**

Veloria WG, Domenico P, LiPuma JJ, Davis JM, Gurzenda E, Kazzaz JA. *In vitro* activity and synergy of bismuth thiols and tobramycin against *Burkholderia cepacia* complex. *J Antimicrob Chemother* 2003; 52: 915–19. **153**

Verdier I, Reverdy ME, Etienne J, Lina G, Bes M, Vandenesch F. *Staphylococcus aureus* isolates with reduced susceptibility to glycopeptides belong to accessory gene regulator group I or II. *Antimicrob Agents Chemother* 2004; 48(3): 1024–7. **133**

Verduyn Lunel FM, Voss A, Kuijper EJ, Gelinck LB, Hoogerbrugge PM, Liem KL, Kullberg BJ, Verweij PE. Detection of the *Candida* antigen mannan in cerebrospinal fluid specimens from patients suspected of having *Candida* meningitis. *J Clin Microbiol* 2004; 42(2): 867–70. **25**

Vermis K, Coenye T, LiPuma JJ, Mahenthiralingam E, Nelis HJ, Vandamme P. Proposal to accommodate *Burkholderia cepacia* genomovar VI as *Burkholderia dolosa* sp. nov. *Int J Syst Evol Microbiol* 2004; 54: 689–91. **144**

Vermis K, Vandamme PA, Nelis HJ. *Burkholderia cepacia* complex genomovars: utilization of carbon sources, susceptibility to antimicrobial agents and growth on selective media. *J Appl Microbiol* 2003; 95: 1191–9. **145**

Vibhagool A, Sungkanuparph S, Mootsikapun P, Chetchotisakd P, Tansuphaswaswadikul S, Bowonwatanuwong C, Ingsathit A. Discontinuation of secondary prophylaxis for cryptococcal meningitis in human immunodeficiency virus-infected patients treated with highly active antiretroviral therapy: a prospective, multicentre, randomised study. *Clin Infect Dis* 2003; 36(10): 1329–31. **252**

Vinh H, Parry CM, Hanh VT, Chinh MT, House D, Tham CT, Thao NT, Diep TS, Wain J, Day NP, White NJ, Farrar JJ. Double-blind comparison of ibuprofen and paracetamol for adjunctive treatment of uncomplicated typhoid fever. *Pediatr Infect Dis J* 2004; 23(3): 226–30. **171**

Viscoli C, Machetti M, Cappellano P, Bucci B, Bruzzi P, Van Lint MT, Bacigalupo A. False-positive galactomannan platelia *Aspergillus* test results for patients receiving piperacillin–tazobactam. *Clin Infect Dis* 2004; 38(6): 913–16. **29**

Voskuil MI, Schnappinger D, Visconti KC, Harrell MI, Dolganov GM, Sherman DR, Schoolnik GK. Inhibition of respiration by nitric oxide induces a *Mycobacterium tuberculosis* dormancy program. *J Exp Med* 2003; 198(5): 705–13. **196**

Waar K, Willems RJ, Slooff MJ, Harmsen HJ, Degener JE. Molecular epidemiology of *Enterococcus faecalis* in liver transplant patients at University Hospital Groningen. *J Hosp Infect* 2003; 55(1): 53–60. **87**

Wagner HJ, Cheng YC, Huls MH, Gee AP, Kuehnle I, Krance RA, Brenner MK, Rooney CM, Heslop HE. Prompt versus preemptive intervention for EBV lymphoproliferative disease. *Blood* 2004; 103(10): 3979–81. **213**

Walsh TJ, Teppler H, Donowitz GR, Maertens JA, Baden LR, Dmoszynska A, Cornely OA, Bourque MR, Lupinacci RJ, Sable CA, dePauw BE. Caspofungin versus liposomal amphotericin B for empiric antifungal therapy in patients with persistent fever and neutropenia. *N Engl J Med* 2004; 351(14): 1391–402. **54**

Wanahita A, Goldsmith EA, Marino BJ, Musher DM. *Clostridium difficile* infection in patients with unexplained leukocytosis. *Am J Med* 2003; 115(7): 543–6. **228**

Warren DK, Nitin A, Hill C, Fraser VJ, Kollef MH. Occurrence of co-colonization or co-infection with vancomycin-resistant enterococci and methicillin-resistant *Staphylococcus aureus* in a medical intensive care unit. *Infect Control Hosp Epidemiol* 2004; 25(2): 99–104. **94**

Warris A, Klaassen CH, Meis JF, De Ruiter MT, De Valk HA,

General index

A

accessory gene regulator (*agr*) type 130, 132–4
ace gene 97, 98
acetazolamide, trial in cryptococcal meningitis 254–5
aciclovir, in prevention of cytomegalovirus infection 211
acute mountain sickness, acetazolamide therapy 254, 255
adenovirus infection
  antiviral therapy 213
    cidofovir 207–8
  detection in HSCT patients with haemorrhagic cystitis 209–11
  effect of alemtuzumab conditioning in HSCT 212–13
  screening after HSCT 204–5
adult bacterial meningitis
  duration of therapy 248–9
  role of dexamethasone 244–7
  see also bacterial meningitis; meningitis
Africa
  incidence of typhoid fever 177
  meningitis belt 241
African tick bite fever 262–3
aggregation substance (AS), as virulence factor 97–9
agr group polymorphism in MRSA 130, 132–4
albumin levels, risk factor in *Clostridium difficile* infection 234–5
alemtuzumab 201
  effect on adenovirus infection after HSCT 212–13
allogeneic stem cell transplantation
  prophylactic antifungal therapy 44–5
  see also haematopoietic stem cell transplantation (HSCT)
Ambisome 42
  see also liposomal amphotericin B
Amblyomma ticks, as vectors of rickettsial infections 262, 263
aminoglycosides, risk of *B. cepacia* colonization 153
p-aminosalicylic acid in MDRTB 190

amoxicillin therapy
  in bacterial meningitis 243, 245
  Clostridium difficile infection 233–4
  in MDRTB 190
  in typhoid fever 163
amphotericin B 41–2
  in combination therapy
    with acetazolamide 254
    for cryptococcal meningitis 42–4, 58
    for invasive mycosis 48
    for orbitocerebral aspergillosis 52–4
  comparison with caspofungin in candidiasis 45–7
  effect on PCR assay in aspergillosis 38–9
  empiric therapy in fever with neutropenia 54–7
  in *Fusarium* infection 50
  susceptibility of *Aspergillus terreus* 4, 5
  susceptibility of *Candida* species 9
ampicillin resistance, *Salmonella typhi* 179
anthrax, cutaneous, differential diagnosis 267
antibiotic resistance *see* antimicrobial resistance
antibiotic therapy *see* antimicrobial therapy
antibiotic use in meningitis 243, 245
antifungal therapy 41–2, 57–9
  in aspergillosis 52–7
  cryptococcal meningitis, combination therapy 42–4
  empiric therapy in neutropenia 54–7
  in *Fusarium* infection, voriconazole therapy 49–51
  in invasive candidiasis 45–7
  invasive mycosis, combination therapy 48
  micafungin 48–9
  prophylactic, in allogeneic stem cell transplantation 44–5
  Scedosporium apiospermum meningitis, voriconazole 51
antigen detection, diagnosis of fungal infections 22
antimannan antibody detection 13
antimicrobial resistance
  in *Burkholderia cepacia* complex 153
  Clostridium. difficile, prophylactic use of resistant strains 220–1, 237

KEEPING UP TO DATE IN ONE VOLUME

Subject matters dealt with in previous volume

The Year in Infection 2003

Mycology
Problems in diagnosis of fungal infection
New antifungal therapies
Issues in haematology
Mycology: nosocomial/intensive therapy unit issues

Human immunodeficiency virus
Adverse effects of antiretrovirals
Antiretroviral drug therapy and metabolism
Human immunodeficiency virus in women
Human immunodeficiency virus in children

Emerging problems with Gram positive bacteria
Vancomycin-resistant enterococci infection control
Staphylococcus aureus bacteraemia
Group B streptococcus
Methicillin-resistant *Staphylococcus aureus*

Emerging and re-emerging infections
Rickettsial diseases
Dengue
Leishmaniasis

Atlas Medical Publishing Ltd
Oxford Centre for Innovation
Mill Street
Oxford OX2 0JX, UK

T: +44 1865 811116
F: +44 1865 251550
E: info@clinicalpublishing.co.uk
W: www.clinicalpublishing.co.uk